Feeding and Nutrition in the Preterm Infant

For Elsevier:

Commissioning Editor: Mary Seager
Development Editor: Rebecca Netemans
Project Manager: Morven Dean
Designer: Judith Wright
Illustrations: Reginald Aloysius

Feeding and Nutrition in the Preterm Infant

Edited by

Elizabeth Jones MPhil RM RN

*Breastfeeding Coordinator, Neonatal Intensive Care, Research Midwife,
University Hospital of North Staffordshire, Stoke-on-Trent, UK*

Caroline King BSc(Hons) SRD

*Chief Dietitian, Paediatrics, Department of Nutrition and Dietetics,
Hammersmith Hospital, London, UK*

Consultant Editor

Andrew Spencer BMedSci BM BS MRCP FRCPCH DM

Forewords by

Tony Williams and Jan Riordan

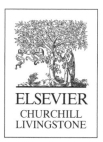

ELSEVIER
CHURCHILL
LIVINGSTONE

EDINBURGH LONDON NEW YORK OXFORD PHILADELPHIA ST LOUIS SYDNEY TORONTO 2005

ELSEVIER
CHURCHILL
LIVINGSTONE

First published 2005

ISBN 0 443 07378 3

British Library Cataloguing in Publication Data
A catalogue record for this book is available from the British Library

Library of Congress Cataloging in Publication Data
A catalog record for this book is available from the Library of Congress

Knowledge and best practice in this field are constantly changing. As new research and experience broaden our knowledge, changes in practice, treatment and drug therapy may become necessary or appropriate. Readers are advised to check the most current information provided (i) on procedures featured or (ii) by the manufacturer of each product to be administered, to verify the recommended dose or formula, the method and duration of administration, and contraindications. It is the responsibility of the practitioner, relying on their own experience and knowledge of the patient, to make diagnoses, to determine dosages and the best treatment for each individual patient, and to take all appropriate safety precautions. To the fullest extent of the law, neither the publisher nor the editors assumes any liability for any injury and/or damage.

The Publisher

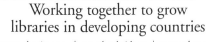

Printed in China by CTPS

Contents

Contributors

Annie Bagnall BSc(Hons) MRCSLT
Specialist Paediatric Speech and Language Therapist, Speech and Language Therapy Department, Hammersmith Hospital, London, UK

Sue C Bell BSc(Hons) SRD
Senior Dietitian, University Hospital of North Staffordshire, Stoke-on-Trent, UK

Peter E Hartmann BRurSc PhD
Professor, School of Biomedical and Chemical Sciences, The University of Western Australia Crawley, Australia

Elizabeth Jones MPhil RM RN
Breastfeeding Co-ordinator, Neonatal Intensive Care, Research Midwife, University Hospital of North Staffordshire, Stoke-on-Trent, UK

Caroline King BSc(Hons) SRD
Chief Dietitian, Paediatrics, Department of Nutrition and Dietetics, Hammersmith Hospital, London, UK

Donna T Ramsay PostGradDip(Sci) PhD
School of Biochemistry and Molecular Sciences, University of Western Australia, Crawley, Australia

Gillian Weaver BSc(Hons) SRD
Milk Bank Manager, Queen Charlotte's and Chelsea Hospital, London, UK

Preface

Providing optimum nutrition to infants who are born preterm is a challenge for those involved in their care. Decision-making has been hampered by the paucity of randomized controlled trials coupled with the large number of studies which are observational or involve only small numbers; the latter can lead to contradictory results. One consistent finding over the last decade has been the growing evidence that breast milk gives many significant advantages over artificial substitutes. Despite this evidence, there are few research-based interventions to guide practice on a combination of issues relating to infant nutrition, lactation and breastfeeding. In addition, many neonatal units lack clinical specialists in nutrition, speech therapy, milk expression and preterm breastfeeding. This has undermined the care given to both mothers and their babies. Staff morale can suffer when a mother's lactation fails and when breastfeeding is not achieved, despite the hard work and best intentions of all health professionals involved. When a women fails in her choice to feed her infant by breast it can often be due to the lack of simple evidence-based advice and support. We hope this book will address these issues by providing clear guidelines on neonatal feeding and milk expression. So often in the past the advice given to families has been generalized from term feeding programmes and not specifically tailored to the specialised needs of preterm infants and their mothers. Infant health has been compromised and many women have failed in their wish both to provide breast milk and to breastfeed their babies.

Elizabeth Jones and Caroline King

Acknowledgements

We would like to thank our colleagues and families for their support throughout this project. We would also like to thank all the authors for their time, help and valuable contributions. In addition, we are especially grateful to Dr Andy Spencer for undertaking the scientific review. We are particularly appreciative of the contribution made to this project by Professor Peter Hartmann. His knowledge, wisdom and generosity has made this book unique, by providing evidence-based guidelines in terms of preterm mammary physiology and milk expression. Without his guidance and patience this project would not have been accomplished.

We have a great debt of gratitude to those of our colleagues who took time in their extremely busy days to read and comment on various chapter: Tony Williams, Sara Wickham, Atul Singhal, Ping Corcoran, Denis Azzopardi and Mike Harrison. Each gave invaluable comments that helped to shape the final drafts.

Finally, we are indebted to the families we have encountered on the Neonatal Unit, whose experiences with feeding have made this book possible. We are especially grateful to the mothers who agreed to be photographed for this book. Thank you for sharing precious and intimate moments with us all.

Elizabeth Jones and Caroline King,
April 2005

Foreword

Advances in care of preterm or low birth weight infants are one of the miracles of our age. Although much has been written about feeding human milk to these special babies, this textbook is the first comprehensive treatment of this topic.

My own personal journey of helping breastfeeding mothers and their babies began about four decades ago, when improvements in technology, notably surfactant and corticosteroids, allowed the survival of babies at earlier gestational ages. Few babies received human milk then, but pediatricians around the world were beginning to recognize its benefits to premature infants, in particular its role in preventing necrotizing enterocolitis.

At that time, despite the fact that human milk was thought to be best for the baby, breastfeeding and maintaining a milk supply were considered too stressful for the mother. Moreover, feeding at the breast made it more difficult to ascertain how much milk the baby had ingested. Parents had limited times they could see their tiny baby in the nursery and felt left out of the care of their child. In those early years, I clearly recall talking to a group of parents of infants in the neonatal intensive care unit about the advantages of breastmilk. After my presentation, one mother took me aside and whispered in my ear, "The truth is that I feel that my baby belongs to the nurses and not to me at all."

Fast forward to 2005. Recognition of the health benefits of human milk for low birth weight infants has accelerated as the result of research worldwide. Parents are not merely encouraged but are expected to assist in the care of their baby, to start pumping their breasts soon after giving birth, and then to put their baby to breast as soon as possible. Kangaroo Care is practised in most countries throughout the world, and premature infants are put to breast earlier thanks to nurse researchers whose careful research found favorable outcomes from these practices.

Technology in neonatology has evolved to the point that adding commercial milk fortifiers to the mothers' own milk to increase infant growth is an accepted practice where it can be supported economically.

The Baby Friendly breastfeeding advertising campaign declares that Every Baby is Born to be Breastfed. Giving of their milk is the one thing that mothers of preterm infants can do that no one else can. Yet many mothers who want to breastfeed their preterm infants will not continue to breastfeed after they leave the birthplace. Lack of consistent information and support from the hospital staff, ineffective breast pumps, and lack of follow-up care following discharge have been long-time barriers to breastfeeding these babies.

Neonatologists, midwives, dieticians, and nurses will appreciate and use the extensive research-based information found in this valuable text. As a result, countless breastfeeding mothers and their preterm babies will receive better and more consistent care free of outdated assumptions and practices. This book, written by experienced clinicians in the United Kingdom and Australia, is a rich and welcome resource that should be available to health care practitioners of all backgrounds who work with preterm infants.

Jan Riordan

Foreword

All babies benefit from being breastfed, yet the vulnerability and potential of preterm babies makes them a group particularly important in this respect. By providing milk mothers make a unique contribution to their welfare, something which professionals have a duty to support. Unfortunately we too often fail to achieve this, usually because we neither understand nor apply in practice the scientific basis of lactation physiology and infant nutrition accumulated over the last half century. Despite growing appreciation of their importance, these are areas of science which have historically been given only cursory attention in medical curricula and sometimes completely omitted.

This book therefore constitutes a major contribution. It puts together expertise from the many disciplines who need to work together effectively in supporting mothers, and does so in a style which those caring professionally for preterm babies will understand. Early chapters explore some of the problems associated with using breastmilk substitutes, and show how the unique biological properties of human milk can be coupled with optimisation of nutrient intake. These are followed by extensive discussion of the physiological basis of human lactation, showing how this knowledge can be applied to maximise the efficiency of milk production after preterm delivery. The structures and processes necessary to provide donor milk for the few babies whose mothers are unable to provide milk in sufficient quantities are also described. Finally the book describes how the process of feeding at the breast develops and can be supported to achieve efficient removal of milk, with the goal of sending home a thriving, breastfeeding baby.

Whilst this book will help to replace folklore and myth with science, it is in the nature of any scientific text that not all readers will agree with the whole content. This is also important: there is still much to be learnt and explained, and the authors will no doubt have helped to stimulate debate and new enquiry in this growing area of neonatal care.

Tony F Williams

Chapter **1**

The benefits of human milk for the preterm baby

Caroline King and Elizabeth Jones

BACKGROUND

Human milk is species-specific and has been adapted throughout evolution to meet the nutritional requirements of the human infant, supporting growth, development and survival.[1] In comparison, artificial substitutes still have to meet many challenges in their evolutionary journey. Many of the studies discussed could be considered to be evaluating the safety of breast-milk substitutes rather than of breast milk itself.

The aim of this chapter is to review the current literature regarding the use of breast milk in the preterm population. Studies are presented to show not only where human milk has proven superior to formula but also its possible detrimental effects; the aim is to give as balanced and unbiased an assessment as possible.

In the last few decades, because of advances in technology and pharmacology, the survival rates of preterm neonates have improved dramatically. Human milk was perceived not to meet all the nutritional requirements of this new and vulnerable population and specialized preterm infant formulas were developed. The trend toward using these new formulas persisted until the late 1980s when an increasing number of studies provided evidence of the benefits of using human milk. Today we have the advantage of a greater insight into the nutritional inadequacies of human milk for the smallest babies and how to remedy most of them; this will be covered in Chapter 3.

Breast milk facilitates a safe adaptation to the extrauterine environment via various mechanisms. The ingestion of breast milk via the close contact of breast-feeding is a unique method of protecting infants from pathogens present in both the maternal and infant environment. Breast milk is highly specialized in its ability to provide protection against infection, for which the baby's active immunity will develop later in life. Preterm infants have the disadvantage both of a significantly immature immune system and the deprivation of placental transfer of valuable protection such as immunoglobulin G (IgG), which occurs predominantly during the third trimester. In addition the endogenous production of many immune factors is delayed in the neonate, leaving these individuals vulnerable to opportunistic infection. This is compounded in the preterm infant since invasive procedures that occur during intensive care on the neonatal unit may lead to an increased risk of infection. Moreover, premature interruption of placental nutrient transfer puts these infants at very high risk of nutrient deficiencies at a time of extremely rapid growth and development. In this respect human milk is an important source of many components which are highly bioavailable compared to artificial substitutes.

The constituents of human milk have three main functions: (1) to provide nutrition; (2) to give immune protection; and (3) to promote development: some constituents accomplish all three. One of the most significant omissions from formula milk is the wide array of anti-infective factors provided by breast milk. Indeed, no currently available formula milk can or does provide any significant immune protection to the vulnerable neonate. In addition breast milk provides growth-regulatory effects in the form of hormones, growth modulators and growth factors that are not present in artificial substitutes (Box 1.1). Breast milk is an extremely complex biological fluid, and as such contains a rich variety of hormones and other complex molecules and cellular material. However it is difficult to be sure which of these components are inherent in the production of breast milk; which are involved in the development, growth and immunological protection of the breast; and which confer benefit to the newborn infant.

The advantages of human milk may extend well beyond the neonatal period. There is evidence for a reduced incidence of cardiovascular risk factors and, in the preterm infant receiving breast milk, neurodevelopment and, in particular, cognitive outcome are improved. However, whether the latter is due to the direct nutritional effect of breast milk or is secondary to a combination of genetic factors, environmental conditions and/or enhanced education levels in mothers who provide breast milk, remains unclear.

Finally, but of equal importance, mothers of preterm infants often report that the provision of milk is the only important positive contribution that they can make for their babies.[8] Failure to provide breast milk may give rise to feelings of maternal helplessness and guilt.[9] When these mothers are unable to provide breast milk or to breast-feed despite their desire to do so, we as health professionals have to look at our practice and evaluate it to find out where we can improve. Whatever the evidence for or against human milk for a sick infant, if it is safe to give it, it is our duty to help mothers in their choice to provide it.

IMMUNOLOGICAL ADVANTAGES OF HUMAN MILK

Human milk provides immunological factors that may be of particular benefit to newborn infants.[10,11]

Many important components of human milk are either scarcely detectable in cow's milk, or are present in very different amounts, for example, lysozyme,[12] epidermal growth factor (EGF),[13] polyamines[4,14] and oligosaccharides[3] (Box 1.1). In addition, whereas secretory IgA is the predominant immunoglobulin in human milk, the predominant immunoglobulin in cow's milk is IgG, reflecting the different needs of the young of each species.[1]

Both well and sick neonates benefit from the provision of breast milk rather than formula milk.[15–17] This effect is probably mediated via a

Box 1.1   Some of the important components of human milk

Antiproteases: antitrypsin and antichymotrypsin may be important to ensure survival of antimicrobial and gut trophic proteins through the gastrointestinal tract

Bifidus factor: a proteolytic product of kappa-casein shown to help promote the growth of beneficial bifidobacteria in the large bowel

Cytokines: such as tumour necrosis factor-alpha and interleukin-1, which can enhance the anti-infective function of leukocytes

Enzymes
  Digestive: bile salt-stimulated lipase and amylase are present; they survive freezing, but not pasteurization. Lipase will release fatty acids which have antimicrobial activity
  Anti-inflammatory: catalase, histaminase and glutathione peroxidase, which protect against oxidant damage. Acetyl hydrolase degrades platelet-activating factor, a factor that is associated with necrotizing enterocolitis

Epidermal growth factor: involved in gut mucosal repair and maturation; epidermal growth factor is stable to freezing and pasteurization

Glycoproteins: these include oligosaccharides (see below). In addition, mucin and lactadherin are associated with the human milk fat globule, respectively: they prevent microbial adhesion to the gut wall and give protection from rotavirus infection[2]

Hormones which may have growth-modulatory effects, e.g. oxytocin, prolactin, cortisol and thyroxine

Immunoglobulins: IgA, IgG, IgM, IgE and IgD. Secretory IgA is present in the highest amounts, particularly in colostrum

Lactoferrin: a protein that binds iron and therefore may not only enhance iron absorption but also withhold iron for bacterial growth in the gut

Lactoperoxidase system: helps to regulate oxidative state

Leukocytes: including lymphocytes, macrophages and neutrophils

Long-chain polyunsaturated fatty acids: e.g. arachidonate and docosahexenoate

Lymphocytes: comprise around 10% of the leukocytes found in breast milk; produce immunoglobulins

Lysozyme: a bactericidal agent

Nucleotides: building blocks of nucleic acid in DNA; they may also enhance leukocyte maturation, considered conditionally essential at times of increased demand, for example during recovery from sepsis or injury

Oligosaccharides: carbohydrate-based compounds that function both as analogues of the binding site of various microbes (and their toxins) and thus reduce their attachment to the gut wall, and as substrate for beneficial bacteria in the large bowel (since they resist digestion in the small bowel[3])

Peroxidase: a bactericidal agent

Polyamines: important triggers of gastrointestinal mucosal growth[4]

Secretory IgA: covalently bonded molecules of IgA that resist digestion and so can retain their antimicrobial activity throughout the bowel[5]

For good reviews, see references 5–7

number of factors present in human milk that play important roles both in gut growth and immunity. The early milk (colostrum) is particularly valuable, despite often being present in low volumes. Figure 1.1 shows a comparison of the composition of some of the immunological components in colostrum versus mature human milk. The immunological protection given by secretory IgA has been likened to an antiseptic paint coating the lining of the gut to protect it from microbial invasion. Due to its altered visual appearance compared to mature milk,

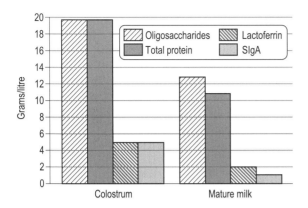

Figure 1.1 Comparison of the major immunological components in colostrum and mature human milk. SIgA, secretory immunoglobulin A. (Adapted from Prentice[18] and Coppa et al.[19])

colostrum has been discarded in some societies and alternatives given before transitional milk comes in. It is therefore important to advise both parents and other health care professionals of the importance of collecting and feeding this early milk despite its appearance and low volume.

A preterm infant's gut can be leaky, allowing absorption of large molecules into the circulation. The long-term effects of this are unknown; however, preterm infants as a group do not appear to be at increased risk of allergy.[20] It is possible that some factors may exert their effects well beyond the gastrointestinal level since they resist digestion and are absorbed by the recipient infant, for example the immunological protein lactoferrin, which has been detected intact in the urine of preterm infants.[21]

It has been suggested that there may be increased levels of anti-infective factors in preterm compared to term milk.[22–24] However, this has not been confirmed by others.[25] Only under conditions of severe malnutrition may the levels of some but not all of these components be reduced: in one study secretory IgA was reduced but lysozyme levels were maintained.[26] Nevertheless, there is evidence that in severe malnutrition milk volume can be significantly reduced.[12]

Human milk may be able to stimulate the functional maturation of the gastrointestinal tract and the baby's immune system; it appears to be important as an educator of the infant's immune system and may be crucial in pro-viding the signals that will lead to appropriate immune responses and immune memory so important for later health.[27] This may be partly due to interactions with the microbial flora that first colonize the gut; in human-milk-fed babies these tend to be less pathogenic than those resulting from the feeding of formula.[7] The concept that nutrition, including the feeding of breast milk, at a critical or sensitive period in early life may influence a wide variety of metabolic, developmental and pathological processes later in life is now widely accepted.[28]

The three major functions of anti-inflammatory agents include: (1) the augmentation of mucosal barriers; (2) the inhibition of non-oxidative systems; and (3) inhibition of oxidative systems.[6] Human milk serves to influence susceptibility to infection in a variety of ways, including augmentation of the gut mucosal barrier. It has recently been shown that milk from mothers of babies born at 23–27 weeks' gestation has significantly higher levels of EGF than milk from older preterm and term babies through to the 4th week of lactation.[30] EGF is thought to have a vital role in surveillance of the gut mucosal surface, initiating repair when necessary[31] and aiding stomach maturation.[32]

NUTRITIONAL AND GASTROINTESTINAL ADVANTAGES OF HUMAN MILK

In addition to the non-nutritive benefits, there is evidence to suggest that the bioavailability of many nutrients is enhanced when presented to the infant as human rather than formula milk. This is of particular importance in preterm infants where digestion and absorption may be compromised by immaturity and illness. Using human milk rather than formula is likely to reduce the time taken to tolerance of full enteral feeds;[33,34] probably aided by more rapid gastric emptying.[35,36] Other gastrointestinal effects include decreased lower gut permeability and improved lactase production;[37,38] the latter is possibly a factor in improved feed tolerance.

Fat in human milk provides up to 50% of its energy content and is the vehicle for fat-soluble vitamins. Fatty acids are more readily absorbed from human milk than from preterm formula in preterm infants[39,40] at a time when fat absorption is compromised.[41–43] There are several reasons for enhanced fat absorption. Breast milk contains bile salt-stimulated lipase,[44] which to a large degree can compensate for the reduced activity of the intestinal lipases in those born preterm. Also, human milk fat digestion is facilitated by the complex organization of the milk fat globule. The distribution of fatty acids on the glycerol backbone molecule helps to explain the high absorption rates of palmitic

acid in human milk[45] (Fig. 1.2). In human milk, unlike in cow's milk fat, the 2 position predominates; fatty acids are preferentially cleaved from the 1 and 3 positions, leaving the monoglyceride of palmitic acid and glycerol, which is then absorbed at the gut surface. This restricts the interaction of free palmitic acid with calcium and the formation of insoluble soaps that lead to large gastrointestinal losses of both calcium and fat.

In addition to improved fat absorption, a number of studies provide evidence for the improved bioavailability of iron,[46] zinc,[47] copper[48] and vitamin E[49] from breast milk compared to formula in preterm infants. Despite good absorption and high biological value, the levels of many nutrients in human milk are insufficient for preterm infants, particularly those below 1500 g; this is addressed in Chapter 3.

PROTECTION FOR PRETERM INFANTS

There is evidence for a reduced risk of sepsis in preterm infants receiving breast milk;[31] a dose-dependent reduction has been shown in some

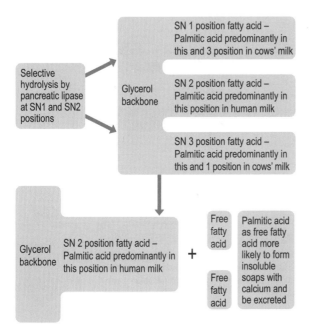

Figure 1.2   Improved absorption of fatty acids from human milk.

studies[7,33,50,51] but not others.[52] The amount of human milk a baby receives may be relevant to these findings. It has recently been shown that a threshold amount of 50 ml/kg of human milk during the first 4 weeks was needed to reduce sepsis significantly.[53]

In addition, babies breast-fed following discharge from the neonatal intensive care unit continue to benefit from a significant decrease in the incidence of sepsis compared to those fed formula.[54] However, it is important to point out that the reduction in sepsis may be due to other confounding factors such as maternal education and social class, which may be unrelated to the properties of the milk itself[55] (see p. 105 in ref 55).[56]

In a review of prospectively collected data on morbidity and diet in premature infants in Houston, Texas, a group of infants were identified who had been fed exclusively on fortified human milk. These infants had a significantly lower incidence of necrotizing enterocolitis (NEC), sepsis and fewer positive blood cultures than infants fed preterm formula or a mixture of fortified human milk and preterm formula.[57] The infants in the group fed exclusively on fortified human milk had significantly more episodes of skin-to-skin contact with their mothers than those fed preterm formula. The results of this study have since been replicated by the same group but only in infants receiving 50 ml/kg fortified human milk or more.[56] Since one of the important protective effects of human milk for an infant may operate via an entero-mammary immune system, skin-to skin contact between the infant and mother may be particularly important. There is evidence that lactating women can be induced to make specific antibodies against the nosocomial pathogens in the neonatal environment and that these antibodies are then secreted in their breast milk (Fig. 1.3). Researchers argue that the lower incidence of infection in the exclusively human milk group strongly suggests that skin-to-skin contact may be a means of providing species-specific antimicrobial protection for both term and premature infants.[5] However, there is a need for a randomized controlled trial to assist in the development of a proper evidence base to test this assumption.

NEC is an acute inflammatory bowel disorder characterized by ischaemic necrosis of the gastrointestinal mucosa, which may lead to perforation and peritonitis. A number of factors have been identified as predisposing an infant to NEC, including fetal hypoxia, unfavourable

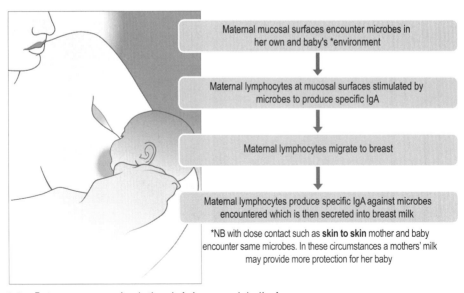

Figure 1.3   Enteromammary circulation. IgA, immunoglobulin A.

gut flora, hypotension and poor bowel perfusion. Enteral feeding, particularly with high-osmolality feeds, and the presence of infection with a range of Gram-negative organisms have also been implicated. Human milk, both the mother's own and donor, has been shown to reduce the risk of NEC in individual studies[51,58,59] and in a recent meta-analysis.[60] The risk of gut perforation in NEC may also be reduced.[61] In one study it appeared that a delay in introducing enteral feeds led to a slight reduction in NEC in formula-fed infants but not in those fed human milk.[58] A study using an animal model showed that feeding of maternal milk was associated with a reduced severity of NEC and increased production of the anti-inflammatory cytokine interleukin-10 in the intestinal epithelium.[62] The benefit of human milk feeding may arise from the presence of the many immunological factors present as well as the fact that it is isotonic to the blood, although it is important to note that its osmolality can be considerably increased by the addition of some medications (see Chapter 7).

NEURODEVELOPMENTAL ADVANTAGES

Early postnatal nutritional influences on the growth and development of the human brain are observed through childhood. The extremely rapid brain growth and development seen during the last part of a full-term pregnancy (Fig. 1.4) are difficult to replicate in infants delivered preterm, putting them at high risk of reduced brain growth.

There is evidence that human milk confers neurodevelopmental advantages. However, due to the ethical constraints of randomizing babies to their own mother's milk or formula, the majority of studies are observational.[63–71]

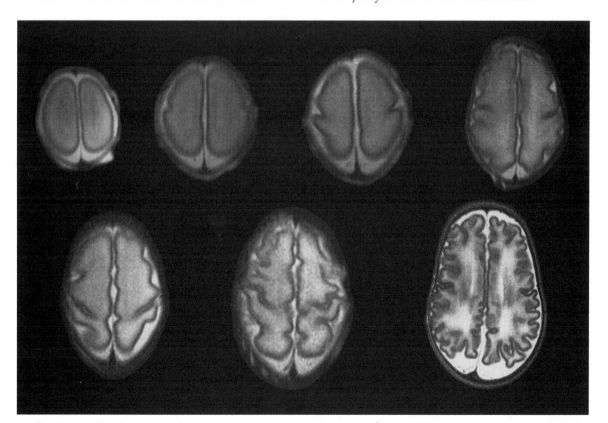

Figure 1.4 Development of the human cortex from 24 weeks to term. (From the Magnetic Resonance Imaging Unit, Hammersmith Hospital, London.)

The observational study of O'Connor et al.[68] demonstrated that those fed predominantly human milk grew less rapidly up to 9 months of age. However, following this period their growth equalled that of infants fed exclusively with preterm formula. Despite their initial slower growth, the breast-fed cohort did at least as well neurodevelopmentally as their formula-fed counterparts.

One paper reported finding no developmental advantage;[72] the authors point out that their cohort was relatively advantaged and homogeneous, and that larger numbers would be required to detect a difference due to breast milk consumption.

All researchers have made some adjustments for confounding variables between groups, e.g. social class and maternal education.[73] However, maternal characteristics associated with successful parenting are difficult to define or quantify. Even randomized controlled trials that stratify data according to infant and maternal characteristics are fraught with difficulties when assessing neurodevelopmental outcome.[74] The type of neurodevelopmental test chosen and its method of administration could alter the results obtained.

The direct relationship between human milk feeding and IQ has been challenged[75] because of the complexity of the many factors which contribute to an infant's neurodevelopmental outcome.[76,77] There is evidence that positive maternal characteristics have a more profound beneficial effect on the development of preterm infants than that of term infants.[78] In addition, Feldman & Eidelman[69] suggest that 'maternal affectionate touch' has both a positive effect on infant motor development and enhances the positive impact of breast milk on mental development.

Despite the above provisos, there are some data suggesting that human milk confers neurodevelopmental advantages independent of maternal characteristics (Fig. 1.5). Randomized allocation of infants to human milk in the form of donated milk is possible but has rarely been done, except by Alan Lucas and colleagues in the UK. In one publication from this group there was a comparison of infants randomized

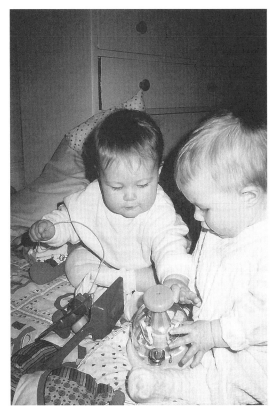

Figure 1.5   Two babies playing.

to donor breast milk or preterm formula either as sole source of nutrition or as a supplement to mother's expressed breast milk. It was shown that at 18 months there was no difference in development despite the far lower nutritional content of the donor milk.[79] In contrast, in a different arm of the trial, those fed a term formula fared significantly worse compared to preterm formula. The advantages seen in this study lend strength to the relationship of optimum brain development via the feeding of breast milk to preterm infants.

Recently there has been much interest in the provision of specific components of neuronal structure, which are thought to be essential for optimum function. Long-chain polyunsaturated fatty acids (LCPs) are essential components of cell membranes and are important in the developing brain and retina. There is a preferential transfer of LCPs across the placenta in the third trimester;[80] thus preterm infants are at a greater risk of deficiency than term infants. Human milk is a relatively consistent source of LCPs despite widely varying maternal diets.[81]

LONG-TERM OUTCOMES

Accumulating evidence shows that the consumption of human milk, both donor and mother's own, in the early neonatal period may help to reduce some cardiovascular risk factors. Although blood pressure, when measured in childhood, was not affected by the type of milk given on the neonatal unit a significant reduction was seen in adolescence in those who had received breast milk as neonates.[82] In addition these individuals had improved lipid ratios and reduced C-reactive protein levels.[83]

RISKS WITH HUMAN MILK

The many positive effects of human milk for preterm infants that have been discussed outweigh most potential disadvantages; however, it is important to be aware of the rare occasions when human milk may be contraindicated.

Many drugs taken by lactating women are secreted into their milk and some of these are considered to be potentially harmful to the recipient baby. A mother's notes should be carefully scrutinized to evaluate any medication she may be on; in addition the mother should be asked directly about any medication she is taking.[84] Personal observation suggests that milk will sometimes be withheld without firm evidence that the drug taken is contraindicated.

There is often confusion about the role of microbes that can be cultured in samples of a woman's breast milk and the potential risk for infection in her infant. It is well known that human milk is not sterile and can grow potential pathogens.[85] However this observation cannot be extrapolated to explain infections in human-milk-fed infants, whether term or preterm.[17,86] When a woman has come into contact with a pathogen in her environment

she will produce anti-infective factors specific to that pathogen, and these factors are then secreted into her milk (see the discussion above). However there are circumstances where the nature of the pathogen could pose a risk to the infant, for example where a woman is human immunodeficiency virus (HIV)-positive.[87,88] In addition, the presence of cytomegalovirus in breast milk and the subsequent infection of babies receiving that milk are well documented.[89] Viral load in the milk can be reduced or eradicated by freezing.[90] A rarer form of infection could be transmitted via group B streptococcus-colonized milk.[91]

There is also a theoretical risk of hepatitis C transmission.[92] The baby of a mother who is hepatitis B-positive should receive both active and passive immunization.[92] In most cases it should be possible for the baby to receive its mother's fresh milk safely.[92]

If hygiene and storage practices are not optimal, human milk is at risk of contamination postexpression: methicillin-resistant *Staphylococcus aureus* (MRSA) has been detected.[93]

The very small risk of adverse effects from contaminated human milk is outweighed by the advantages discussed in the preceding part of this chapter. However, it is important to ensure that mothers who are at high risk of having infected milk are identified and that all are given clear instructions on clean collection and storage of their milk.[94]

SUMMARY

Further systematic reviews and meta-analyses would help to provide definitive evidence in respect of the benefits of human milk for preterm infants; this type of evidence does exist but is limited to the reduced risk of NEC.[60] In a recent systematic review of studies seeking to examine preterm feeding with respect to other outcomes, many studies were excluded because of serious methodological flaws both in design and execution.[95] Although the reviewers could not find conclusive evidence of advantage for the use of human milk for preterm babies because of the weaknesses in the studies that currently form the body of literature, they are not denying that benefit exists. They are simply stating that larger studies with more stringent attention to design must be performed. Nevertheless, the cumulative advantages outlined above suggest that preterm babies will benefit from provision of human milk, particularly their own mother's milk. Although optimal nutrition for preterm infants remains controversial, many neonatologists prefer human milk because it is better tolerated and the advantages of breast milk outweigh the few risks that are associated with it.[96]

In conclusion, human milk contains immunologic factors that potentially reduce the incidence of sepsis in preterm infants. It provides advantages that span the digestion and assimilation of key nutrients through to the reduction in risk of life-threatening conditions such as NEC.

There is strong evidence that the absorption rate of nutrients from human milk is better than from breast-milk substitutes; in addition, its enzymes, hormones and growth factors play important roles in gastrointestinal growth and maturation. It is better tolerated than cow's milk formula and human milk often helps accelerate establishment of enteral feeding. There is convincing evidence that prevention of infection can be enhanced by close physical contact between a mother and her baby. This will enable the production of specific antibodies which will be secreted in maternal milk to give each baby unique protection from infection. When a mother wishes to provide breast milk for her infant and she is helped to succeed, it is not only the mother and baby who benefit – the health professionals involved also benefit.

Thus, fresh human milk from a baby's own mother, given along with the appropriate supplements, is undoubtedly the feed of choice for a preterm infant.

However, human milk can only be given if adequate volumes are produced. In the following chapters, we will discuss the long-term management of milk expression and feeding for mothers and babies following admission to a neonatal intensive care unit. Throughout this book evidence-based guidelines on starting and maintaining lactation have been formulated: it is the authors' hope that the numbers of preterm babies receiving their mother's own expressed milk will increase. In turn this will enable large studies to be carried out to advance our knowledge of the many benefits of human milk.

References

1. Goldman AS, Chheda S, Garofalo R. Evolution of immunologic functions of the mammary gland and the postnatal development of immunity. Pediatr Res 1998; 43:155–162.

2. Peterson JA, Patton S, Hamosh M. Glycoproteins of the human milk fat globule in the protection of the breastfed infant against infection. Biol Neonate 1998; 74(2):143–162.

3. Brand Miller JB, McVeagh P. Human milk oligosaccharides: 130 reasons to breast-feed. Br J Nutr 1999; 82:333–335.

4. Capano G, Bloch KJ, Carter EA et al. Polyamines in human and rat milk influence intestinal cell growth in vitro. J Pediatr Gastroenterol Nutr 1998; 27(3):281–286.

5. Hanson LA, Korotkova M. The role of breastfeeding in prevention of neonatal infection. Semin Neonatol 2002; 7:275–281.

6. Hamosh M. Bioactive factors in human milk. Pediatr Clin North Am 2001; 48:69–86.

7. Xanthou M. Immune protection of human milk. Biol Neonate 1998; 74(2):121–133.

8. Kavanaugh K, Meier P, Zimmermann B et al. The rewards outweigh the efforts: breastfeeding outcomes for mothers of preterm infants. J Hum Lact 1997; 13:15–21.

9. Meier PP, Brown LP, Hurst NM. Breast feeding the preterm infant. In: Jones and Bartlett, eds. Breast feeding and human lactation. Boston: 1999:456.

10. Hawkes JS, Neumann MA, Gibson RA. The effect of breast feeding on lymphocyte subpopulations in healthy term infants at 6 months of age. Pediatr Res 1999; 45:648–651.

11. Goldman AS, Garza C, Nichols BL et al. Immunologic factors in human milk during the first year of lactation. J Pediatr 1982; 100:563–567.

12. Hennart PF, Brasseur DJ, Delogne-Desnoeck JB et al. Lysozyme, lactoferrin, and secretory immunoglobulin A content in breast milk: influence of duration of lactation, nutrition status, prolactin

status, and parity of mother. Am J Clin Nutr 1991; 53:32–39.

13. IaCopetta BJ, Griell F, Horisberger M et al. Epidermal growth factor in human and bovine milk. Acta Paediatr Scand 1992; 81:287–291.

14. Romain N, Dandrifosse G, Jeusette F et al. Polyamine concentration in rat milk and food, human milk, and infant formulas. Pediatr Res 1992; 32:58–63.

15. Howie PW, Forsyth JS, Ogston SA. Protective effect of breast feeding against infection. Br Med J 1990; 300:11–16.

16. Ashraf RN, Fehmida J, Zaman S. Breast feeding protection against neonatal sepsis in a high risk population. Arch Dis Child 1991; 66:488–490.

17. Narayanan I, Prakash K, Pratharkar. A planned prospective evaluation of the anti-infective property of varying quantities of expressed human milk. Acta Paediatr Scand 1982; 71:441–445.

18. Prentice A. Constituents of human milk. Food Nutr Bull 1996; 17 number 4.

19. Coppa GV, Gabrielli O, Pierani P et al. Changes in carbohydrate composition in human milk over 4 months of lactation. Pediatrics 1993; 91(3):637–641.

20. Buhrer C, Grimmer I, Niggemann B et al. Low 1-year prevalence of atopic eczema in very low birthweight infants. Lancet 1999; 353:1674.

21. Hutchens TW, Henry JF, Yip TT et al. Origin of intact lactoferrin and its DNA-binding fragments found in the urine of human milk-fed preterm infants. Evaluation by stable isotopic enrichment. Pediatr Res 1991; 29:243–250.

22. Goldman AS, Garza C, Nichols B et al. Effects of prematurity on the immunologic system in human milk. J Pediatr 1982; 101:901–905.

23. Mathur NB, Dwarkadas AM, Sharma VK et al. Anti-infective factors in preterm human colostrum. Acta Paediatr Scand 1990; 79:1039–1044.

24. Straussberg R, Sirota L, Hart J et al. Phagocytosis-promoting factor in human colostrum. Biol Neonate 1995; 68:15–18.

25. Velona T, Abbiati L, Beretta B et al. Protein profiles in breast milk from mothers delivering term and preterm babies. Pediatr Res 1999; 45:658–663.

26. Miranda R, Saravia NG, Ackerman R et al. Effect of maternal nutritional status on immunological substances in human colostrum and milk. Am J Clin Nutr 1983; 37:632–640.

27. Kelly D, Coutts AG. Early nutrition and the development of immune function in the neonate. Proc Nutr Soc 2000; 59:177–185.

28. Lucas A. Does early diet program future outcome? Acta Paediatr Scand 1990; 365 (suppl.):58–67.

29. Dvorak B, Fituch CC, Williams CS et al. Increased epidermal growth factor levels in human milk of mothers with extremely premature infants. Pediatr Res 2003; 54:15–19.

30. Playford RJ, Wright NA. Why is epidermal growth factor present in the gut lumen? Gut 1996; 38:303–305.

31. el-Mohandes AE, Picard MB, Simmens SJ et al. Use of human milk in the intensive care nursery decreases the incidence of nosocomial sepsis. J Perinatol 1997; 17:130–134.

32. Kelly EJ, Newell SJ, Brownlee KG et al. Role of epidermal growth factor and transforming growth factor alpha in the developing stomach. Arch Dis Child Fetal Neonatal Ed 1997; 76:F158–F162.

33. Uraizee F, Gross SJ. Improved feeding tolerance and reduced incidence of sepsis in sick very low birth weight (VLBW) infants fed maternal milk. Pediatr Res 1989; 25:298A.

34. Simmer K, Metcalf R, Daniels L. The use of breastmilk in a neonatal unit and its relationship to protein and energy intake and growth. J Paediatr Child Health 1997; 33:55–60.

35. Ewer AK, Durbin GM, Morgan ME et al. Gastric emptying in preterm infants. Arch Dis Child Fetal Neonatal Ed 1994; 71:F24–F27.

36. Van Den Driessche M, Peeters K, Marien P et al. Gastric emptying in formula-fed and breast-fed infants measured with the C-13-octanoic acid breath test. J Pediatr Gastroenterol Nutr 1999; 29:46–51.

37. Shulman RJ, Schanler RJ, Lau C et al. Early feeding, feeding tolerance, and lactase activity in preterm infants. J Pediatr 1998; 133:645–649.

38. Shulman RJ, Schanler RJ, Lau C et al. Early feeding, antenatal glucocorticoids, and human milk decrease intestinal permeability in preterm infants. Pediatr Res 1998; 44:519–523.

39. Armand M, Hamosh M, Mehta NR et al. Effect of human milk or formula on gastric function and fat digestion in the premature infant. Pediatr Res 1996; 40:429–437.

40. Morgan C, Stammers J, Colley J et al. Fatty acid balance studies in preterm infants fed formula milk containing long-chain polyunsaturated fatty acids (LCP) II. Acta Paediatr 1998; 87:318–324.

41. Rings E, Minich D, Fetter W et al. Fat malabsorption in preterm and term neonates is not due to insufficient lipolysis, but to impaired uptake of long chain fatty acids from the intestinal lumen. Pediatr Res 1999; 45:290A.

42. Hamosh M. Lipid metabolism in premature infants. Biol Neonate 1987; 52 (suppl. 1):50–64.

43. Boehm G, Braun W, Moro G et al. Bile acid concentrations in serum and duodenal aspirates of healthy preterm infants: effects of gestational and postnatal age. Biol Neonate 1997; 71:207–214.

44. Hernell O and Olivecrona T. Human milk lipases II Bile salt stimulated lipase. Biochem, Biophys Acta 1974; 369:234–244.

45. Carnielli VP, Luijendijk IH, van Goudoever JB et al. Feeding premature newborn infants palmitic acid in amounts and stereoisomeric position similar to that of human milk: effects on fat and mineral balance. Am J Clin Nutr 1995; 61:1037–1042.

46. Bosscher D, Caillie-Bertrand M, Robberecht H et al. In vitro availability of calcium, iron, and zinc from

first-age infant formulae and human milk. J Pediatr Gastroenterol Nutr 2001; 32:54–58.

47. Wauben I, Gibson R, Atkinson S. Premature infants fed mothers' milk to 6 months corrected age demonstrate adequate growth and zinc status in the first year. Early Hum Dev 1999; 54:181–194.

48. Ehrenkranz RA, Gettner PA, Nelli CM et al. Zinc and copper nutritional studies in very low birth weight infants: comparison of stable isotopic extrinsic tag and chemical balance methods. Pediatr Res 1989; 26:298–307.

49. Woodruff CW, Latham CB, James EP et al. Vitamin A status of preterm infants: the influence of feeding and vitamin supplements. Am J Clin Nutr 1986; 44:384–389.

50. el-Mohandes AE, Picard MB, Simmens SJ. Human milk utilization in the ICN decreases the incidence of bacterial sepsis. Pediatr Res 1995; 37:306A.

51. Schanler RJ, Shulman RJ, Lau C et al. Feeding strategies for premature infants: randomized trial of gastrointestinal priming and tube-feeding method [see comments]. Pediatrics 1999; 103:434–439.

52. Hylander MA, Strobino DM, Dhanireddy R. Human milk feedings and infection among very low birth weight infants. Pediatrics 1998; 102:E38.

53. Furman L, Taylor G, Minich N et al. The effect of maternal milk on neonatal morbidity of very low-birth-weight infants. Arch Pediatr Adolesc Med 2003; 157:66–71.

54. Blaymore Bier JA, Oliver T, Ferguson A et al. Human milk reduces outpatient upper respiratory symptoms in premature infants during their first year of life. J Perinatol 2002; 22:354–359.

55. Schanler RJ. Clinical benefits of human milk for premature infants. In: Zeigler EE, Lucas A, Moro GE, eds. Nutrition of the very low birthweight infant, vol. 43. Nestle Nutrition Workshop series. Philadelphia, PA: Nestec,Vevey/Lippincott Williams & Wilkins; 1999:95–106.

56. Schanler RJ, Shulman RJ, Lau C. Feeding strategies for premature infants: beneficial outcomes of feeding fortified human milk versus preterm formula. Pediatrics 1999; 103:1150–1157.

57. Schanler RJ, Shulman RJ, Lau C. Fortified human milk improves the health of the premature infant. Pediatr Res 1996; 40:551A.

58. Lucas A, Cole TJ. Breast milk and neonatal necrotising enterocolitis. Lancet 1990; 336:1519–1523.

59. Beeby PJ, Jeffrey H. Risk factors for necrotising enterocolitis: the influence of gestational age. Arch Dis Child 1992; 67:432–435.

60. McGuire W, Anthony MY. Donor human milk versus formula for preventing necrotising enterocolitis in preterm infants: systematic review. Arch Dis Child Fetal Neonatal Ed 2003; 88:F11–F14.

61. Covert RF, Barman N, Domanico RS et al. Prior enteral nutrition with human milk protects against intestinal perforation in infants who develop necrotising enterocolitis. Pediatr Res 1995; 37:305A.

62. Dvorak B, Halpern MD, Holubec H et al. Maternal milk reduces severity of necrotizing enterocolitis and increases intestinal IL-10 in a neonatal rat model. Pediatr Res 2003; 53:426–433.

63. Morley R, Cole TJ, Powell R et al. Mother's choice to provide breast milk and developmental outcome. Arch Dis Child 1988; 63:1382–1385.

64. Amin SB, Merle KS, Orlando MS et al. Brainstem maturation in premature infants as a function of enteral feeding type. Pediatrics 2000; 106:318–322.

65. Turner-McKinley L, Thorpe J, Tucker R et al. Outcomes at 18 months corrected age of very low birth weight (VLBW) infants who received human milk during hospitalisation. Pediatr Res 2000; 47:291A.

66. Horwood L, Darlow B, Mogridge N. Breast milk feeding and cognitive ability at 7–8 years. Arch Dis Child: Fetal Neonatal Edn 2001; 1:7.

67. Bier JA, Oliver T, Ferguson AE et al. Human milk improves cognitive and motor development of premature infants during infancy. J Hum Lact 2002; 18:361–367.

68. O'Connor DL, Jacobs J, Hall R et al. Growth and development of premature infants fed predominantly human milk, predominantly premature infant formula, or a combination of human milk and premature formula. J Pediatr Gastroenterol Nutr 2003; 37:437–446.

69. Feldman R, Eidelman AI. Direct and indirect effects of breast milk on the neurobehavioral and cognitive development of premature infants. Dev Psychobiol 2003; 43:109–119.

70. Elwood PC, Pickering L, Davies DP et al. The long term effect of breast feeding: cognitive function in the Caerphilly cohort. Arch Dis Child 2003; 88 (suppl. 1):A12.

71. Smith MM, Durkin M, Hinton VJ et al. Influence of breastfeeding on cognitive outcomes at age 6–8 years: follow-up of very low birth weight infants. Am J Epidemiol 2003; 158:1075–1082.

72. Pinelli J, Saigal S, Atkinson SA. Effect of breastmilk consumption on neurodevelopmental outcomes at 6 and 12 months of age in VLBW infants. Adv Neonatal Care 2003; 3:76–87.

73. Jacobson JL, Jacobson SW. Breast-feeding and gender as moderators of teratogenic effects on cognitive development. Neurotoxicol Teratol 2002; 24:349–358.

74. Singer L. Randomized clinical trials in infancy: methodologic issues. Semin Neonatol 2001; 6:393–401.

75. Jacobson SW, Chiodo LM, Jacobson JL. Breastfeeding effects on intelligence quotient in 4- and 11-year-old children. Pediatrics 1999; 103:e71.

76. Burgard P. Critical evaluation of the methodology employed in cognitive development trials. Acta Paediatr 2003; 92 (suppl.):6–10.

77. Rey J. Breastfeeding and cognitive development. Acta Paediatr 2003; 92 (suppl.):11–18.

78. Rassin DK, Smith KE. Nutritional approaches to improve cognitive development during infancy:

antioxidant compounds. Acta Paediatr 2003; 92 (suppl.):34–41.

79. Lucas A, Morley R, Cole TJ, Gore. A randomised multicentred study of human milk vs formula and later development in preterm infants. Arch Dis Child 1994; 70:F141–F146.

80. Carlson SE. Docosahexaenoic acid and arachidonic acid in infant development. Semin Neonatol 2001; 6:437–449.

81. Koletzko B, Thiel I, Abiodun PO. The fatty acid composition of human milk in Europe and Africa. J Pediatr 1992; 120:S62–S70.

82. Singhal A, Cole TJ, Lucas A. Early nutrition in preterm infants and later blood pressure: two cohorts after randomised trials. Lancet 2001; 357:413–419.

83. Singhal A, Cole TJ, Fewtrell M et al. Breastmilk feeding and lipoprotein profile in adolescents born preterm: follow-up of a prospective randomised study. Lancet 2004; 363:1571–1578.

84. Hale TW. Medications and mother's milk, 11th edn. Amarillo, USA: Pharmsoft; 2004.

85. Carrol L, Osman M, Davies DP et al. Bacteriological criteria for feeding raw breast milk to babies on neonatal units. Lancet 1979; 2:732–733.

86. Law BJ, Urias BA, Lertzman J et al. Is ingestion of milk-associated bacteria by premature infants fed raw human milk controlled by routine bacteriologic screening? J Clin Microbiol 1989; 27:1560–1566.

87. Nicoll A, Newell ML, Van Praag E et al. Infant feeding policy and practice in the presence of HIV-1 infection. AIDS 1995; 9:107–119.

88. Coutsoudis A, Rollins N. Breast-feeding and HIV transmission: the jury is still out. J Pediatr Gastroenterol Nutr 2003; 36:434–442.

89. Bryant P, Morley C, Garland S et al. Cytomegalovirus transmission from breast milk in premature babies: does it matter? Arch Dis Child Fetal Neonatal Ed 2002; 87:F75–F77.

90. Dworsky M, Stagno S, Pass RF et al. Persistence of cytomegalovirus in human milk after storage. J Pediatr 1982; 101:440–443.

91. Arias-Camison JM. Late onset group B streptococcal infection from maternal expressed breast milk in a very low birth weight infant. J Perinatol 2003; 23:691–692.

92. Balmer SE, Nicol A, Weaver G et al. Guidelines for the collection, storage and handling of mother's breast milk to be fed to her own baby on a neonatal unit. United Kingdom Association for Milk Banking 2001.

93. Novak FR, Da Silva AV, Hagler AN et al. Contamination of expressed human breast milk with an epidemic multiresistant *Staphylococcus aureus* clone. J Med Microbiol 2000; 49:1109–1117.

94. United Kingdom Association for Milk Banking. Guidelines for the collection, storage and handling of breast milk for a mother's own baby in hospital, 2nd edn. London: Queen Charlotte's and Chelsea Hospital; 2001.

95. McGuire W, Anthony MY. Formula milk versus preterm human milk for feeding preterm or low birth weight infants. Cochrane Database Syst Rev 2001; 3:CD002972.

96. Schanler RJ, Hurst NM. Human milk for the hospitalised preterm infant. Semin Perinatol 1994; 18:476–484.

Chapter 2

Nutritional requirements

Caroline King

SUMMARY OF RECOMMENDATIONS

See Table 2.1: levels of nutrients suggested by Klein are recommended

Energy
- Most stable growing babies will require 110–120 kcal (460–500 kJ)/kg per 24 h
- During an acute-phase response, energy requirements may be temporarily reduced

Protein
- In formula: Between 3.0 and 4.3 g/kg per 24 h with energy levels as above

Fat-soluble vitamins
Vitamin A
- If supplements are given, adequate zinc status must be ensured

Vitamin D
- 400 IU/24 h; best as vitamin D3 Avoid use of 1α vitamin D unless there is severe deficiency

Vitamin E
- Supplementation beyond current recommendations may be useful when more than 2 mg/kh per 24 h of iron is given

Iron
- Ensure 2 mg/kg per 24 h from 4 weeks, independently of transfusion history
- Consider starting earlie and using higher dose in infants on erythropoietin

For other nutrients see text

Table 2.1   Comparison of recommendations

Nutrients	Tsang et al.[2] per 100 ml[a] based on 80 kcal/100 ml	Tsang et al.[2] per 100 kcal[a]	Klein[1] per 100 kcal[a]
Energy (kcal)	110–120/kg	110–120/kg 67–80/100 ml	110–135/kg 67–94/100 ml
Protein (g/kg)	< 1000 g 3.6–3.8 > 1000 g 3.0–3.6	< 1000 g 3.0–3.16 > 1000 g 2.5–3.0	2.5–3.6
Fat (g)	3. 5–4.8 (tentative)		4.4–5.7
Medium-chain triglycerides (maximum % total fat)	NS	NS	50
Long-chain polyunsaturated acids (maximum % total fat)[27]	Conditionally essential	Conditionally essential	AA 0. 6 (0.4) DHA 0.35 (0.35)
AA: DHA	NS	NS	1.5–2.0
EPA (maximum % DHA)	NS	NS	30
Linoleic acid (LA)(g)	0.35–1.36	0.44–1.7	% total FA 8–25
α-Linolenic acid (ALA)(g)	0.09–0.35	0.11–0.44	% total FA 1.75–4
LA:ALA (minimum–maximum)	NS	NS	6:1 16:1
Carbohydrate (g)	NS	NS	9.6–12.3
Lactose (g)	2.4–7.6	3–9.5	4–12.5
Minerals			
Sodium (mg)	30–46	37–57	39–63
Potassium (mg)	52–80	65–100	60–160
Chloride (mg)	47–71	59–89	60–160
Calcium (mg)	80–154	100–193	123–185
Phosphorus (mg)	48–112	50–117	82–109
Ca:P ratio (by mass)	NS	NS	1.7:1 to 2:1
Magnesium (mg)	5–10	6.3–12.5	6.8–17
Iron (mg)	2.0 (/kg)	1.56	1.7–3
Zinc (mg)	0.7	0.85	1.1–1.5
Copper (μg)	80–100	100–125	100–250
Iodine (μg)	20–40	25–50	6–35
Manganese (μg)	5	6.3	6.3–25
Selenium (μg)	0.9	1.0–2.5	1.8–5.0
Fluoride (μg)	NS	NS	Maximum 25
Chromium (μg)	NS	NS	NS
Molybdenum (μg)	NS	NS	NS
Vitamins			
Vitamin A (μg)[b]	CLD: 450–840 μg/kg No CLD: 210–450 μg/kg		204–380 μg
Vitamin D[b]	2.4–6.4 Minimum 10/day =400 IU	3–8 μg 120–320 IU	1.9–7 μg 75–270 IU
Vitamin E (TE) (mg)[b]	4–8 IU (maximum 25 IU/day)	5–10	2–8 (alpha-tocopherol equivalent) mg: PUFA g >1.5:1
Vitamin K (μg)	5.3–6.7	6.6–8.4	4–25
Thiamin B_1 (mg)	0.12–0.16	0.15–0.2	0.03–0.25
Riboflavin B_2 (mg)	0.16–0.24	0.20–0.3	0.08–0.62

(Continued)

Table 2.1　Continued

Nutrients	Tsang et al.[2] per 100 ml[a] based on 80 kcal/100 ml	Tsang et al.[2] per 100 kcal[a]	Klein[1] per 100 kcal[a]
Vitamins			
Niacin (mg)	2.4–3.2	3–4	0.55–5
Pantothenic acid (mg)	0.8–1.2	1.0–1.5	0.3–1.9
Pyridoxine B_6 (mg)	0.1–0.14	0.125–0.175	0.03–0.25
Folic acid (µg)	17–34	21.2–42.5	30–45
Vitamin B_{12} (µg)	0.2	0.25	0.08–0.7
Biotin (µg)	2.4–4.0	3–5	1–37
Vitamin C (mg)	12–16	15–20	8.3–37
Other			
Choline (mg)	10–15	12–18	7–23
Taurine (mg)	3–6	3.75–7.5	5–12
Inositol (mg)	22–54	27–67	4–44
Carnitine (mg)	~ 2.4	1.2–2.4	2–5.9
Nucleotides	NS	NS	NS
Beta-carotene (µg)	NS	NS	NS
Oligosaccharides (g)	NS	NS	NS
Osmolality (mosmol/kg per H_2O)	NS	NS	NS
Potential renal solute load (mosmol/100 kcal)	NS	NS	22–32

[a]Unless otherwise stated.
[b]Conversion factors: vitamin A: µg ÷ 0.3 = IU; vitamin D: µg × 40 = IU. 1 IU vitamin E = 1 mg d, Lα tocopherol acetate.
NS, not specified; AA, arachidonic acid; DHA, docosahexaenoic acid; EPA, eicosapentaenoic acid; FA, fatty acid; CLD, chronic lung disease; PUFA, polyunsaturated fatty acids

Table 2.2　Energy requirements

kcal/kg per day (multiply by 4.18 for kJ)	Acute phase	Intermediate phase	Convalescence
Resting energy expenditure (REE)[a]	45	50–60	50–70
Cold stress	0–10	0–10	5–10
Activity/handling[b]	0–10	5–15	5–15
Stool losses[c]	0–10	10–15	10–15
Specific dynamic action[d]	0	0–5	10
Growth	0	20–30	20–30
Total	50–80	85–135	105–150[e]

[a]The lower level applies to babies with normal REE and the upper limit to those with diseases associated with increased REE, e.g. cardiac abnormalities/chronic lung disease.
[b]Zero if paralysed/heavily sedated.
[c]Zero if on total parenteral nutrition.
[d]10% of calories infused if on total parenteral nutrition.
[e]The upper limit may not be physiological and should rarely be necessary.

INTRODUCTION

Human milk is the feed of choice for preterm infants both for nutritional and non-nutritional reasons (see Chapter 1). The high bioavailability of many of its nutritional components means that there cannot be the same recommendations for levels of intake as formula. In addition, due to the variability of human milk, close attention is needed to ensure that all nutrients are provided in adequate amounts. Chapter 3 gives a discussion of the nutritional management of preterm babies fed on human milk.

Comprehensive recommendations for both breast-milk and formula-fed babies are available in the form of a book.[2] A recent recommendation for the nutritional composition of preterm formulas is also available and contains much general background information: it can be printed free from the internet.[1] A comparison of the two is summarized in Table 2.1. As can be seen, there is a great deal of overlap; however Klein[1] reviews more recent studies and thus is the preferred set of recommendations.

These most recent recommendations[1,2] supersede European ones from 1987.[3] Tables 2.3 and 2.4 show the composition of current preterm formulas in the USA and UK.

The following is a summary of some of the above guidelines, incorporating more recent data where it may lead to a different recommendation to Klein.[1] However, it is a brief discussion and reference to the original texts is recommended for more detailed background information.

ENERGY

Theoretical energy requirements have been calculated,[4] but because of the many different factors influencing energy expenditure it is impossible to prescribe the exact requirements for each infant. Instead an estimate must be made, taking into consideration relevant factors (Table 2.2; see also Brooke et al.[5]).

In general energy expenditure increases with age, intake and growth rate[2,6] and has been found to be closely related to energy intake.[7]

Tsang et al.[2] recommend 110–120 kcal/kg (460–500 kJ) while Klein[1] recommends 110–135 kcal/kg. At the time of publication Tsang et al. felt that there were insufficient data to suggest a different level for sick infants. However, there is some evidence that when infants undergo a stress response with raised C-reactive protein levels, i.e. when septic or postsurgery, they may require less energy until the stress is resolved.[8,9] This may be because the energy cost of growth is considerably reduced.[10] A recent review of the energy needs of critically ill neonates has given similar recommendations to those of Tsang et al., which are to feed to the energy requirements of the individual in a non-stressed state.[11]

Some have suggested that well infants weighing below 1000 g have average requirements of around 130 kcal/kg.[12] However, in practice, when excessive energy expenditure is kept at a minimum, levels much above 120 kcal/kg are rarely needed (Table 2.2). It should be borne in mind that the recommendations of expert committees apply to populations and individual variations can be high.[13,14]

PROTEIN

The recommendations of Tsang et al.[2] stratify intake according to gestation and birth weight whereas Klein[1] gives one recommended figure (Table 2.1). The latter guideline is recommended as it is clinically more practical.

Numerous balance studies are summarized in Tsang et al.,[2] showing that the in utero protein accretion rate of around 2 g/kg per day in 27–35-week fetuses can be achieved with protein intakes around 3–4 g/kg as long as energy intake is at least 110 kcal/kg (400 kJ). It has been suggested that there is incomplete utilization of protein at > 3 g/100 kcal.[15] Protein accretion increases in a linear fashion up to 4 g protein/kg intakes, and thereafter there is no further accretion[2,15] (see Chapter 3). At lower intakes there is a significant correlation with weight gain.[16–18] The capacity to accrete nitrogen above the intrauterine rate may be useful when catch-up growth is occurring.

Table 2.3 Composition of preterm formulas in the USA

Nutrients per 100 ml	Enfamil Premature 20 (Mead Johnson)	Enfamil Premature 24 (Mead Johnson)	Similac Special Care 20 (Ross)	Similac Special Care 24 (Ross)
Energy (kcal)	68	81	67	80
Protein (g)	2	2.4	2	2.4
Fat (g)	3.4	4.1	3.6	4.4
Medium-chain triglycerides (% total fat)	40	40	50	50
AA, DHA	✓	✓	✓	✓
Linoleic acid (g)	0.55	0.66	0.47	0.56
Linolenic acid (g)	0.06	0.07	✓	✓
Carbohydrate (g)	7.4	9	6.9	8.3
Minerals				
Sodium (mg)	39	47	29	35
Potassium (mg)	66	80	87	104
Chloride (mg)	61	73	54	66
Calcium (mg)	112	134	121	146
Phosphorus (mg)	56	67	67	81
Ca:P ratio (by weight)	2:1	2:1	1.8:1	1.8:1
Magnesium (mg)	6.1	7.3	8.1	9.7
Iron (mg)	0.34 (with Fe 1.22)	0.41 (with Fe 1.46)	0.2 (with Fe 1.2)	0.3 (with Fe 1.4)
Zinc (mg)	1	1.22	1	1.2
Copper (μg)	81	97	168	202
Iodine (μg)	17	20	4	5
Manganese (μg)	4.3	5.1	8.1	9.7
Selenium (μg)	1.89	2.3	1.2	1.4
Vitamins				
Vitamin A (μg)[a]	255	303	375	375
Vitamin D (μg)[a]	4	4.8	2.5	3
Vitamin E (TE) (mg)	4.3	5.1	2.7	3.2
Vitamin K (μg)	5.4	6.5	8.1	9.7
Thiamin B_1 (mg)	0.13	0.16	0.16	0.20
Riboflavin B_2 (mg)	0.2	0.24	0.41	0.50
Niacin (mg)	2.7	3.2	3.3	4
Pantothenic acid (mg)	0.8	0.97	1.28	1.5
Pyridoxine B_6 (mg)	0.1	0.12	0.17	0.2
Folic acid (μg)	27	32	25	30
Vitamin B_{12} (μg)	0.17	0.2	0.37	0.44
Biotin (μg)	2.7	3.2	25	30
Vitamin C (mg)	13.5	16.2	25	30
Other				
Choline (mg)	13.5	16.2	6.7	8
Taurine (mg)	4.1	4.9	NS	NS
Inositol (mg)	30	36	27	32
Carnitine (mg)	1.6	1.9	NS	NS
Nucleotides (mg)	2.8	3.36	NS	NS
Beta-carotene (μg)	–	–	NS	NS

(Continued)

Table 2.3 Continued

Nutrients per 100 ml	Enfamil Premature 20 (Mead Johnson)	Enfamil Premature 24 (Mead Johnson)	Similac Special Care 20 (Ross)	Similac Special Care 24 (Ross)
Osmolality (mosmol/kg per H$_2$0)	260	310	235	280
Estimated renal solute load (mosmol/l)	125	150	NS	NS

_ Not present.
[a]Conversion factors: vitamin A: µg ÷ 0.3 = IU; vitamin D: µg × 40 = IU. 1 IU vitamin E= 1 mg d, Lα tocopherol acetate.
AA, arachidonic acid; DHA, docosahexaenoic acid; NS, not specified.

This information is correct at the time of publication but may change: please check with the manufacturers

Table 2.4 Composition of preterm formulas in the UK

Nutrients per 100ml	Nutriprem (Cow & Gate)	Osterprem (Farley's)	Pre-Aptamil (Milupa)	LBW (SMA)	Pre Nan (Nestle)
Energy (kcal)	80	80	80	82	80
Protein (g)	2.4	2.0	2.4	2.0	2.3
Fat (g)	4.4	4.6	4.4	4.4	4.2
Medium-chain triglycerides % total fat	4.4 –	4.6 –	4.4 –	4.4 15%	4.2 26%
Long-chain polyunsaturated fatty acids	AA/DHA/GLA	DHA/GLA	AA/DHA/GLA	AA/DHA	AA/DHA/GLA
Linoleic acid (g)	0.6	0.54	0.59	0.7	0.64
Linolenic acid (g)	0.04	0.06	0.08	0.07	0.07
Carbohydrate (g)	7.9	7.6	7.7	8.6	8.6
Minerals					
Sodium (mg)	41	42	40	35	33
Potassium (mg)	80	72	90	85	95
Chloride (mg)	48	60	47	60	51
Calcium (mg)	100	110	100	80	99
Phosphorus (mg)	50	63	53	43	53
Ca:P ratio (by weight)	2:1	1.7:1	2:1	1.9:1	1.8:1
Magnesium (mg)	10	5	10	8	8.3
Iron (mg)	0.9	0.04	0.9	0.8	1.2
Zinc (mg)	0.7	0.9	0.7	0.8	0.6
Copper (µg)	80	96	80	83	70
Iodine (µg)	25	8	25	10	20
Manganese (µg)	10	3	7.2	10	5.2
Selenium (µg)	1.9	–	1.9	–	–

(Continued)

Table 2.4 Continued

Nutrients per 100ml	Nutriprem (Cow & Gate)	Osterprem (Farley's)	Pre-Aptamil (Milupa)	LBW (SMA)	Pre Nan (Nestle)
Vitamins					
Vitamin A (µg)*	227	100	147	74	84
Vitamin D (µg)*	5	2.4	2.4	1.5	2
Vitamin E (TE) (mg)	3	10	3	1.2	1.4
Vitamin K (µg)	6.6	7.0	8	8.0	6.4
Thiamin B_1 (mg)	0.14	0.1	0.14	0.12	0.56
Riboflavin B_2 (mg)	0.2	0.18	0.2	0.2	0.12
Niacin (mg)	3.0	1.0	2.9	1.3	0.8
Pantothenic acid (mg)	1.0	0.5	1.0	0.45	0.36
Pyridoxine B_6 (mg)	0.12	0.1	0.12	0.07	0.06
Folic acid (µg)	48	50	37	49	56
Vitamin B_{12} (µg)	0.2	0.2	0.2	0.3	0.24
Biotin (µg)	3	2	3	2.4	1.8
Vitamin C (mg)	16	28	16	11	13
Other					
Choline (mg)	10	5.6	13	13	12
Taurine (mg)	5.5	5.1	5.5	7	6.4
Inositol (mg)	30	3.2	30	4.5	5.2
Carnitine (mg)	2	1	2	2.9	1.7
Nucleotides(mg)	1.8	–	–	–	–
Beta-carotene (µg)	6.7	24	7.2	2.5	–
Osmolality (mosmol/kg per H_2O)	310	300	305	277	325
Estimated renal solute load (mosmol/l)	148	134	150	134	143

*Conversion factors: vitamin A: µg ÷ 0.3 = IU; vitamin D: µg × 40 = IU; 1 IU vitamin E= 1 mg d, Lα tocopherol acetate.
_ Not present; AA, arachidonic acid; DHA, docosahexaenoic acid; GLA, gamma-linolenic acid.

This information is correct at the time of publication but may change: please check with the manufacturers

However if a baby is not able or needing to make catch-up growth, protein intakes above 4 g/kg will be associated with increased nitrogenous byproducts exerting an increased metabolic stress and could be harmful (see Chapter 3).

LIPID

Percentage fat absorption is higher in human-milk-fed compared to formula-fed babies (see Chapters 1 and 3).

Longer-chain unsaturated fats tend to be absorbed less efficiently from formula in pre-term infants.[13] This is likely to be due to a reduction in bile salt pool,[19,20] reduced pancreatic lipase activity[21,22] and pancreatic immaturity.[23] There is an increasing net absorption of dietary energy with advancing maturation, and this may be a reflection of improving fat absorption.[24]

Medium-chain triglycerides (MCT) have been added to preterm formulas to improve fat absorption. However a recent systematic review concluded that there was no proof of its advantage[25] and therefore its use is not recommended. Despite this review, Klein[1] does not discourage the use of MCT: this is one area where Klein's recommendations are not endorsed.

All human-milk-fed infants receive a supply of the preformed long-chain polyunsaturated fatty acids (LCPs) docosahexanoic acid (DHA) and arachidonic acid (AA). A positive relationship has been found in some studies between these fatty acids and visual development,[26] and they have now been added to preterm formulas. While Klein[1] and experts in the field[27] suggest that both LCPs should be added preformed (Table 2.1), a recent systematic review could find no significant benefits of LCP supplementation.[28] Many studies were not eligible for scrutiny because of design faults and it was remarked that those that were eligible tended to look at healthy and fairly mature preterm infants. Neverthless, as no harm has been found, it is recommended that preterm infants are given a feed containing these fatty acids at the levels suggested (Table 2.1) if they cannot receive human milk.

WATER-SOLUBLE VITAMINS

The content of water-soluble vitamins in a mother's milk may vary with her daily consumption of these nutrients, so all mothers producing milk for their babies should be advised to include fruit and vegetables in their diet every day (see Chapter 3); however large doses of vitamin supplements are not recommended.

Infants who are no longer on a parenteral supply of vitamins and who are receiving breast milk but have not yet started on breast-milk fortifier should have a multivitamin supplement containing the major water-soluble vitamins.

On many neonatal units in the UK additional folic acid is still given to infants on preterm formula despite the more-than-adequate level in current formulas.[29] This is not recommended.

FAT-SOLUBLE VITAMINS

Vitamin A

Human milk does not supply sufficient vitamin A for the preterm infant; however, it is not clear exactly how much is needed as a supplement. Thus guidelines for the amount recommended for formula-fed infants should be followed.

There is recent evidence for a higher enteral dose than that recommended in Table 2.1 in order to attain normal serum levels in formula-fed infants. This is because most preterm infants appear to be born with poor stores[30] and there is evidence for significant vitamin A malabsorption in very-low-birth-weight infants.[31] This may be linked to the impaired fat absorption seen in preterm infants (see above). Levels around 4000–5000 IU/day have resulted in normal serum levels,[32,33] although these have not been recommended by Klein.[1]

Interest in achieving an adequate vitamin A status has arisen due to the association between vitamin A status and lung disease. A meta-analysis of observational studies has shown that poor vitamin A status is associated with adverse respiratory outcome,[34] although individual studies have not found a relationship.[35]

Although the mechanisms are not understood, effective vitamin A supplementation may help to reduce the incidence of chronic lung disease.[36–38] In these studies the intramuscular route was used to overcome the variable response to enteral supplementation. A systematic review acknowledges that intramuscular vitamin A leads to a reduction in death and oxygen requirements at 1 month; however, it is recommended that the intravenous route should be investigated as a less invasive therapy.[39] Not all studies employing vitamin A prophylaxis have noted a reduction in chronic lung disease.[40]

Vitamin D

All preterm infants will require a supplement containing 400 IU vitamin D per day: higher doses have not been found to be beneficial.[41,42] In the UK it has been reported that there is a resurgence of neonatal vitamin D deficiency. This has led to a call for all high-risk women to receive supplements during pregnancy, as this would help prevent poor status in their infants.[43] Those mothers who are at high risk of deficiency should be identified on the neonatal unit and it should be ensured that they are on supplemental vitamin D.

In infants, the active 1α form of vitamin D should be restricted to cases of proven deficiency as it is a potent hormone-like compound influencing metabolism in tissues other than bone, and may lead to calcium resorption from bone when given in excess.[44]

Vitamin E

Healthy infants around 1500 g birth weight appear to maintain vitamin E status with unsupplemented human milk,[45] so it is unclear whether preterm infants on human milk require a supplement. Nevertheless most breast-milk fortifiers contain vitamin E, which will ensure that the smaller more vunerable infant will receive additional supplies.

Although high requirements have been shown in those below 1250 g birth weight,[46] pharmacological serum levels have been associated with an increased risk of sepsis and necrotizing enterocolitis. As a result a systematic review concludes that supplementation with pharmacological doses is not recommended.[47] There is evidence that supplemental iron may depress serum vitamin E levels.[48,49] If an infant requires > 2 mg/kg iron, as may occur in an infant who is becoming iron-deficient on erythropoietin therapy, it may be wise to give additional vitamin E.

CALCIUM, PHOSPHORUS AND MAGNESIUM

During the last trimester mineral accretion by the fetus is at its peak. An infant born at 26 weeks' gestation will have acquired approximately 6 g calcium, which rises to 30 g in one who is born at term.[50] Requirements for bone substrate are very high in growing preterm

infants and it is now recognized that mineral rather than vitamin D deficiency is the major cause of osteopenia of prematurity,[41] although lack of physical activity may also be more important than was previously realized (see below).

The management of the mineral needs of preterm infants on human milk is covered in Chapter 3.

Radiological rickets has been found to be associated with normal vitamin D levels but a low serum phosphorus level.[51] A serum phosphate < 1.8 mmol/l in formula-fed and < 1.2 mmol/l in breast-milk-fed babies was found in a group of infants developing rickets.[52] Thus serum levels should guide phosphate supplementation whatever the mode of feeding.

Table 2.1 outlines current recommendations for calcium intake. Although in the past more emphasis was placed on achieving higher calcium intakes, this led to problems with calcium soap intestinal bolus obstruction.[53] In addition intakes above those recommended by Klein[1] are unlikely to give a long-term benefit with respect to bone mineralization as this improves in all preterm infants over the first year (see Chapter 8).

If additional calcium is considered it should be borne in mind that calcium given as an oral supplement significantly decreases fat absorption both from human milk and formula[54] (1.5–2 mmol/kg per day was given).

Also if iron supplements are prescribed to be given at the same time during the day as phosphorus[55] and calcium,[56] there is the risk that insoluble compounds will be formed, rendering the mineral unavailable to the infant. Shake bottles of ready-to-feed formula vigorously before feeding to ensure mixing of the sediment.

A novel approach to bone health for these infants may be the promotion of physical activity as this has been shown to promote a higher rate of mineral accretion.[57,58]

IRON

Without an exogenous source of iron the preterm infant becomes depleted by about 8 weeks.[59]

The early anaemia of prematurity is not influenced by iron supplementation,[60,61] whereas the late anaemia is.

Tsang et al.[2] recommend enteral iron supplementation at any time from birth to 8 weeks postnatally. In contrast, Klein[1] recommends that all preterm formula should contain sufficient iron to cover needs once full enteral feeds have been achieved. There is evidence that leaving supplementation to 8 weeks may put some infants at risk of iron deficiency.[62] However, giving iron within the first 4 weeks when enteral feeds have only barely begun to be tolerated may put an infant at risk of gastrointestinal disturbance. Iron supplements tend to be of high osmolality when given undiluted, and if mixed with breast milk, there may be disruption of the anti-infective properties.[63]

It is recommended that iron supplements are started between 4 and 6 weeks postnatally. This would both avoid the problems of giving iron too early and ensure that those well infants who are discharged before 8 weeks do not miss out.

The recommend enteral intake is around 2 mg/kg per day.[1,2,64] Preterm formula should contain 1.3 mg/100 ml in order to ensure 2 mg/kg when fed at 150 ml/kg; for those below this level an iron supplement is needed.

Infants undergoing erythropoietin therapy may require a larger dose, started at an earlier date, but no firm recommendations exist.

Iron should not be given at the same time as calcium[56] or phosphorus supplements[55] as insoluble compounds may be formed, reducing the bioavailability of each mineral.

For further reading on iron requirements for preterm infants, Kling & Winzerling[65] and Rao & Georgieff[66] are good review articles.

TRACE ELEMENTS

Selenium

Selenium is a component of numerous selenoproteins, including glutathione peroxidase, which is involved in protecting cell membranes from oxidative damage.[67]

Preterm infants appear to have significantly lower selenium status at birth, and without supplementation, levels continue to drop.[68] There is some evidence that poor selenium status correlates with poor respiratory outcome in preterm infants[69] and that supplementation of formula-fed infants leads to significantly less sepsis,[70] although not all supplementation studies show clinical benefit.[71] It is recommended that formula-fed infants receive a formula which is selenium-supplemented to the levels recommended by Klein.[1]

Zinc

Zinc is an essential cofactor for many enzymes and is essential for optimal immune function.[72] It is an important growth regulator; in a longitudinal study of preterm infants, length at 3 months was best predicted by length at birth and zinc intake.[73]

One group has found that in preterm infants fed unsupplemented human milk, zinc was highly bioavailable and status was normal.[74] However there have been many reports of zinc deficiency in human-milk-fed preterm infants.[75–78] Thus zinc-containing human milk fortifiers are recommended, with a provision of 0.5 mg/kg per day after the first 4–6 weeks.[1]

Despite zinc/iron interactions, formulas supplemented to a high zinc-to-iron ratio have not been shown to reduce iron absorption,[79] whereas a higher zinc formula has led to lower serum copper levels.[80]

Copper

Levels in human milk are adequate for low-birth-weight infants, although it is possible that large supplements of iron[81] and zinc[80] may reduce copper absorption.

Iodine

Iodine is needed for optimal brain development and production of thyroid hormones. Although levels depend on maternal status, early human milk should supply iodine needs; however, later on a supplement will be required to achieve the 30–60 µg/kg per day recommended.[2] The relative levels of iodine found in human milk depending on geographical location are discussed in Klein.[1]

Preterm infants fed formula with inadequate supplementation have been shown to be at risk of deficiency;[82] hence formula containing recommended amounts should be given.[1]

NUCLEOTIDES

Humans are capable of de novo synthesis of nucleotides; however, a salvage pathway exists that reuses preformed nucleotides taken in the diet. It is thought that during times of high demand the salvage path becomes important, and thus a good dietary supply is required.[83]

Human milk is a rich source both of nucleic acid and nucleotides:[84–86] unsupplemented infant formulas contain very little of either.

Evidence for the advantages of nucleotides comes mainly from studies in term infants which show reduced diarrhoea,[87] improved growth[88] and immunological advantages.[89]

Improved growth with nucleotides has not been replicated in preterm infants.[90] This study and a lack of other evidence for benefit has led to neither Klein[1] nor Tsang et al.[2] giving recommendations for supplementation of preterm formula.

β-CAROTENE

No recommendation is made for β-carotene intake; however, it is attracting attention because of its antioxidant and provitamin A activity and has been added to some preterm formulas. Unlike vitamin A, β-carotene and other carotenoids have antioxidant effects.

Carotenoids such as β-carotene may be necessary for optimal immune function.[91,92] Although the addition of β-carotene brings formula composition a little closer to human milk, it remains very different. β-Carotene is one of many carotenoids present in human milk, and it comprises only about 25% of the total.[93] Lutein is present in larger amounts than β-carotene and there is evidence that it is actively transferred into breast milk.[94] In addition the amount of carotenoids found in human milk varies considerably between individuals, depending also on time from initiation of lactation and number of previous lactations. The levels increase with increasing numbers of lactations, suggesting a possible role in the protection of the mammary gland rather than purely a nutritional role. Early milk can contain as much as 200 µg/100 ml, decreasing to as little as 4 µg/100 ml within the first week.[93] A single dose of β-carotene does not lead to a dose-dependent increase in human milk levels, but is more dependent on initial levels.[95] In this latter study levels of other major carotenoids in the milk were not affected, but in a chronic supplementation study (in non-lactating adults) serum lycopene was decreased.[96] This suggests possible competitive inhibition of absorption between carotenoids.

So far no randomized controlled trials have been published on the effect of β-carotene supplementation on the preterm infant; despite this, many preterm formulas now contain this carotenoid in isolation. Such trials are vitally important for two reasons: firstly, to demonstrate benefit, and secondly to show a lack of harm. Several trials of β-carotene supplementation in adults have been stopped early because of increased total and cancer deaths.[97] Possible mechanisms have been discussed[98] and explored using animal models.[99] The risk of harm has led to government guidelines advising against supplementation in the general population.[100]

References

1. Klein CJ. Nutrient requirements for preterm infant formulas. J Nutr 2002; 132 (suppl. 1):1395S–1577S.
2. Tsang RC, Lucas A, Uauy R et al. Nutritional needs of the preterm infant: scientific basis and practical guidelines. Williams & Wilkins; 1993.
3. ESPGAN. Nutrition and feeding of preterm infants. Acta Paediatr Scand 1987; suppl. 336.
4. Brooke OG. Energy expenditure in the fetus and neonate: sources of variability. Acta Paediatr Scand 1985; 319 (suppl.):128–134.
5. Brooke OG, Alvear J, Arnold M. Energy retention, energy expenditure, and growth in healthy immature infants. Pediatr Res 1979; 13:215–220.
6. Leitch CA, Denne SC. Energy expenditure in the extremely low-birth weight infant. Clin Perinatol 2000; 27:181–viii.
7. Bauer K, Laurenz M, Ketteler J et al. Longitudinal study of energy expenditure in preterm neonates <30 weeks' gestation during the first three postnatal weeks. J Pediatr 2003; 142:390–396.
8. Chwals WJ, Lally KP, Woolley MM et al. Measured energy expenditure in critically ill infants and young children. J Surg Res 1988; 44:467–472.
9. Garza JJ, Shew SB, Keshen TH et al. Energy expenditure in ill premature neonates. J Pediatr Surg 2002; 37:289–293.
10. Chwals WJ. Metabolism and nutritional frontiers in pediatric surgical patients. Surg Clin North Am 1992; 72:1237–1266.
11. Schwarzenberg S, Kovacs A. Metabolic effects of infection and postnatal steroids. Clin Perinatol 2002; 29:295–312.
12. Denne SC. Protein and energy requirements in preterm infants. Semin Neonatol 2001; 6:377–382.
13. Spencer SA, McKenna S, Stammers J et al. Two different low birth weight formulae compared. Early Hum Dev 1992; 30:21–31.
14. Cooke RJ, Ford A, Werkmans SH. Postnatal growth in infants born between 700-1500g. J Pediatr Gastroenterol Nutr 1993; 16:130–135.
15. Kashyap S, Schulze KF, Forsyth M et al. Growth, nutrient retention, and metabolic response in low birth weight infants fed varying intakes of protein and energy. J Pediatr 1988; 113:713–721.
16. Simmer K, Metcalf R, Daniels L. The use of breastmilk in a neonatal unit and its relationship to protein and energy intake and growth. J Paediatr Child Health 1997; 33:55–60.
17. Berry MA, Abrahamowicz M, Usher RH. Factors associated with growth of extremely premature infants during initial hospitalization. Pediatrics 1997; 100:640–646.
18. Faerk J, Petersen S, Peitersen B et al. Diet and growth in premature infants. Pediatr Res 1998; 44:450A.
19. Signer E, Murphy GM, Edkins S et al. Role of bile salts in fat malabsorption of premature infants. Arch Dis Child 1974; 49:174–180.
20. Katz L, Hamilton JR. Fat absorption in infants of birth weight less than 1300 g. J Pediatr 1974; 85:608–614.
21. Hamosh M. Lipid metabolism in premature infants. Biol Neonate 1987; 52 (suppl. 1):50–64.
22. Boehm G, Bierbach U, DelSanto A et al. Activities of trypsin and lipase in duodenal aspirates of healthy preterm infants: effects of gestational and postnatal age. Biol Neonate 1995; 67:248–253.
23. Forget P, Van den Neucker A, Degraeuwe P et al. Steatorrhea in premature infants is linked with functional pancreatic immaturity. Pediatr Res 1995; 37.
24. Brooke OG. Energy balance and metabolic rate in preterm infants fed with standard and high-energy formulas. Br J Nutr 1980; 44:13–23.
25. Klenoff-Brumberg HL, Genen LH. High versus low medium chain triglyceride content of formula for promoting short term growth of preterm infants. Cochrane Database Syst Rev 2003; 1:CD002777.
26. Carlson SE. Docosahexaenoic acid and arachidonic acid in infant development. Semin Neonatol 2001; 6:437–449.
27. Koletzko B, Agostoni C, Carlson SE et al. Long chain polyunsaturated fatty acids (LC-PUFA) and perinatal development. Acta Paediatr 2001; 90:460–464.
28. Simmer K, Patole S. Longchain polyunsaturated fatty acid supplementation in preterm infants. Cochrane Database Syst Rev 2004; 1:CD000375.
29. Ek J, Behncke L, Halvorsen KS et al. Plasma and red cell folate values and folate requirements in formula fed premature infants. Eur J Pediatr 1984; 142:78–82.
30. Mupanemunda RH, Lee DS, Fraher LJ et al. Postnatal changes in serum retinol status in very low birth weight infants. Early Hum Dev 1994; 38:45–54.
31. Ojeda F, Carver JD, Torres BA et al. Retinyl palmitate [RP] absorption in preterm [PT] infants. Pediatr Res 1994; 35:317A.
32. Landman J, Sive A, De V et al. Comparison of enteral and intramuscular vitamin A supplementation in preterm infants. Early Hum Dev 1992; 30:163–170.
33. Schwarz KB, Cox JM, Sharma S et al. Possible antioxidant effect of vitamin A supplementation in premature infants. J Pediatr Gastroenterol Nutr 1997; 25:408–414.
34. Inder TE, Graham PJ, Winterbourn CC et al. Plasma vitamin A levels in the very low birthweight infant - relationship to respiratory outcome. Early Hum Dev 1998; 52:155–168.
35. Rugolo A Jr, Miranda AFM, Rugolo LMSS et al. Blood retinol levels of very low birthweight infants and its relationship with bronchopulmonary dysplasia. Pediatr Res 2003; 53:408A.
36. Papagaroufalis C, Cairis M, Pantazatou E et al. A trial of vitamin A supplementation for the

prevention of bronchopulmonary dysplasia (BPD) in very low birth weight (VLBW) infants. Pediatr Res 1988; 23:518A.

37. Robbins ST, Fletcher AB. Early vs delayed vitamin A supplementation in very-low-birth- weight infants. J Parenter Enteral Nutr 1993; 17:220–225.

38. Tyson JE, Wright LL, Oh WOM et al. Vitamin A supplementation for extremely-low-birth-weight infants. N Engl J Med 1999; 340:1962–1968.

39. Darlow BA, Graham PJ. Vitamin A supplementation for preventing morbidity and mortality in very low birthweight infants. Cochrane Database Syst Rev 2002; 4:CD000501.

40. Chauhan S, Ostrea Jr EM, Ambat MT et al. Vitamin A prophylaxis for bronchopulmonary dysplasia: is it effective? Pediatr Res 2003; 53:471A.

41. Evans JR, Allen AC, Stinson DA et al. Effect of high-dose vitamin D supplementation on radiographically detectable bone disease of very low birth weight infants. J Pediatr 1989; 115:779–786.

42. Backstrom MC, Maki R, Kuusela AL et al. Randomised controlled trial of vitamin D supplementation on bone density and biochemical indices in preterm infants. Arch Dis Child 1999; 80:F161–F166.

43. Shaw NJ, Pal BR. Vitamin D deficiency in UK Asian families: activating a new concern. Arch Dis Child 2002; 86:147–149.

44. Raisz LG, Trummel CL, Holick MF et al. 1,25-dihydroxycholecalciferol: a potent stimulator of bone resorption in tissue culture. Science 1972; 175:768–769.

45. Woodruff CW, Latham CB, James EP et al. Vitamin A status of preterm infants: the influence of feeding and vitamin supplements. Am J Clin Nutr 1986; 44:384–389.

46. Bhutani VK, Johnson L, Sivieri E et al. Micronutrient profile for vitamins E, A and Zn in <1250g BW infants: hypoproteinemia as an index of subnormal values and their interrelationships. Pediatr Res 1998; 43:256A.

47. Brion L, Bell E, Raghuveer T. Vitamin E supplementation for prevention of morbidity and mortality in preterm infants. Cochrane Database Syst Rev 2003; 4:CD003665.

48. Gross SJ, Gabriel E. Vitamin E status in preterm infants fed human milk or infant formula. J Pediatr 1985; 106:635–639.

49. Rudolph N, Allen L, Colindres J et al. Early iron supplementation in prematures: an advantage or not? Pediatr Res 1994; 35:319A.

50. Ziegler EE, O'Donnell AM, Nelson SE et al. Body composition of the reference fetus growth. Growth 1976; 40:329–341.

51. Koo WW, Sherman R, Succop P et al. Serum vitamin D metabolites in very low birth weight infants with and without rickets and fractures. J Pediatr 1989; 114:1017–1022.

52. Aiken CG, Sherwood RA, Lenney W. Role of plasma phosphate measurements in detecting rickets of prematurity and in monitoring treatment. Ann Clin Biochem 1993; 30:469–475.

53. Koletzko B, Tangermann R, von Kries R et al. Intestinal milk-bolus obstruction in formula-fed premature infants given high doses of calcium. J Pediatr Gastroenterol Nutr 1988; 7:548–553.

54. Chappell JE, Clandinin MT, Kearney VC et al. Fatty acid balance studies in premature infants fed human milk or formula: effect of calcium supplementation. J Pediatr 1986; 108:439–447.

55. Peters T Jr, Apt L, Ross JF. Effect of phosphates upon iron absorption studied in normal human subjects and in an experimental model using dialysis. Gastroenterology 1971; 61:315–322.

56. Cook JD, Dassenko SA, Whittaker P. Calcium supplementation: effect on iron absorption [see comments]. Am J Clin Nutr 1991; 53:106–111.

57. Moyer-Mileur L, Luetkemeir M, Boomer L et al. Effect of physical activity on bone mineralization in premature infants. Pediatr Res 1994; 35:317A.

58. Miller ME. The bone disease of preterm birth: a biomechanical perspective. Pediatr Res 2003; 53:10–15.

59. Olivares M, Llaguno S, Marin V et al. Iron status in low-birth-weight infants, small and appropriate for gestational age. A follow-up study. Acta Paediatr 1992; 81:824–828.

60. Shaw JCL. Iron absorption by the premature infant. The effect of transfusion and iron supplements on the serum ferritin levels. Acta Paediatr Scand 1982; (suppl. 299):83–89.

61. Simes MA, Heikinheimo M. Regulation of erythropoiesis during early infancy. Pediatr Hematol Oncol 1991; 8(1):ix–xii.

62. Franz AR, Mihatsch WA, Sander S et al. Prospective randomized trial of early versus late enteral iron supplementation in infants with a birth weight of less than 1301 grams. Pediatrics 2000; 106:700–706.

63. Chan GM. Effects of powdered human milk fortifiers on the antibacterial actions of human milk. J Perinatol 2003; 23:620–623.

64. Ehrenkranz RA. Iron requirements of preterm infants. Nutrition 1994; 10:77–78.

65. Kling PJ, Winzerling JJ. Iron status and the treatment of the anemia of prematurity. Clin Perinatol 2002; 29:283–294.

66. Rao R, Georgieff MK. Neonatal iron nutrition. Semin Neonatol 2001; 6:425–435.

67. Daniels LA. Selenium metabolism and bioavailability. Biol Trace Elem Res 1996; 54:185–199.

68. Lockitch G, Jacobson B, Quigley G et al. Selenium deficiency in low birth weight neonates: an unrecognized problem [see comments]. J Pediatr 1989; 114:865–870.

69. Darlow BA, Inder TE, Graham PJ et al. The relationship of selenium status to respiratory outcome in the very low birth weight infant. Pediatrics 1995; 96:314–319.

70. Darlow BA, Winterbourn CC, Inder TE et al. The effect of selenium supplementation on outcome in very low birth weight infants: a randomized controlled trial. The New Zealand Neonatal Study Group. J Pediatr 2000; 136:473–480.

71. Huston R, Jelen BJ, Ray LK et al. Parenteral and enteral selenium supplementation in low birthweight preterm infants. Pediatr Res 1996; 39 311A.

72. Doherty CP, Weaver LT, Prentice AM. Micronutrient supplementation and infection: a double-edged sword? J Pediatr Gastroenterol Nutr 2002; 34:346–352.

73. Friel JK, Gibson RS, Kawash GF et al. Dietary zinc intake and growth during infancy. J Pediatr Gastroenterol Nutr 1985; 4:746–751.

74. Wauben I, Gibson R, Atkinson S. Premature infants fed mothers' milk to 6 months corrected age demonstrate adequate growth and zinc status in the first year. Early Hum Dev 1999; 54:181–194.

75. Aggett PJ, Atherton DJ, More J et al. Symptomatic zinc deficiency in a breast-fed preterm infant. Arch Dis Child 1980; 55:547–550.

76. Stapleton KM, O'Loughlin E, Relic JP. Transient zinc deficiency in a breast-fed premature infant. Australas J Dermatol 1995; 36:157–159.

77. Heinen F, Matern D, Pringsheim W et al. Zinc deficiency in an exclusively breast-fed preterm infant. Eur J Pediatr 1995; 154:71–75.

78. Stevens J, Lubitz L. Symptomatic zinc deficiency in breast-fed term and premature infants. J Paediatr Child Health 1998; 34:100.

79. Friel JK, Serfass RE, Fennessey PV et al. Elevated intakes of zinc in infant formulas do not interfere with iron absorption in premature infants. J Pediatr Gastroenterol Nutr 1998; 27:312–316.

80. Diaz-Gomez NM, Domenech E, Barroso F et al. The effect of zinc supplementation on linear growth, body composition, and growth factors in preterm infants. Pediatrics 2003; 111:1002–1009.

81. Haschke F, Ziegler EE, Edwards et al. Effect of iron fortification of infant formula on trace mineral absorption. J Pediatr Gastroenterol Nutr 1986; 5:768–773.

82. Ares S, Quero J, Duran S et al. Iodine content of infant formulas and iodine intake of premature babies: high risk of iodine deficiency. Arch Dis Child Fetal Neonatal Ed 1994; 71:F184–F191.

83. Rudolph FB. Symposium: dietary nucleotides: a recently demonstrated requirement for cellular development and immune function. J Nutr 1994; 124 (suppl.):1431S–1432S.

84. Leach JL, Baxter JH, Molitor BE et al. Total potentially available nucleosides of human milk by stage of lactation. Am J Clin Nutr 1995; 61:1224–1230.

85. Thorell L, Sjoberg LB, Hernell O. Nucleotides in human milk: sources and metabolism by the newborn infant. Pediatr Res 1996; 40:845–852.

86. Schlimme E, Martin D, Meisel H. Nucleosides and nucleotides: natural bioactive substances in milk and colostrum. Br J Nutr 2000; 84 (suppl. 1):S59–S68.

87. Pickering L, Masor M, Granoff D et al. Human milk [HM] levels of nucleotides in infant formula reduce incidence of diarrhea. FASEB J 1996; 10:A554.

88. Cosgrove M, Davies DP, Jenkins HR. Nucleotide supplementation and the growth of term small for gestational age infants. Arch Dis Child Fetal Neonatal Ed 1996; 74:F122–F125.

89. Pickering LK, Granoff DM, Erickson JR et al. Modulation of the immune system by human milk and infant formula containing nucleotides. Pediatrics 1998; 101:242–249.

90. DeCastor LA, Brans YW. The effects of super premie SMA with nucleotides on the growth and development of very low birth weight infants. Pediatr Res 1992; 31:287A.

91. Bendich A. Carotenoids and the immune response. J Nutr 1989; 119:112–115.

92. Jyonouchi H, Sun S, Gross M. Effect of carotenoids on in vitro immunoglobulin production by human peripheral blood mononuclear cells: astaxanthin, a carotenoid without vitamin A activity, enhances in vitro immunoglobulin production in response to a T-dependent stimulant and antigen. Nutr Cancer 1995; 23:171–183.

93. Patton S, Canfield LM, Huston GE et al. Carotenoids of human colostrum. Lipids 1990; 25:159–165.

94. Gossage CP, Deyhim M, Yamini S et al. Carotenoid composition of human milk during the first month postpartum and the response to beta-carotene supplementation. Am J Clin Nutr 2002; 76:193–197.

95. Canfield LM, Giuliano AR, Neilson EM et al. Beta-carotene in breast milk and serum is increased after a single beta-carotene dose. Am J Clin Nutr 1997; 66:52–61.

96. Gaziano JM, Johnson EJ, Russell RM et al. Discrimination in absorption or transport of beta-carotene isomers after oral supplementation with either all-trans- or 9-cis-beta-carotene. Am J Clin Nutr 1995; 61:1248–1252.

97. Rowe PM. Beta-carotene takes a collective beating (news) [see comments]. Lancet 1996; 347:249.

98. Russell RM. The vitamin A spectrum: from deficiency to toxicity. Am J Clin Nutr 2000; 71:878–884.

99. McCarthy M. Beta-carotene supplements linked to cancer. Lancet 1999; 353:215.

100. COMA Department of Health. Nutritional aspects of the development of cancer. London: HMSO; 1998.

Background reading

Rennie J, Roberton NRC. Textbook of neonatology. Churchill Livingstone; 1999.

Tsang RC, Uauy R, Koletzko B et al., eds. Nutritional needs of the preterm infant. Scientific basis and practical guidelines, 2nd edn. Cincinnati, OH: Digital Educational; 2004.

Chapter 3

Ensuring nutritional adequacy of human–milk–fed preterm babies

Caroline King

CHAPTER CONTENTS

SUMMARY OF RECOMMENDATIONS

Factors affecting breastmilk composition
- For most nutrients, maternal diet has little effect on breast milk composition, with the exception of fatty acids and some vitamins
- If a woman is very malnourished she may need dietetic advice to improve her nutritional status and ensure adequate milk production
- A dietary source or supplement of vitamin B_{12} is advisable for vegan mothers
- Women at risk of vitamin D deficiency should have a vitamin D supplement
- Milk expressed in the first week or so may be higher in protein. This effect may be accentuated when only small volumes are expressed
- Milk should be handled and processed as little as possible to avoid nutrient loss:
  - Fat adheres to containers and tubing
  - Fat delivery may be adversely affected by freezing
  - Some vitamins and immunological components are lost on refrigeration, freezing, pasteurization and excessive light exposure
  - In addition lipase is destroyed by pasteurization, leading to poor fat absorption

Limiting nutrients in breast milk for infants weighing less than 1500 g*
(*This is an arbitrary cut-off point and some infants of above 1500 g may still need additional nutrients, as above)

- See also Chapter 2 and fortification (below) in conjunction with this section
- The risk of insufficient energy will be reduced if each breast is fully emptied at each expression to obtain all the hindmilk
- Protein concentration may be sufficient for growth in preterm expressed milk but will fall to levels found in mature milk and may become limiting after approximately 2 weeks
- Calcium and phosphorus levels in human milk are insufficient for most infants. However phosphorus alone can be given as a supplement initially as it is the most limiting of the two at this stage. Be guided by approximately twice-weekly serum estimations of phosphorus over the first few weeks
- Sodium levels are variable and can be raised as a result of breast inflammation and poor lactation. However, in general, levels are too low. With respect to supplementation be guided by a baby's serum levels; aim to keep > 133 mmol/l
- Iron levels are insufficient and a supplement will be necessary from 8 weeks postnatally at the latest
- There is a risk of insufficient zinc and a supplement is recommended; this is usually given as part of a breast-milk fortifier (BMF: see below)
- As a safety net the major trace elements should be supplemented for those infants with the highest requirements; these are usually given as part of a BMF (see below)
- Most fat-soluble vitamins will need to be provided in higher levels than are found in human milk. Particular attention should be paid to ensuring vitamin D 200 IU/kg to a maximum of 400 IU/day and vitamin A around 1500 IU/kg to a maximum of 5000 IU/day
- The water-soluble vitamin content of human milk will vary considerably with maternal diet so it is recommended that a supplement be given
- Infants on a BMF that does not contain a range of water- and fat-soluble vitamins may need a multivitamin supplement

Hindmilk

- Ensure that breasts are completely emptied to obtain the fat-rich hindmilk at each expression
- When serum urea is > 2 mmol/l and the baby is on maximum volume of enteral feed but not showing satisfactory weight gain, consider feeding hindmilk preferentially
- Obtaining a creamatocrit will help to identify optimal milk for an individual baby; however, if this is not possible and there is sufficient milk, simply dividing each milk expression, using the second part and storing the first, should ensure a higher fat intake
- Protein nutritional status should be carefully evaluated during the use of hindmilk, particularly in those infants who are not yet receiving a BMF
- If creamatocrits are carried out there should be a strict protocol guiding sampling technique to avoid spurious results
- Care must be taken to ensure an adequate protein intake while feeding predominantly hindmilk; in practice creamatocrits over 8% should not be necessary and may contain excessive energy from fat

Breast-milk fortification (BMF)

- All infants < 1500 g birth weight should be considered for fortification when on human milk
- Supplemental iron will be needed by 8 weeks postnatally at the latest
- Do not administer iron at same time of day as any calcium or phosphorus supplements
- All infants should be on full enteral feeds before fortifier is considered; this means the maximum tolerated. However, aim for a minimum of 180 ml/kg
- In general fortification should only be considered after 2 weeks of mother's milk
- When serial measurements have shown a steady decline, a serum urea of 2 mmol/l can be used to assess when additional protein and thus fortifier is needed, assuming no other factors besides nutritional ones are affecting urea levels
- In the first 21 days some infants < 31 weeks' gestation may have low ureas despite adequate protein

- Fortify at half-strength for first 24 h, going on to full-strength if tolerated
- Fortify the minimum amount of milk as close as possible to feeding time
- Never make up more than the minimum amount of fortified milk at a time
- Obtain weekly serum alkaline phosphatase in addition to routine biochemistry
- Monitor serum sodium at least weekly
- Consider stopping fortifier if formula makes up > 50% total feeds
- Use fortifier cautiously in infants who are on dexamethasone therapy
- Never add fortifier to formula
- If there is a very strong family history of atopy and cow's milk protein is to be avoided, use hypoallergenic formula powder instead of fortifier, and monitor carefully for signs of nutritional adequacy

FACTORS AFFECTING BREAST MILK COMPOSITION

Naturally occurring variability

The nutritional variability of expressed milk, particularly with respect to protein and fat, can be great.[1–8] Much of this variability may be due to sampling techniques and timing as the nutritional profile of human milk is known to vary within and between feeds, as well as within and between women, between breasts and with the stage of lactation. There may be a wide range of other nutrients, although how far this is due to genetic variation and how much is due to maternal dietary differences is not clear. For good reviews concerning nutrient variability see *Handbook of Milk Composition*[9] and Picciano.[10]

Diet

Most components are not affected by maternal diet despite wide variations in nutritional intake.[11] However the type of fat eaten is reflected in the milk: there is higher polyunsaturated fatty acid (PUFA) content when the diet is rich in PUFA. When the diet is very low in fat the amount of non-essential fatty acids increases due to conversion of dietary carbohydrate to fatty acids.[12] In addition, despite widely differing intakes of arachidonic and docosahexaenoic acids, these appear in all breast milk in similar amounts.[13]

In general the water-soluble vitamin content of human milk is more dependent on maternal diet than the fat-soluble vitamin content. The latter will be stored in maternal depots of relatively well-nourished mothers;[11] however, marginal maternal diets can compromise vitamin content.[10]

There is some evidence for a regulatory process during the transfer of water-soluble vitamins into the milk, thus ensuring that supraphysiological doses in the mother's diet are not reflected in her breast milk. This has not been demonstrated so well for fat-soluble vitamins.[11] For this reason supplements above the recommended intake are not currently advised. However women who are at high risk of vitamin D deficiency should take a supplement of this vitamin.[14] During extended lactation the maternal diet may become relatively more important, as seen in a study where folic acid-supplemented women maintained their folate status better than unsupplemented women.[15] Vegan and possibly strict vegetarian mothers may produce milk with suboptimal vitamin B_{12},[16] so a dietary source or supplement may be needed.

Of the trace elements, the selenium and iodine content of the maternal diet seems most closely reflected in breast milk.[10] A good review of the area is available.[17]

Effect of preterm delivery

Some groups have shown a higher than expected level of fat in preterm expressed milk.[18–20] This has not been seen by others, but could be the result of fully emptying a breast of hindmilk. Studies looking at protein and fat levels in preterm milk found very high variability between and within individuals.[8] The wide variation in fat levels could be explained both by degree of breast emptying and therefore amount of hindmilk collected and possibly differences in sampling technique (see below for a discussion of hindmilk).

Many observers have found that preterm milk is higher than term milk in protein[2,4,20,21] and sodium,[22] with levels generally declining towards those of mature term milk over the first few weeks (Fig. 3.1). Although other studies have found no difference in average protein levels between term and preterm milk,[23] there was high variability in the preterm milk.[8,24] An inverse relationship between volume of milk expressed and protein levels has been shown by several groups[2] (Fig. 3.2).[25] Of the other nutrients, calcium levels have been found to be significantly lower in preterm than term milk,[26] although the reduction is not clinically significant.

Expression technique

As discussed above, full expression of the breast with removal of all the fat rich hindmilk will result in a much higher-energy milk than partial expression, when only the lower-fat foremilk is removed. However, when a baby is breast-feeding these differences may be balanced out over a few feeds as the partially emptied breast may have a higher fat content at the beginning of the next feed. How this relates to mothers expressing milk is uncertain. The milk which sometimes drips from one breast when the other is being expressed is called drip milk, and is usually predominantly foremilk. Table 3.1 shows approximate levels of some nutrients in drip milk compared to expressed mature milk, highlighting the greatly reduced fat level.

Mastitis, whether due to breast trauma with poor expression technique or to other causes, may lead to increased sodium content.[27]

Postexpression processing

Postexpression milk can be fed fresh and unprocessed to the baby. If not, it must be refrigerated or frozen; if it is to be donated to a milk bank it must be pasteurized. In some units mother's own milk is pasteurized, although this is not recommended.[28] In addition, expressed

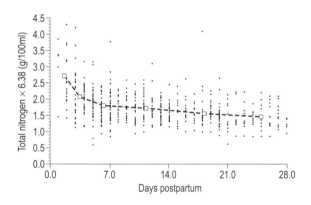

Figure 3.1   Protein content of preterm milk relative to time postdelivery. (Reproduced with permission from the BMJ Publishing Group: Lucas A, Hudson GJ. Preterm milk as a source of protein for low birth weight infants. Arch Dis Child 1984; 59:831–836.[2])

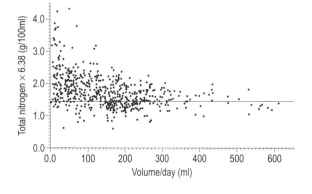

Figure 3.2   Protein content of human milk relative to volume expressed. (Reproduced with permission from the BMJ Publishing Group: Lucas A, Hudson GJ. Preterm milk as a source of protein for low birth weight infants. Arch Dis Child 1984; 59:831–836.[2])

breast milk may have individual nutrients or a multinutrient fortifier added, and this will be discussed in more detail later.

Many immunological components become inactive after refrigeration, freezing and pasteurization.[29–31] In addition milk frozen for 21 days compared to 2 min allowed significantly greater bacterial growth at 8 h.[32] However freezing reduces the viral load if cytomegalovirus is present (see Chapter 1). Other effects of freezing are disruption of milk fat globules with an increase in triglyceride hydrolysis,[33] and poorer fat delivery compared to refrigerated milk.[34] For this reason it is preferable to feed fresh milk whenever possible.

Pasteurization is an essential part of the processing of donor expressed breast milk (DEBM); however it leads to the denaturation of bile salt-stimulated lipase,[35] which reduces fat digestion. This in turn leads to increased gastrointestinal loss of fat, which can result in poor weight gain, and the loss of sodium, calcium and phosphorus as insoluble soaps.[36,37] Pasteurization also leads to a reduction in levels of folate, vitamin B_6 and B_{12} and vitamin C[38,39] (Table 3.2). Human milk should also be protected from excessive light to avoid vitamin loss.[40]

Even when the fat content of human milk is adequate there is a risk of fat loss on the journey from breast to baby as fat adheres to containers and tubing,[41] particularly with continuous feeding. A significant loss of protein has also been seen with this method of feeding.[41]

As milk fat is prone to separation from the aqueous portion, and fortifier may sediment when left standing, feeds should be regularly mixed.

LIMITING NUTRIENTS

The following nutrients may be present in limiting amounts for many infants of less than 2000 g, although some well infants who can tolerate large volumes of enteral feeds will not need supplements.

Energy

With respect to energy, the poor fat absorption from DEBM will lead to insufficient energy after long-term feeding (see above) and both drip and foremilk are intrinsically too low in fat for preterm energy requirements. If feeding DEBM for longer than a few weeks it should be fortified as for mother's own milk; however an additional energy source may also be needed.

Table 3.1 Nutritional composition of drip milk and expressed mature human milk[158]

Per 100 ml	Drip human milk	Mature human milk
Protein (g)	1.0	1.07
Sodium (mmol)	0.5	0.6
Fat (g)	0.5–1.0	4
Calcium (mmol)	0.4	0.8
Phosphorus (mmol)	0.5	0.5
Energy (kcal)	46	70
(×4.18 = kJ)		

Table 3.2 Effect of pasteurization

	Approximate percentage survival at 62.5°C for 30 min			
Immunological components		Vitamins		
IgA	67–99	C		64
IgM IgE	0	Folate		69
Lysozyme	75-95	B_6		85
Lactoferrin	40	B_{12}		90

Ig, immunoglobulin.
Adapted from Ford et al.[29] and Evans et al.[30]

Milk from a fully emptied breast is likely to provide more than enough energy because of its high fat content. As part of a study on human milk fortification the creamatocrit was calculated on a daily basis in each of 38 women.[42] The mean was found to be 6.6% (1.2% SD), giving a mean of 73 kcal/100 ml (range 65–81). Even though they were not instructed to collect hindmilk preferentially, these women produced milk of adequate energy profile. At this energy level infants will receive 120 kcal/kg when given 170 ml/kg milk; in practice many infants tolerate 180–200 ml/kg.

Protein

Human milk protein has a higher biological value than alternatives as it has evolved to meet the needs of the human infant. However term and mature unfortified expressed milk are not nutritionally equipped to support growth in infants of less than 1500 g because of inadequate protein levels.[43,3]

For those babies receiving (early) mother's own milk, levels of protein should be sufficient for theoretical needs during the first 2–3 weeks.[2,44] However after the first weeks of lactation inadequate protein intake due to declining levels may lead to poor growth.[3,45] Weight gain may be partly maintained when sufficient energy is provided; however, body composition will be skewed towards increased fat deposition.[46] A strong correlation between protein intake and weight gain up to a maximum of 3 g protein/kg and with energy intake up to 120 kcal/kg has been shown.[3] Another group has shown that the nitrogen accreted from an intake of 3 g protein/kg is not enhanced when more than 120 kcal/kg is fed.[46] Protein supplementation should be considered after the first 2–3 weeks.[4,47,48]

Sodium

Breast milk sodium can be raised in mastitis[27] and when milk production is declining, e.g. when the breast tissue is involuting on weaning from the breast.[49] However, in general, sodium levels are insufficient to match the high requirements of the very-low-birth-weight infant; clinicians should be guided by serum estimations and aim to keep levels > 133 mmol/l while avoiding hypernatraemia.

Vitamins

All preterm infants on human milk will need a supplement of water- and fat-soluble vitamins – most importantly an intake of 200 IU/kg vitamin D to a maximum of 400 IU/day[50] and around 1500 IU/kg vitamin A.[51,52] A maximum of 5000 IU/day vitamin A may be required to normalize levels (see Chapter 2). Many multi-vitamin supplements do not contain folic acid; however there is insufficient evidence to warrant its addition separately before a BMF is started. Most BMFs contain folic acid; for those that do not, a supplement of 50 µg/day has been suggested.[51]

Trace elements

Iodine levels in human milk are variable depending on maternal status. When status is good early human milk may supply iodine needs; however later on a supplement will be required to achieve the 30–60 µg/kg per day recommended.

Although there is evidence that human milk provides the zinc requirements of many preterm infants,[53] zinc status can become marginal,[54,55] so supplementation is recommended.

Copper levels in human milk are adequate, although there is the possibility that large supplements of iron may reduce copper absorption.[56] Selenium levels are usually sufficient but may become marginal where the selenium status of the population is marginal.[52] Infants are unlikely to become selenium-deficient unless their mothers are, therefore supplements are not necessary.

Iron

Preterm infants fed human milk will need an additional source of iron by 6–8 weeks or on doubling of their birth weight, whichever is first. Most human milk fortifiers do not contain iron so a supplement is usually needed.[57] A fortifier with iron added is not recommended as it may predispose to increased bacterial growth.[58] Iron should not be given at the same time as calcium or phosphate as an insoluble compound may be formed, reducing bioavailability.[59,60]

Calcium and phosphorus

Calcium and phosphorus are well absorbed from human milk – up to 70% of total calcium[61] and 95% of phosphorus.[62] However they are not present in adequate levels to support a desirable accretion rate for infants born below around 1500 g and 32 weeks' gestation. Absorption may be reduced from donor milk.[36] Phosphorus becomes the rate-limiting substrate for bone mineralization as it is used preferentially for lean body requirements when the infant is in positive nitrogen balance. Thus a lower calcium-to-phosphorus ratio is required for preterm infants compared to term infants.[63] A phosphorus supplement early on may help prevent calciuria[64] (Table 3.3).

A phosphorus supplement of approximately 0.5 mmol/100 ml human milk for all babies below 1500 g fed human milk has been suggested.[65] In practice a supplementation of 0.5 mmol twice daily appears to work well.[66] When supplementation of very small volumes of milk is needed, 0.5 mmol should be added to a minimum of 10 ml. This will keep the osmolality below 460 mOsm/kg,[67] the level recommended to avoid the risk of necrotizing enterocolitis (NEC).[68,69] However, trends in

serum calcium and phosphorus should always be observed before supplementation is started. Excessive phosphate supplementation can lead to depression of serum ionized calcium levels[70] and secondary hyperparathyroidism,[64] which may result in calcium wasting rather than accretion. Additional calcium will be needed eventually; however by this time most infants will go on to have their mother's milk fortified with a multinutrient fortifier containing calcium. A weekly serum alkaline phosphatase may help to monitor bone health, although occasionally the liver isoenzyme can be considerably raised during an infection. A bone-derived serum alkaline phosphatase above around 900 IU should be avoided as it may indicate osteopenia. It has been observed that failure to meet protein requirements may result in poor utilization of dietary calcium leading to calciuria.[71] Serum levels should normally be kept within the following ranges: calcium 2.15–2.65 mmol/l, phosphorus 1.5–2.2 mmol/l, with Ca > P.

Paradoxically, unsupplemented human milk during the neonatal period was associated with greater bone mineral density at 5 years than in children of similar size born at term.[72] However, the prime aim must remain the prevention of short-term morbidity such as severe osteopenia and fractures; this aim is best served by some degree of human milk mineral supplementation.

Whatever the mineral input, the clinical condition of the baby may affect bone mineralization. Passive exercise may show benefits (see Chapter 2).

Table 3.3 Early calcium and phosphorus economy in preterm infants

	Calcium (mmol/kg)	Phosphorus (mmol/kg)
Daily intrauterine accretion (last trimester)	3.5	2.4
Human milk fed at 200 ml/kg	1.6	1.0
Maximum absorbed from milk	1.0	0.9
Protoplasmic requirements	Minimal	0.6
Remaining for bone	1.0	0.3
Used for bone formation	0.5	0.3
Excreted in urine	0.5	0

Magnesium

The magnesium content of human milk seems adequate, with up to 89% being absorbed.[73] A maximum of 4 mmol/l in formula and fortified human milk has been suggested.[51]

HINDMILK

Definition of hindmilk

The energy provided by human milk is largely dependent on the fat content which, as discussed previously, can be highly variable between expressions.

When a breast has been fully emptied at the previous expression, the first milk removed at the next expression is likely to be low in fat (foremilk) and the milk at the end of the expression, as the breast becomes empty, will be high in fat (hindmilk). This means that if the breast is only partially emptied there is a risk that only low-fat foremilk is extracted, which will not provide the infant's energy needs.[74,75] Thus it is possible that different degrees of breast expression explain some of the large differences in fat levels quoted in different papers. However there is some evidence that there is little variation in percentage fat within individuals' breast milk when a full breast expression is analysed.[19]

Hindmilk and growth

Feeding predominantly hindmilk has been used to improve weight gain;[76–78] however this will not remedy protein insufficiency as hindmilk has a higher energy content than foremilk but similar nitrogen levels. In one study hindmilk feeding did not always improve weight gain.[79]

Another study, which enlisted a large cohort, including preterm infants, found that the fat level in mother's milk did not correlate with growth rates.[80] However in these studies the protein content was not evaluated, nor was fat malabsorption excluded (preterm infants are at high risk of fat malabsorption: see Chapter 2). It is important to evaluate protein nutrition during hindmilk feedings and ensure that it is adequate (see below). Hindmilk feeding should be a relatively short-term measure as the aim is to educate each mother on the appropriate expression technique in order to ensure that all her milk is of an adequate fat content. In theory, feeding above 50% kcal as fat could lead to ketosis, although this has not been investigated in preterm infants.

Creamatocrit

The fat and therefore energy content of hindmilk can be calculated via the creamatocrit,[81] which has been evaluated by others.[82,83] This process involves centrifuging a well-mixed sample of milk in a haematocrit tube and measuring the fat layer produced. This measurement corresponds to a calculated energy level.[81] In a small group of women the efficacy of mothers estimating the creamatocrit of their own milk has been evaluated and found to be accurate and acceptable.[84] In addition the procedure was well accepted by the women in this study. However it is possible that a request for some mothers to carry out this procedure themselves may create an additional burden, particularly if the creamatocrit is low. An alternative method has been evaluated where the first part of the milk expression is separated and stored while the last part is fed to the baby.[85] Milk collected by these methods was tested via the creamatocrit and all such milk was found to contain 2 g/100 ml more fat than the foremilk. In one study, where women were not given specific instructs on hindmilk collection, the mean creamatocrit was found to be 6.6% (1.2% SD), giving a mean of 73 kcal/100 ml (range 65–81).[42]

See Table 3.4 for the relationship between creamatocrit and milk energy value and the volume of milk needed at various creamatocrit values to provide 115 kcal/kg.

BREAST MILK FORTIFICATION

Growth on unfortified milk

During the initial few weeks of feeding mother's own preterm milk, preterm babies have been shown to grow satisfactorily.[86–90]

Table 3.4   Creamatocrit values

ml/kg	Creamatocrit (%)	kcal /100ml	% calories from fat
140	8	82	56
150	7	76	52
160	6	69	48
170	6	69	48
180	5	62	44
190	5	62	44
200	4	56	37

Creamatocrit necessary to achieve approximately 115 kcal/kg at various volumes assuming protein content of human milk of 1.2 g/100 ml. (Adapted from data of Liz Jones and Sue Bell.)

In another study weight and length were poor on unsupplemented human milk, although head circumference was maintained compared to protein-supplemented human milk.[4] In this study approximately half the babies were fed their mother's own milk and half donor milk with no separate analysis of growth for each group. This makes it difficult to evaluate whether babies fed their mother's own unsupplemented milk would have done as well as those fed donor milk with a protein supplement.

Despite the reports that some infants below 2000 g birth weight grow well on human milk alone beyond the first few weeks, many eventually require additional supplies of the limiting nutrients discussed above, especially infants below 1500 g. Larger well infants may tolerate up to 220 ml/kg, precluding the need for supplementary protein; it is therefore recommended that the maximum tolerated volume of milk is achieved before fortification is considered. However these infants will still need vitamin and iron supplements once parenteral nutrition has finished. They may also need additional phosphorus and sodium.

Various methods have been used to decide when additional protein is given, as is discussed below.

Analysis of human milk protein

The preferred option would be to analyse the nutritional composition of mother's milk and add the desired amount of protein.[6,91]

In one study the trial design was of fixed fortification versus fortification adjusted according to the infant's serum urea nitrogen.[91] However on the adjustment scheme the range of the amount of fortifier added was very small and, although these infants received more protein, there was no significant difference in weight gain. Due to the crucial role of protein in neonatal growth it would be useful to see the results of further larger trials similar to those discussed here. However, as they stand these results make it hard to justify the high frequency of serum urea estimations necessary.[91]

In another study Polberger et al.[6] concluded that, while waiting for the results of milk analysis, the infants' requirements changed so that the babies were always getting slightly less protein than they needed; the results were taking around 1 week. Laboratory techniques already in use to analyse other fluids (e.g. cerebrospinal fluid protein and serum lipids) have been investigated.[92] However they are also subject to delay in delivering results and may be more suited to analysing milk either when there is a surplus supply or for donor milk. It is hoped that in the near future an accurate validated portable human milk analyser will be developed, enabling rapid cotside results.

It has been pointed out that, with the very high variation in milk composition, it is virtually impossible to get a good estimate of infants' overall intake via their mother's milk.[8] To do so would require that every expression be pooled for analysis, which again in some cases would deny a baby its mother's fresh milk, as in the study of Polberger et al.[6] With improved support for mothers and therefore larger milk supplies it is hoped that analysis of stored milk will become more feasible.

Empirical addition of protein

Some units partially replace human milk with preterm formula once a set enteral volume is given to an infant. This has been shown to improve formula fat absorption, possibly via the effect of human bile salt-stimulated lipase on formula fat digestion.[93] However, there are also many disadvantages; the risk of sepsis may become the same as that for formula-fed babies if human milk provides less than < 50 ml/kg of the baby's intake.[94] It has also been shown that adding formula to human milk leads to significant decreases in lysozyme[95] and transforming growth factor-alpha.[96] Finally the mother may feel undermined and that it is less crucial for her to provide milk, leading to a reduction in volume produced.

In addition, rather than assessing the adequacy of protein intake, it is the practice in many centres to start fortification once the infant reaches a set volume of milk, irrespective of serum biochemistry: 100 ml/kg is most often quoted in individual studies and national recommendations.[52,97,98]

The drawbacks of substituting human milk with formula or early fortification, coupled with the fact that additional protein is not usually nutritionally necessary in the first 2–3 weeks, suggests that an alternative approach should be considered (see below). The advantages of human milk (which are often dose-dependent; see Chapter 1) suggest that all efforts should be directed towards maintaining maternal lactation.

Using a surrogate to assess protein nutrition

An alternative to the methods discussed above is to use an indirect measure of protein adequacy. If there is a decline in serum urea during the first few weeks postnatally and it eventually drops below 1.6 mmol/l, there is a good chance that an infant's protein intake is < 3 g/kg per day[99] (however, see discussion below). In a study by Polberger et al.,[99] mother's milk was analysed and then the amount of added dried human milk powder was adjusted to give a fixed level of protein. However, later on during recovery in well, growing infants, a serum urea < 2 mmol/l is probably a sign of protein economy similar to the low serum amino acid levels seen in term infants in similar circumstances.[100]

The relationship between protein intake and serum urea has also been described in animal studies[101] and in infancy,[102] but other studies suggest that this indicator of protein adequacy needs to be interpreted carefully. In very preterm infants depression of serum urea may occur independently of protein intake due to immaturity of the urea synthetic pathway.[103] In the study by Boehm et al.,[103] infants > 31/40 weeks' gestation at birth showed a dose-related response in urea to protein intake, whereas those < 31 weeks' gestation did not at day 8 but did by day 21 (the only two points at which the infants were studied, indicating that maturation occurs between days 8 and 21). For this reason fortification may be not be clinically indicated in infants below 1500 g in the first 2–3 weeks of ingesting their mother's own milk, even if the serum urea is below 1.6 mmol/l. However, often when serial measurements are available a clear decline is seen over time.

It has been suggested that in some infants there may be an elevation of serum urea independently of protein intake due to immaturity of the renal system,[104] with some backing from an observational study.[105] Unfortunately no other serum proteins have been found to reflect protein status in preterm infants accurately.

Prevention of poor weight gain due to inadequate protein is the primary aim, thus fortification is recommended when serial measurements show a steady decline but before serum urea drops below 1.6 mmol/l (i.e. at around 2 mmol/l). In the absence of any other obvious influential factors, e.g. dehydration, impaired renal function and steroid administration, it is probably useful to aim to keep the serum urea between 2 and 8 mmol/l.[102]

A systematic review of protein supplementation concluded that there is increased short-term growth (weight, length and head circumference) but that there are insufficient data to indicate long-term effects.[106]

Single versus multinutrient fortification

If each nutrient is added separately (e.g. protein, phosphorus, calcium, sodium, trace elements and vitamins) there is an increased risk of dose error, milk contamination and unacceptably high osmolality (> 460 mOsm/kg; see Chapter 7). In addition, it may not be an economical use of nursing and medical time.

A recent editorial discusses this problem and suggests that fortification with a commercial multinutrient product, while not ideal, is probably the most practical route at the present.[107] However, this method can be enhanced by close monitoring of serum biochemistry (not only of urea but also of sodium, calcium, phosphorus and alkaline phosphatase). A systematic review has looked at studies of multinutrient fortification and concluded that there are short-term growth benefits but insufficient evidence for other conclusions.[108]

Fortification may not be needed when human milk makes up less than 50% total volume and the rest is preterm formula,[109] although individuals making catch-up growth may continue to benefit.

Outcome of feeding fortified milk

The primary outcomes are to preserve any benefits of human milk, while optimizing nutritional status and growth (note that optimal growth may not be fastest growth: see Chapter 8).

Most papers have not found any significant problems with tolerance of fortified breast milk.[109–112] One study did suggest that it led to feed intolerance[113] and in another study there were increased signs of intolerance; however, the authors felt that the doubling of feed volumes over the observation period may have been a more likely culprit.[114] Studies looking specifically at gastric emptying have been contradictory – one found no effect[115] while another showed a delay.[116]

In some studies there has been found to be poorer fat absorption with fortified compared to unfortified milk.[117] This appeared to be associated with the calcium content of the particular brand of fortifier used, leading to the formation of insoluble soaps which are then not absorbed.[111,117,118] This is supported by the observation that fortifiers containing less calcium and more moderate calcium supplementation allow higher fat absorption.[119,120]

Recent studies have shown no significant difference in growth between infants given multinutrient-fortified human milk or milk supplemented with minerals alone.[121] However, infants fed human milk supplemented with minerals alone received a larger volume and therefore more protein per kilogram, precluding direct comparison of the groups. In contrast, another group showed improved growth when the fortified milk provided over 50% of the enteral intake.[109] Others have shown poorer weight gain but equivalent length and head growth in infants fed human milk with fortifier compared to preterm formula[113,122–124] (head circumference alone, as length was not reported). Fortified milk led to improved length but not weight compared to unfortified milk.[125]

Bone mineralization has been shown to be equivalent in infants fed fortified human milk compared to preterm formula.[126]

In two large observational studies, infants fed fortified milk grew more poorly than those fed preterm formula but volumes were not stated.[45,127] In the paper by O'Connor et al.[127] neurodevelopment was assessed at 12 months and found not to be compromised in those on fortified breast milk compared to infants fed a preterm formula, despite the poorer growth. In fact those with chronic lung disease showed neurodevelopmental advantage with human milk. In this study although head circumference, length and weight were all lower at discharge, there was no difference at 4, 6 and 9 months between human-milk-fed and formula-fed infants.

In an observational study infants who received > 80% breast milk while hospitalized had significantly lower weight at discharge and lower height at 1 year;[128] however the authors point out that the data were collected when their unit's policy restricted the use of fortifier for economic reasons.

One group has looked at giving protein supplementation in addition to already fortified milk and found that it led to improved weight gain. The infants received a total of 1.5 g protein (0.7 g from fortifier, 0.8 g in addition: EE Ziegler, personal communication 2004) added to 100 ml breast milk.[129] As discussed above, the large variability in measured human milk protein means that many infants will receive well in excess of requirements when as much as 1.5 g/100 ml protein is added to early preterm human milk which could potentially already contain 3–4 g protein/100 ml.

More work is needed on the optimal amount of protein with which to supplement human milk.

Fortification with human milk–based fortifier

This has been studied and carried out in some Scandinavian countries, mainland Europe, North America and Japan.[3,4,6,91,119,130–134] It has been shown to improve weight gain, but has resulted in lower serum phosphorus and higher calciuria than the unfortified group.[134] The authors speculated that the increased weight gain led to higher phosphorus demands, which could not be met by feeding dried skimmed human milk powder alone without giving additional mineral.

Growth and biochemical responses were not significantly different between babies fed with human milk in comparison to protein-fortified cow's milk[135] and nitrogen assimilation is similar with the two sources of protein.[119] However human milk protein should give advantages as large amounts of active secretory immunoglobulin A are preserved.[136]

Whether this form of fortification will ever become commercially available is uncertain as there are difficulties in obtaining sufficient donated milk. However it would be useful where there is a strong family history of allergy

and should be investigated further as and when lactation rates improve on neonatal units.

Infants at high risk of atopy

If there is a strong family history of atopy and it is deemed advisable to avoid cow's milk-based products, a hypoallergenic formula powder instead of fortifier may be advisable. One of the scoops present in the formula tin per 100 ml of breast milk is a suggested amount to use. A graded introduction would be advisable, i.e. half a scoop/100 ml milk for the first 24 h and, if tolerated, increased to one scoop/100 ml. Serum biochemistry should be observed for additional requirements of protein and minerals (particularly phosphorus). A vitamin supplement would be useful, providing 200 IU vitamin D/kg to a maximum of 400 IU/day.

Commercially available fortifiers

Multinutrient fortifiers are available in Europe, Australia and North America: in North America they are available both in liquid and powder form. The composition of fortifiers is outlined in Tables 3.5 and 3.6. Term formula powder has been used in the past but is unacceptable because of its low protein-to-energy ratio.

Eoprotin

An earlier formulation of Eoprotin was one of the first available in Europe and was widely used for many years in Germany and France, following trials there showing satisfactory growth without adverse metabolic sequelae.[137] It was often used to fortify banked donor milk. Recently it has been reformulated and it is now identical to Cow & Gate's Nutriprem BMF (see below).

Nutriprem breast-milk fortifier

This product, manufactured by Cow & Gate, most closely follows the nutritional guidelines of Tsang et al.[51] Recent work shows that it allows good growth, with no adverse side-effects.[138]

Table 3.5 Composition of human milk fortifiers in the UK and continental Europe

Composition of recommended dose	Nutriprem breast–milk fortifier (Cow & Gate)	Eoprotin (Milupa)	SMA breast–milk fortifier (SMA)[a][b]	FM85 (Nestle)
Recommended dose (g/100 ml)	4.2	4.2	4	5
Protein (g)	0.8[c]	0.8[c]	1.0	0.8[c]
Casein : whey	50:50	50:50	0:100	0:100
Energy (kcal)[d]	15	15	15	18
Minerals (mg)				
Calcium	64	64	90	51
Phosphorus	44	44	45	34
Magnesium	6	6	3	2
Sodium	10	10	18	27
Potassium	8	8	27	11.5
Chloride	6	6	17	18.5
Trace elements (µg)				
Zinc	400	400	260	–
Copper	30	30	–	–
Manganese	8	8	4.6	–
Iodine	11	11	–	–
Vitamins (µg)				
Vitamin A[e]	130	130	270	–
Vitamin C (mg)	12	12	40	–
Vitamin D[e]	5	5	7.6	–
Vitamin E (mg)[e]	2.6	2.6	3	–
Vitamin K	6.3	6.3	11	–
Biotin	2.5	2.5	1.5	–
Folic acid	50	50	30	–
Niacin	2500	2500	3600	–
Vitamin B_{12}	0.2	0.2	0.3	–
Pyridioxine B_6	110	110	260	–
Riboflavin B_2	170	170	260	–
Thiamin	130	130	220	–
Pantothenic acid B_5	750	750	900	–
Presentation	2.1-g sachets: powder	200-g tins: powder	2-g sachets: powder	200-g tins: powder

[a]Available on request to company.
[b]SMA breast-milk fortifier contains beta-carotene.
[c]Hydrolysed protein.
[d]All contain carbohydrate only as energy source.
[e]Conversion factors are as follows: vitamin A: µg ÷ 0.3 = IU; vitamin D: µg × 40 = IU; 1 IU vitamin E = 1 mg d, Lα tocopherol acetate.

This information is correct at the time of publication but may change: please check with the manufacturers

Table 3.6 Composition of human milk fortifiers in the USA

Composition of recommended dose	Enfamil (Mead Johnson)	Similac (Ross)	Similac Natural Care[a] (Ross)
Recommended dose (g/100 ml)	4	3.6 (4 sachets)	100ml (Dilute half and half with breast milk)
Protein (g)	1.1	1	2.4
Casein : whey	60:40	60:40	60:40
Carbohydrate	<0.4	1.8	8.3
Fat	1[b]	0.36	4.4
Energy (kcal)	14	14	81
Minerals (mg)			
Calcium	90	117	170
Phosphorus	50	67	94
Magnesium	1	7	9.7
Sodium	16	15	35
Potassium	29	63	104
Chloride	13	38	66
Trace elements (µg)			
Iron (mg)	1.44	0.4	0.3
Zinc	720	1000	1200
Copper	44	170	203
Manganese	10	7	9.7
Iodine	–	–	4.9
Vitamins (µg)			
Vitamin A[c]	285	186	304
Vitamin C (mg)	12	25	30
Vitamin D[c]	3.75	3	3
Vitamin E (mg)[c]	4.6	3.2	3.2
Vitamin K	4.4	8	9.7
Biotin	2.7	26	30
Folic acid	25	23	30
Niacin	3000	3580	4057
Vitamin B_{12}	0.18	0.64	0.44
Pyridoxine B_6	115	212	203
Riboflavin B_2	220	418	503
Thiamin B_1	150	234	203
Pantothenic acid B_5	730	1504	1541
Presentation	1-g sachets: powder	0.9-g sachets: powder	liquid

[a]Contains taurine, inositol, choline.
[b]70% medium-chain triglycerides.
[c]Conversion factors are as follows: vitamin A µg ÷ 0.3 = IU; vitamin D: µg × 40 = IU: 1 IU vitamin E= 1 mg d, Lα tocopherol acetate.

This information is correct at the time of publication but may change: please check with the manufacturers

However, sodium may become limiting when levels drop in breast milk, as late hyponatraemia has been associated with Enfamil human milk fortifier, which has the same sodium content.[139] If subsequent work indicates a benefit for large doses of vitamin A in particular, a supplement may be necessary.[140,141] Nutriprem contains calcium glycerophosphate, an organic salt, theoretically more bioavailable because of its high solubility compared to the inorganic salts.[142] So far, only the phosphorus component has been shown to be more soluble.[143] One study has shown that gastric emptying is unaffected by addition of this fortifier to expressed breast milk.[115] The protein source is hydrolysed casein and whey but its allergenicity has not been evaluated.

Enfamil human milk fortifier

Enfamil has been widely used in North America. It is of interest as it has been used in one of the largest trials of human milk fortification, in which it was compared with milk supplemented with minerals only.[109] Short-term growth was improved in the Enfamil fortified group when breast milk comprised > 50% of intake, but there was no significant effect on development at 18 months. There were two points of concern: one was a non-significant increase in infection and NEC; this was discussed in a corresponding editorial[144] in which it was pointed out that levels of NEC remained similar to those found in other studies of infants fed human milk. In this study, milk was fortified up to 24 h before use.[109] However, where possible milk should be fortified just before feeding as subsequent storage could result in higher bacterial counts.[145] A second concern raised by this study was indirect evidence of poorer bone mineralization. This may be a reflection of the high calcium-to-phosphorus ratio in the formulation used in this study as more infants experienced hypercalcaemia in the fortified group. This high calcium level may reduce fat absorption, as demonstrated in another study of infants fed milk fortified with Enfamil BMF[111] (see above). As discussed in Chapter 2, a lower calcium-to-phosphorus ratio than previously thought may be required for preterm infants.

Use of this fortifier has also been associated with late hyponatraemia, which is a reflection of its low sodium content.[139] However, during reformulation the calcium : phosphorus has been reduced and more sodium has been added. Recently it was reformulated to provide iron, giving 2 mg/kg when at full concentration and fed at 150 ml/kg. However there are concerns over the effect of adding iron to breast milk on bacterial growth.[58]

Similac human milk fortifier

This product is used in North America and Australia but is not available in Europe. It is a powder and should not require mineral or vitamin supplemention. Levels of calcium and phosphorus are the highest of all the fortifiers and may be more than required, potentially bringing the disadvantages of fatty acid/calcium soap formation, as described above. It has been compared to Similac Natural Care (liquid) in a randomized study. In this study it was found to be less well tolerated than Similac Natural Care but the duration of breast-feeding was significantly longer in relation to the mother's initial plan compared to Natural Care.[147]

Similac Natural Care

This is a liquid product designed to be added to mother's milk when there is insufficient to provide all her baby's needs. It is uncertain how much of an advantage it is over simply using preterm formula. There is a theoretical danger that it may be used in larger proportions than 1:1 with breast milk, leading to an unbalanced nutritional intake. In addition it has been suggested that this fortifier leads to a lower protein intake and retention when compared with Enfamil fortifier.[97] In a randomized controlled trial comparing this product with the Enfamil fortifier it was found to lead to higher serum alkaline phosphatase and lower serum calcium, indicating that vitamin D levels may have been insufficient (they were approximately one-third of the Enfamil vitamin D levels).[110]

See above for a study comparing this fortifier with Similac human milk fortifier, in which randomization to Natural Care led to a shorter duration of breast-feeding compared to the mother's initial plans.

SMA breast-milk fortifier

This product is only available by special arrangement with the company in the UK and is not available in North America. Several B-vitamins, including folate, appear low and may need supplementing. SMA breast-milk fortifier contains similar amounts of calcium and phosphorus as Enfamil and therefore may have similar drawbacks (see above).

FM 85

This is the Nestlé BMF and it is available in continental Europe but not the UK. The protein source is hydrolysed cow's milk protein but there are no data on its allergenicity. It does not contain any trace elements or vitamins and therefore will need at least a multivitamin supplement. In one study using this product a large number of infants remained hypercalciuric, suggesting the need for more phosphorus.[148] *Please check with individual manufacturers for most recent formulations and research.

Precautions

Fortifier should be added to human milk as close as possible to the time of feeding, as storage reduces the effectiveness of some of the anti-infective components.[95,149] After 24 h bacterial growth was significantly higher in fortified compared to unfortified milk,[145] despite the fact that both were refrigerated. In the same study fortified milk stored for 4 h at ambient temperature led to a significant increase in bacterial count.

The addition of iron and fortifier containing iron to human milk has been shown to decrease its antibacterial properties.[58]

In addition, prolonged storage of fortified milk may lead to an unacceptably high increase in osmolality.[150,151] Avoidance of osmolality

above 460 mOsm/kg has been advocated to reduce the risk of NEC (see Chapter 7). Osmolality probably increases with hydrolysis of BMF dextrins by human milk amylase.[150] Jocson et al.[145] found that fortified milk had an osmolality of around 400 mOsm/kg compared to 300 mOsm/kg in unfortified milk; however it only increased by 4% after 24 h storage. Despite this relatively low increase during storage, in practice the minimum amount of milk possible should be fortified and used as soon as possible to avoid further increases in osmolality.

Adding a fortifier to early high-protein expressed breast milk, as discussed above, could lead to excessive protein intakes for some preterm infants, providing intakes well above their needs. For example, some milk may contain up to 4 g protein/100 ml (Figs 3.1 and 3.2).[2] If such milk is fortified, protein content will be increased to approximately 5 g protein/100 ml. This is unlikely to give any nutritional advantage, as shown in Tsang et al.,[51] where a summary of 21 separate studies shows that weight gain reaches a plateau at protein intakes of > 4 g/kg. Not only will these levels of protein be of no advantage but also there are potential risks. For example, hyperaminoacidaemia may occur: this has previously been associated with developmental delay.[152,153] Poor oral feeding with lethargy has also been reported.[154] An early study found that babies taking more than 8 g protein/kg had poorer weight gain than those fed between 3 and 8 g/kg, and this poor growth continued postdischarge, suggesting nutritional programming.[155] Although these data are from studies of formula-fed infants, they serve as a warning that protein intakes above requirements may not have benign effects.

When an infant is fed a mixture of human milk and formula, great care should be taken to ensure that the fortifier is only added to the human milk. Accidental addition to formula may increase the risk of gastrointestinal calcium bolus obstruction if intakes exceed 4 mmol calcium/100 ml.[156] In addition, with continuous feeding it is vital to ensure complete mixing of powdered fortifiers as there can be poor delivery of many minerals.[157]

References

1. Hibberd CM, Brooke O, Carter ND. Variations in the composition of breast milk during the first five weeks lactation: implications for the feeding of preterm infants. Arch Dis Child 1982; 57:658–662.

2. Lucas A, Hudson GJ. Preterm milk as a source of protein for low birth weight infants. Arch Dis Child 1984; 59:831–836.

3. Polberger SK, Axelsson IA, Raiha NC. Growth of very low birth weight infants on varying amounts of human milk protein. Pediatr Res 1989; 25:414–419.

4. Ronnholm KA, Perheentupa J, Simes MA. Supplementation with human milk protein improves growth of small premature infants fed human milk. Pediatrics 1986; 77:649–653.

5. Michaelsen KF, Skafte L, Badsberg JH et al. Variation in macronutrients in human bank milk: influencing factors and implications for human milk banking. J Pediatr Gastroenterol Nutr 1990; 11:229–239.

6. Polberger S, Raiha NC, Juvonen P et al. Individualized protein fortification of human milk for preterm infants: comparison of ultrafiltrated human milk protein and a bovine whey fortifier. J Pediatr Gastroenterol Nutr 1999; 29:332–338.

8. Weber A, Loui A, Jochum F et al. Breast milk from mothers of very low birthweight infants: variability in fat and protein content. Acta Paediatr 2001; 90:772–775.

9. Handbook of milk composition. San Diego, CA: Academic Press; 1995.

10. Picciano MF. Nutrient composition of human milk. Pediatr Clin North Am 2001; 48:53–67.

11. Atkinson SA. Feeding the normal term infant: human milk and formula. In: Sinclair, Bracken, eds. Effective care of the newborn infant. Oxford University Press; 1992:73–93.

12. Insull W, Hirsch T, Ahrens E. The fatty acids of human milk. II Alterations produced by manipulation of caloric balance and exchange of dietary fats. J Clin Invest 1959; 38:443–450.

13. Koletzko B, Thiel I, Abiodun PO. The fatty acid composition of human milk in Europe and Africa. J Pediatr 1992; 120:S62–S70.

14. Shaw NJ, Pal BR. Vitamin D deficiency in UK Asian families: activating a new concern. Arch Dis Child 2002; 86:147–149.

15. Mackey AD, Picciano MF. Maternal folate status during extended lactation and the effect of supplemental folic acid. Am J Clin Nutr 1999; 69:285–292.

16. Johnson PR, Raloff JS. Vitamin B_{12} deficiency in an infant strictly breast fed by a mother with latent pernicious anaemia. J Pediatr 1982; 187:917–919.

17. Renner E. Micronutrients in milk and milk based food products. London: Elsevier Applied Science; 1989.

18. Anderson GH, Atkinson S. Energy and macronutrient content of human milk during early lactation from mothers giving birth prematurely and at term. Am J Clin Nutr 1981; 34:258–265.

19. Jennings T, Meier P, Meier W. High lipid and caloric content in milk from mothers of preterm infants. Pediatr Res 1997; 41:233A.

20. Faerk J, Skafte L, Petersen S et al. Macronutrients in milk from mothers delivering preterm. In: Newburg, ed. Bioactive components of human milk. New York: Kluwer Academic/Plenum Publishers; 2001:409–413.

21. L'Abbe MR, Friel JK. Superoxide dismutase and glutathione peroxidase content of human milk from mothers of premature and full-term infants during the first 3 months of lactation. J Pediatr Gastroenterol Nutr 2000; 31:270–274.

22. Gross SJ, David RJ. Nutritional composition of milk produced by mothers delivering preterm. J Pediatr 1980; 96:641–644.

23. Dvorak B, Fituch CC, Williams CS et al. Increased epidermal growth factor levels in human milk of mothers with extremely premature infants. Pediatr Res 2003; 54:15–19.

24. Velona T, Abbiati L, Beretta B et al. Protein profiles in breast milk from mothers delivering term and preterm babies. Pediatr Res 1999; 45:658–663.

25. Anderson DM, Williams FH, Merkatz RB et al. Length of gestation and nutritional composition of human milk. Am J Clin Nutr 1983; 37:810–814.

26. Friel JK, Andrews WL, Jackson SE et al. Elemental composition of human milk from mothers of premature and fulllterm infants during the first 3 months of lactation. Biol Trace Elem Res 1999: Mar:67(3):225–247.

27. McKiernan J, Hull D. The constituents of neonatal milk. Pediatr Res 1982; 16:60–64.

28. Balmer SE, Nicol A, Weaver G et al. Guidelines for the collection, storage and handling of mothers breast milk to be fed to her own baby on a neonatal unit. United Kingdom Association for Milk Banking; 2001.

29. Ford JE, Law BA, Marshall VM et al. Influence of the heat treatment of human milk on some of its protective constituents. J Pediatr 1977; 90:29–35.

30. Evans TJ, Ryley JC, Neale LM. Effect of storage and heat on antimicrobial proteins in human milk. Arch Dis Child 1978; 53:239–241.

31. Xanthou M. Human milk cells [comment]. Acta Paediatr 1997; 86:1288–1290.

32. Hernandez J, Lemons P, Lemons J et al. Effect of storage processes on the bacterial growth-inhibiting activity of human breast milk. Pediatrics 1979; 63:597–601.

33. Waddell JM, Hill CM, D'Souza SW. Effect of pasteurization and of freezing and thawing human milk on its triglyceride content. Acta Paediatr Scand 1981; 70(4):467–471.

34. Lavine M, Clark RM. The effect of short-term refrigeration of milk and addition of breast-milk fortifier on the delivery of lipids during tube feeding. J Pediatr Gastroenterol Nutr 1989; 8:496–499.

35. Henderson TR, Fay TN, Hamosh M. Effect of pasteurization on long chain polyunsaturated fatty acid levels and enzyme activities of human milk. J Pediatr 1998; 132:876–878.

36. Williamson S, Finucane E, Ellis H. Effect of heat treatment of human milk absorption of nitrogen, fat, sodium, calcium and phosphorus by preterm infants. Arch Dis Child 1978; 53:553–563.

37. Stein H, Cohen D, Herman AA et al. Pooled pasteurized breast milk and untreated own mother's milk in the feeding of very low birth weight babies: a randomized controlled trial. J Pediatr Gastroenterol Nutr 1986; 5:242–247.

38. Van Zoeran D, Schrijver J, Van den berg H et al. Vitamin losses from expressed human milk. Pediatr Res 1986; 20:1051 (abstract).

39. Bank MR, Kirksey A, West K et al. Effect of storage time and temperature on folacin and vitamin C levels in term and preterm human milk. Am J Clin Nutr 1985; 41:235–242.

40. Bates CJ, Liu DS, Fuller NJ et al. Susceptibility of riboflavin and vitamin A in breast milk to photodegradation and its implications for the use of banked breast milk in infant feeding. Acta Paediatr Scand 1985; 74:40–44.

41. Stocks RJ, Davies DP, Allen F et al. Loss of breast milk nutrients during tube feeding. Arch Dis Child 1985; 60:164–166.

42. Warner JT, Linton HR, Dunstan FD et al. Growth and metabolic responses in preterm infants fed fortified human milk or a preterm formula. Int J Clin Pract 1998; 52:236–240.

43. Lucas A, Gore SM, Cole TJ et al. Multicentre trial on feeding low birthweight infants: effects of diet on early growth. Arch Dis Child 1984; 59:722–730.

44. Donovan SM, Atkinson SA, Whyte RK et al. Partition of nitrogen intake and excretion in low-birth-weight infants. Am J Dis Child 1989; 143:1485–1491.

45. Simmer K, Metcalf R, Daniels L. The use of breastmilk in a neonatal unit and its relationship to protein and energy intake and growth. J Paediatr Child Health 1997; 33:55–60.

46. Boehm G, Melichar V, Senger H et al. Effects of varying energy intakes on nitrogen retention and growth in very low birthweight infants fed fortified human milk. Acta Paediatr Scand 1990; 79:228–229.

47. Kashyap S, Schulze KF, Forsyth M et al. Growth, nutrient retention, and metabolic response of low-birth-weight infants fed supplemented and unsupplemented preterm human milk. Am J Clin Nutr 1990; 52:254–262.

48. Schanler RJ, Garza C, Nichols BL. Fortified mother's milk for very low birth weight infants.

    Results of growth and nutrient balance studies. J Pediatr 1985; 107:437–445.

49. Neville MC, Morton J. Physiology and endocrine changes underlying human lactogenesis II. J Nutr 2001; 131:3005S–3008S.

50. Backstrom MC, Maki R, Kuusela AL et al. Randomised controlled trial of vitamin D supplementation on bone density and biochemical indices in preterm infants. Arch Dis Child 1999; 80:F161–F166.

51. Tsang RC, Lucas A, Uauy R et al. Nutritional needs of the preterm infant: scientific basis and practical guidelines. Williams & Wilkins; 1993.

52. Klein CJ. Nutrient requirements for preterm infant formulas. J Nutr 2002; 132 (suppl. 1):1395S–1577S.

53. Wauben I, Gibson R, Atkinson S. Premature infants fed mothers' milk to 6 months corrected age demonstrate adequate growth and zinc status in the first year. Early Hum Dev 1999; 54:181–194.

54. Aggett PJ, Atherton DJ, More J et al. Symptomatic zinc deficiency in a breast-fed preterm infant. Arch Dis Child 1980; 55:547–550.

55. Heinen F, Matern D, Pringsheim W et al. Zinc deficiency in an exclusively breast-fed preterm infant. Eur J Pediatr 1995; 154:71–75.

56. Haschke F, Ziegler EE, Edwards et al. Effect of iron fortification of infant formula on trace mineral absorption. J Pediatr Gastroenterol Nutr 1986; 5:768–773.

57. Ehrenkranz RA. Iron requirements of preterm infants. Nutrition 1994; 10:77–78.

58. Chan GM. Effects of powdered human milk fortifiers on the antibacterial actions of human milk. J Perinatol 2003; 23:620–623.

59. Cook JD, Dassenko SA, Whittaker P. Calcium supplementation: effect on iron absorption [see comments]. Am J Clin Nutr 1991; 53:106–111.

60. Peters T Jr, Apt L, Ross JF. Effect of phosphates upon iron absorption studied in normal human subjects and in an experimental model using dialysis. Gastroenterology 1971; 61:315–322.

61. Hillman LS, Johnson LS, Lee DZ et al. Measurement of true absorption, endogenous fecal excretion, urinary excretion, and retention of calcium in term infants by using a dual-tracer, stable-isotope method. J Pediatr 1993; 123:444–456.

62. Senterre J, Putet G, Salle B et al. Effects of vitamin D and phosphorus supplementation on calcium retention in preterm infants fed banked human milk. J Pediatr 1983; 103:305–307.

63. Mize CE, Uauy R, Waidelich D et al. Effect of phosphorus supply on mineral balance at high calcium intakes in very low birth weight infants. Am J Clin Nutr 1995; 62:385–391.

64. Senterre J, Salle B. Renal aspects of calcium and phosphorus metabolism in preterm infants. Bio Neonate 1988; 53:220–229.

65. Bishop NJ. Bone disease in preterm infants. Arch Dis Child 1989; 64 (10):1403–1409.

66. Holland P, Wilkinson A, Diez J et al. Prenatal deficiency of phosphate, phosphate supplementation and rickets in very low birth weight infants. Lancet 1990; 335:697–701.

67. Srinivasan L, Bokiniec R, King C et al. Increased osmolality of breast milk with therapeutic additives. Arch Dis Child Fetal Neonat Ed 2004; Nov:89(6):F514–517.

68. Barness LA, Mauer AM, Holliday MA et al. Commentary on breast feeding and infant formulas, including proposed standards for formulas. Pediatrics 1976; 57:278–285.

69. Willis DM, Chabot J, Radde IC et al. Unsuspected hyperosmolality of oral solutions contributing to necrotizing enterocolitis in very-low-birth-weight infants. Pediatrics 1977; 60:535–538.

70. Rowe JC, Wood DH, Rowe DW et al. Nutritional hypophosphatemic rickets in a premature infant fed breast milk. N Engl J Med 1979; 300:293–296.

71. Hillman LS, Salmons SS, Erickson MM et al. Calciuria and aminoaciduria in very low birth weight infants fed a high-mineral premature formula with varying levels of protein. J Pediatr 1994; 125:288–294.

72. Bishop NJ, Dahlenburg SL, Fewtrell MS et al. Early diet of preterm infants and bone mineralization at age five years. Acta Paediatr 1996; 85:230–236.

73. Liu YM, Neal P, Ernst J et al. Absorption of calcium and magnesium from fortified human milk by very low birth weight infants. Pediatr Res 1989; 25:496–502.

74. Daly SE, Di Rosso A, Owens RA et al. Degree of breast emptying explains changes in the fat content, but not fatty acid composition, of human milk. Exp Physiol 1993; 78:741–755.

75. Neville MC, Keller RP, Seacat J et al. Studies on human lactation. I. Within-feed and between-breast variation in selected components of human milk. Am J Clin Nutr 1984; 40:635–646.

76. Valentine C, Hurst NM, Schanler RJ. Hindmilk improves weight gain in low birth weight infants fed human milk. J Pediatr Gastroenterol Nutr 1994; 18:474–477.

77. Vasan U, Meier P, Meier W et al. Individualizing the lipid content of own mothers milk:effect of weight gain for extremely low birth weight (ELBW) infants. Pediatr Res 2004; 43:270A.

78. Slusher T, Hampton R, Bode-Thomas F et al. Promoting the exclusive feeding of own mother's milk through the use of hindmilk and increased maternal milk volume for hospitalized, low birth weight infants (< 1800 grams) in Nigeria: a feasibility study. J Hum Lact 2003; 19:191–198.

79. Spencer SA, Hendrickse W, Roberton D et al. Energy intake and weight gain of very low birthweight babies fed raw expressed breast milk. Br Med J Clin Res Ed 1982; 285:924–926.

80. Chatterjee R, Chatterjee S, Datta T et al. Longitudinal study of human milk creamatocrit and weight gain in exclusively breastfed infants. Ind Pediatr 1997; 34:901–904.

81. Lucas A, Gibbs JA, Lyster RL et al. Creamatocrit: simple clinical technique for estimating fat concentration and energy value of human milk. Br Med J 1978; 1:1018–1020.

82. Wang CD, Chu PS, Mellen BG et al. Creamatocrit and the nutrient composition of human milk. J Perinatol 1999; 19:343–346.

83. Meier PP, Engstrom JL, Murtaugh MA et al. Mothers' milk feedings in the neonatal intensive care unit: accuracy of the creamatocrit technique. J Perinatol 2002; 22:646–649.

84. Griffin TL, Meier PP, Bradford LP et al. Mothers' performing creamatocrit measures in the NICU: accuracy, reactions, and cost. J Obstet Gynecol Neonatal Nurs 2000; 29:249–257.

85. Lalari VV, Innis SM. Fractionation of expressed milk for the selective collection of hind-milk by mothers who deliver premature infants. Pediatr Res 2003; 53:488A.

86. Chessex P, Reichman B, Verellen G et al. Quality of growth in premature infants fed their own mothers' milk. J Pediatr 1983; 102:107–112.

87. Atkinson SA, Radde IC, Anderson GH. Macromineral balances in premature infants fed their own mothers' milk or formula. J Pediatr 1983; 102:99–106.

88. Hendrickse WA, Spencer SA, Roberton DM et al. The calorie intake and weight gain of low birth weight infants fed on fresh breast milk or a special formula milk. Eur J Pediatr 1984; 143:49–53.

89. McGuinness J, Bryan H, Myhr T et al. Unfortified EBM should be fed to very low birthweight infants. Pediatr Res 1995; 37:313A.

90. Faerk J, Petersen S, Peitersen B et al. Diet and bone mineral content at term in premature infants. Pediatr Res 2000; 47:148–156.

91. Moro GE, Minoli I, Ostrom M et al. Fortification of human milk: evaluation of a novel fortification scheme and of a new fortifier. J Pediatr Gastroenterol Nutr 1995; 20:162–172.

92. Lynch PL, O'Kane MJ, O'Donohoe J et al. Determination of the total protein and triglyceride content of human breast milk on the Synchron CX7 Delta analyser. Ann Clin Biochem 2004; 41:61–64.

93. Alemi B, Hamosh M, Scanlon JW et al. Fat digestion in very low-birth-weight infants: effect of addition of human milk to low-birth-weight formula. Pediatrics 1981; 68:484–489.

94. Furman L, Taylor G, Minich N et al. The effect of maternal milk on neonatal morbidity of very low-birth-weight infants. Arch Pediatr Adolesc Med 2003; 157:66–71.

95. Quan R, Yang C, Rubinstein S et al. The effect of nutritional additives on anti-infective factors in human milk. Clin Pediatr Phila 1994; 33:325–328.

96. Lessaris KJ, Forsythe DW, Wagner CL. Effect of human milk fortifier on the immunodetection and

molecular mass profile of transforming growth factor-alpha. Biol Neonate 2000; 77:156–161.

97. Schanler RJ. The use of human milk for premature infants. Pediatr Clin North Am 2001; 48:207–219.

98. Ziegler EE, Thureen PJ, Carlson SJ. Aggressive nutrition of the very low birthweight infant. Clin Perinatol 2002; 29:225–244.

99. Polberger SKT, Axelsson IE, Raitia NCR. Urinary and serum urea as indicators of protein metabolism in very low birth weight infants fed varying human milk protein intakes. Acta Paediatr Scand 1990; 79:737–742.

100. Scott PH, Berger HM, Wharton BA. Growth velocity and plasma amino acids in the newborn. Pediatr Res 1985; 19:446–450.

101. Eggum BO. Blood urea measurement as a technique for assessing protein quality. Br J Nutr 1970; 24:983–988.

102. Kashyap S, Heird WC. Protein metabolism during infancy. Nestle Nutrition Services 1994; 6:139a.

103. Boehm G, Muller DM, Beyreiss K et al. Evidence for functional immaturity of the ornithine-urea cycle in very low birth weight infants. Biol Neonate 1988; 54:121–125.

104. Wilkins BH. Renal function in sick very low birthweight infants: 2. Urea and creatinine excretion. Arch Dis Child 1992; 67:1146–1153.

105. Ridout E, Melara D, Thureen PJ. Amino acid intake is a poor predictor of blood urea nitrogen (BUN) concentrations in ventilated and ill neonates in the first days of life. Pediatr Res 2004; 53:405A.

106. Kuschel CA, Harding JE. Protein supplementation of human milk for promoting growth in preterm infants. Cochrane Database Syst Rev 2001; 2:CD000433.

107. Ziegler EE. Breast-milk fortification. Acta Paediatr 2001; 90:720–723.

108. Kuschel CA, Harding JE. Multicomponent fortified human milk for promoting growth in preterm infants. Cochrane Database Syst Rev 2004; 1:CD000343.

109. Lucas A, Fewtrell MS, Morley R. Randomised outcome trial of human milk fortification and developmental outcome in preterm infants. Am J Clin Nutr 1996; 64:142–151.

110. Sankaran K, Papageorgiou A, Ninan A et al. A randomized, controlled evaluation of two commercially available human breast-milk fortifiers in healthy preterm neonates. J Am Diet Assoc 1996; 96:1145–1149.

111. Schanler RJ, Shulman RJ, Lau C. Feeding strategies for premature infants: beneficial outcomes of feeding fortified human milk versus preterm formula. Pediatrics 1999; 103:1150–1157.

112. Barrett-Reis BB, Hall RT, Schanler RJ et al. Enhanced growth of preterm infants fed a new powdered human milk fortifier: a randomized, controlled trial. Pediatrics 2000; 106:581–588.

113. Metcalf R, Dilena B, Gibson R et al. How appropriate are commercially available human milk fortifiers? J Paediatr Child Health 1994; 30:350–355.

114. Moody GJ, Schanler RJ, Shulman RJ et al. The addition of human milk fortifier does not affect feeding tolerance in premature infants. Pediatr Res 1998; 43:265A.

115. McClure RJ, Newell SJ. Effect of fortifying breast milk on gastric emptying. Arch Dis Child 1996; 74:F60–F62.

116. Ewer AK, Yu VY. Gastric emptying in pre-term infants: the effect of breast-milk fortifier. Acta Paediatr 1996; 85:1112–1115.

117. Schanler R, Henderson TR, Hamosh M. Fatty acid soaps may be responsible for poor fat absorption in premature infants fed fortified human milk(FHM). Pediatr Res 1999; 45:290A.

118. Katz L, Hamilton JR. Fat absorption in infants of birth weight less than 1300 gm. J Pediatr 1974; 85:608–614.

119. Boehm G, Muller DM, Senger H et al. Nitrogen and fat balances in very low birth weight infants fed human milk fortified with human milk or bovine milk protein. Eur J Pediatr 1993; 152:236–239.

120. Salle B, Senterre J, Putet G et al. Effects of calcium and phosphorus supplementation on calcium retention and fat absorption in preterm infants fed pooled human milk. J Pediatr Gastroenterol Nutr 1986; 5:638–642.

121. Wauben IP, Atkinson SA, Grad TL et al. Moderate nutrient supplementation of mother's milk for preterm infants supports adequate bone mass and short-term growth: a randomized, controlled trial. Am J Clin Nutr 1998; 67:465–472.

122. Bullough C, Chan M, Graves C et al. Growth rates in very low birth weight infants fed preterm formula or fortified human milk. Pediatr Res 1998; 43:256A.

123. Faerk J, Petersen S, Peitersen B et al. Diet and growth in premature infants. Pediatr Res 1998; 44:450A.

124. Pieltain C, De Curtis M, Gerard P et al. Weight gain composition in preterm infants with dual energy X-ray absorptiometry. Pediatr Res 2001; 49:120–124.

125. Kokinopoulos D, Photopoulos SVN, Kafegidakis L et al. The effect of human milk, protein-fortified human milk and formula on immunologic factors of newborn infants. In: Mestecky JEA, ed. Immunology of milk and the neonate. New York: Plenum Press; 1991:77–85.

126. Lapillonne AA, Glorieux FH, Salle BL et al. Mineral balance and whole body bone mineral content in very low-birth-weight infants. Acta Paediatr 1994; 405 (suppl.):117–122.

127. O'Connor DL, Jacobs J, Hall R et al. Growth and development of premature infants fed predominantly human milk, predominantly premature infant formula, or a combination of human milk and premature formula. J Pediatr Gastroenterol Nutr 2003; 37:437–446.

128. Pinelli J, Saigal S, Atkinson SA. Effect of breastmilk consumption on neurodevelopmental outcomes at 6 and 12 months of age in VLBW infants. Adv Neonatal Care 2003; 3:76–87.

129. Carlson SJ, Johnson K, Cress G et al. Higher protein intake improves growth of VLBW infants fed fortified breast milk. Pediatr Res 2004; 45:278A.

130. Moro GE, Minoli I, Fulconis F et al. Growth and metabolic responses in low-birth-weight infants fed human milk fortified with human milk protein or with a bovine milk protein preparation. J Pediatr Gastroenterol Nutr 1991; 13:150–154.

131. Schanler RJ, Garza C, Smith EO. Fortified mothers' milk for very low birth weight infants: results of macromineral balance studies. J Pediatr 1985; 107:767–774.

132. dos Santos M, Martinez FE, Seiber V et al. Nitrogen, fat, Ca, P, Mg and Cu plasma levels and balance of VLBW-infants fed with formula or mother's own milk enriched with evaporated human milk or commercial human milk fortifier (HMF). Pediatr Res 1998; 43:258A.

133. Lucas A, Lucas PJ, Chavin SI et al. A human milk formula. Early Hum Dev 1980; 4:15–21.

134. Itabashi K, Hayashi T, Tsugoshi T et al. Fortified preterm human milk for very low birth weight infants. Early Hum Dev 1992; 29:339–343.

135. Hagelberg S, Lindblad BS, Persson B. Amino acid levels in the critically ill preterm infant given mother's milk fortified with protein from human or cow's milk. Acta Paediatr Scand 1990; 79:1163–1174.

136. Hagelberg S, Lindblad BS, Lundsjo A et al. The protein tolerance of very low birth weight infants fed human milk protein enriched mother's milk. Acta Paediatr Scand 1982; 71:597-601.

137. Product information booklet. Eoprotin – human milk fortifier for preterm and low birth weight infants. Milupa; 1994.

138. Nicholl R, Gamsu H. Changes in growth and metabolism in very low birthweight infants fed with fortified breast milk. Acta Paediatr 1999; 88:1056–1061.

139. Kloiber LL, Winn NJ, Shaffer SG et al. Late hyponatremia in very-low-birth-weight infants: incidence and associated risk factors. J Am Diet Assoc 1996; 96:880–884.

140. Kennedy KA, Stoll BJ, Ehrenkranz RA et al. Vitamin A to prevent bronchopulmonary dysplasia in very-low-birth-weight infants: has the dose been too low? The NICHD neonatal research network. Early Hum Dev 1997; 49:19–31.

141. Tyson JE, Wright LL, Oh WOM et al. Vitamin A supplementation for extremely-low-birth-weight infants. N Engl J Med 1999; 340:1962–1968.

142. Wauben IP, Atkinson SA, Grad TL et al. Calcium glycerophosphate as Ca/P source in a new powdered fortifier for preterm mother's milk: measurement of mineral balances, bone mineralization and growth. Pediatr Res 1994; 35:322A.

143. Schanler RJ, Schulman RJ, Lau C. Early feeding increases mineral absorption in preterm infants. Pediatr Res 1995; 37:319A.

144. Schanler RJ. Human milk fortification for premature infants. Am J Clin Nutr 1996; 64:249–250.

145. Jocson MA, Mason EO, Schanler RJ. The effects of nutrient fortification and varying storage conditions on host defense properties of human milk. Pediatrics 1997; 100:240–243.

147. Fenton TR, Tough SC, Belik J. Breast milk supplementation for preterm infants: parental preferences and postdischarge lactation duration. Am J Perinatol 2000; 17:329–333.

148. Raupp P, von Kries R, Schmidt E et al. Human milk fortification. Lancet 1988; 1:1160–1161.

149. Wagner CL, Forsythe D. Effect of human milk fortifier on the immunodetection of TGF alpha within human milk. Pediatr Res 1997; 41:88A.

150. De Curtis M, Candusso M, Pieltain C et al. Effect of fortification on the osmolality of human milk. Arch Dis Child 1999; 81:F141–F143.

151. Fenton TR, Belik J. Routine handling of milk fed to preterm infants can significantly increase osmolality. J Pediatr Gastroenterol Nutr 2002; 35:298–302.

152. Goldman HI, Goldman JS, Kaufman I et al. Late effects of early dietary protein intakes on low birth weight infants. J Pediatr 1974; 85:764–796.

153. Mamunes P, Prince PE, Thornton NH. Intellectual deficits after transient tyrosinaemia in the term neonate. Pediatrics 1976; 57:675–680.

154. Goldman HI, Freudenthal R, Holland B et al. Clinical effects of two different levels of protein intake on low-birth-weight infants. J Pediatr 1969; 74:881–889.

155. Omans WB, Barness LA, Rose CS et al. Prolonged feeding studies in premature infants. J Pediatr 1961; 59:951–957.

156. Koletzko B, Tangermann R, von Kries R et al. Intestinal milk-bolus obstruction in formula-fed premature infants given high doses of calcium. J Pediatr Gastroenterol Nutr 1988; 7:548–553.

157. Bhatia J, Rassin DK. Human milk supplementation. Delivery of energy, calcium, phosphorus, magnesium, copper, and zinc. Am J Dis Child 1988; 142:445–447.

158. Department of Health and Social Security report. Artificial feeds for the young infant. Report of the working party on the composition of foods for infants and young children, Committee on Medical Aspects of Food Policy. London: DHSS; 1977:1–104.

Chapter 4

Mammary anatomy and physiology

Peter E Hartmann and Donna T Ramsay

Summary of key points

- The growth of the breast during pregnancy and the onset of lactogenesis I with respect to the implications of premature delivery are discussed
- The initiation of lactation and its delay in mothers of premature infants are considered
- The large variation in milk composition is examined along with implications for fortification of mother's milk for preterm infants
- The importance of the milk ejection reflex during the expression of milk in preterm mothers is discussed
- Factors affecting milk synthesis are examined with respect to endocrine and autocrine control

ACKNOWLEDGEMENTS

The authors thank Medela AG, the Women's and Infants' Research Foundation, National Human Milk Resource Centre (NHMRC) and the University of Western Australia for their support. In addition we greatly appreciate the co-operation of the volunteer mothers and the support of the Western Australian branch of the Australian Breastfeeding Association.

INTRODUCTION

Lactation is the final phase of the reproductive cycle in mammals and in almost all species mother's milk is essential for the survival of the young during the critical period of early postnatal life. However, the composition of milk varies greatly, even between closely related species,[1] and it is now clear that the composition of milk of each species is uniquely adapted to meet the specific metabolic, developmental and host defence requirements of its young. Furthermore, there are large differences in the maturity of mammals at birth, ranging from the guinea pig that is relatively mature at birth and soon able to consume solid foods, to the marsupials such as the kangaroo and quokka that are very immature at birth. Many marsupials, for example kangaroo, tammar wallaby and quokka, remain permanently attached to the nipple in the pouch for long periods of time and increase their body weight more than 1000-fold during the period of exclusive breastfeeding. To facilitate this lengthy extrauterine development there is extensive growth of the suckled mammary gland and the composition of the milk changes markedly as the exclusively breast-fed young grows.[2] In contrast, during the same period of human lactation, breast growth is usually complete by parturition and milk composition changes little after the transition from colostrum to mature milk[1] (that is, after the first 2 weeks of lactation). Furthermore, the body weight of the human infant merely doubles during the recommended period of 6 months of exclusive breastfeeding.[3]

Over recent years medical science has greatly improved the viability of infants born preterm such that babies born a little over halfway through gestation may survive and develop outside the protective and physiologically regulated environment of the gravid uterus. Thus very preterm infants may need to increase their birth weight almost 10-fold to reach the birth weight of normal term babies. In the past preterm infants did not survive, therefore it cannot be assumed that the composition of breast milk produced by the preterm mother has been adapted to meet the special nutritional and host defence needs of these infants. Indeed, clinical experience and comparison with the progressive changes in the composition of marsupial milk suggest that some modification (fortification) of mother's own milk is required for the optimal nutrition of the preterm human infant.[4–7] Nevertheless, current research has led national and international medical bodies as well as companies marketing infant formula[8] to acknowledge the benefits of breast milk as the principal nutrient for preterm infants.[9] Indeed, the American Academy of Paediatrics[10] states that 'Extensive research, especially in recent years, documents diverse and compelling

advantages to infants, mothers, families, and society from breastfeeding and the use of human milk for infant feeding.' Furthermore, preterm mothers often report that the provision of milk is the only important positive contribution that they can make for their babies[11] and failure to provide breast milk may give rise to maternal feelings of helplessness and guilt.[12]

Birth in women can occur either at term (>36 weeks' gestation) or preterm (22–36 weeks). In term mothers the initiation of lactation includes the growth of glandular tissue of the breast (mammogenesis) and the differentiation of the glandular epithelial cells into lactocytes (mammary secretory epithelial cells) capable of synthesizing specific milk products during pregnancy (lactogenesis I). After birth the transition from colostrum to mature milk represents the onset of copious milk secretion (lactogenesis II) and the mechanism controlling this transition is closely coupled to that controlling the timing of birth.[13] Therefore, it is important to consider the effects that the premature cessation of pregnancy may have on the structure and functional development of the human breast and the ability of mothers to provide milk for their preterm babies.

BREAST ANATOMY

Glandular tissue

The breast is composed of glandular (secretory) and adipose (fatty) tissue held together by a loose framework of fibrous connective tissue called Cooper's ligaments. There is a tendency for glandular tissue to be more abundant in the lateral portion of the breast, with a greater concentration of adipose tissue in the medial portion. Before pregnancy the glandular tissue in the breast consists of small lobules containing a network of branching ducts, lined by one or two layers of cuboidal epithelial cells, separated by loose connective tissue, with dense fibroconnective tissue between the lobules.[14]

The glandular tissue and milk ducts in the breast are normally well developed at term. During lactation there is a decrease in the amount of adipose tissue relative to glandular tissue.[15] The glandular tissue is composed of lobes that drain independently to the nipple.[16,17] The lobes are composed of lobules consisting of 10–100 alveoli of approximately 0.12 mm diameter.[18,19] Within a lobe, small ducts drain the alveoli and coalesce, forming larger ducts and eventually joining to form a single milk duct of approximately 2 mm diameter that drains towards the nipple, where it narrows as it opens on to the surface of the nipple at the nipple orifice. The orifices of the ducts are 0.4–0.7 mm in diameter[20] and are surrounded by circular muscle fibres.[17]

The current descriptions as well as textbook diagrams of the anatomy of the lactating breast show milk ducts leading from the nipple to enlarged lactiferous sinuses and little or no secretory tissue close to the nipple and areola area.[17] This structure of the lactating breast is based on the interpretation of Cooper's detailed dissections in 1840.[21] However, recently Ramsay et al. carried out ultrasound examinations of the breasts of 21 lactating women and questioned the classical portrayal of the anatomy of the lactating breast.[22,23,97] Ramsay et al. observed that on average there were nine functional milk ducts leading from the nipple and that all of these ducts branched close to the nipple and within the boundary of the areola. The milk ducts were convoluted and displayed increased

diameter at points of branching but became smaller as the degree of branching increased (Figs 4.1 and 4.2). Milk duct diameter remained constant over time, only increasing at milk ejection.[24] This increase in duct diameter persisted for only 2 min, even when no milk was

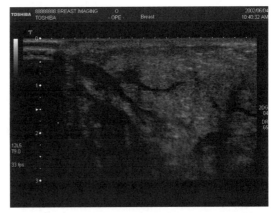

Figure 4.1 Ultrasound image of the anatomy of a lactating breast. A main milk duct (↗) that is anechoic (black, absent of echoes) is seen coursing toward the nipple (N). Note the early branching of this milk duct very close to the nipple. The skin (S) is a thin echogenic (bright echoes) layer at the top of the image and below the skin a small amount of subcutaneous fat (F) is seen as a hypoechoic layer (fewer echoes, less bright). The glandular tissue (G) is highly echogenic; note the large peripheral duct (↑) that is as large as a main milk duct (↗) near the nipple.

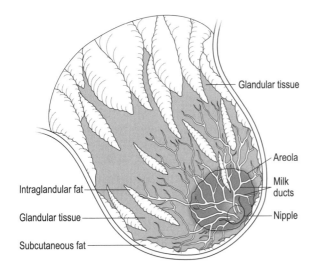

Figure 4.2 Diagram of the gross anatomy of the lactating breast as imaged by ultrasound,[22] showing the branching of the milk ducts beneath the areola and the distribution of the secretory and fatty tissue within the breast.

expressed from the breast. Furthermore, small branches of the milk ducts drained glandular tissue situated adjacent to the nipple and immediately beneath the areola. The average diameter of the main milk duct prior to initial branching was about 2–3 mm, ranging from 1 to 8 mm. Since the average diameter of the milk ducts of lactating women was similar to that reported for non-lactating women, it is unlikely that the structure of the major milk ducts would be underdeveloped in mothers who deliver preterm.

Storage capacity

The storage capacity of a breast is a functional concept and is defined as the maximum amount of milk that can be stored in the breast and that is available to the infant under normal patterns of breastfeeding. It can be determined by measuring the progressive changes in the volume of a mother's breast before and after each breastfeed over a period of 24 h.[25] Breast volume decreased when the baby removed milk from the breast and increased as the mother synthesized milk between feeds. The breast storage capacity was determined by subtracting the minimum breast volume from the maximum breast volume observed over the 24-h period. There is a wide variation in the storage capacity of women's breasts, ranging from 60 to 600 ml, and breasts with larger storage capacities have the potential to deliver more milk at either a feed or pumping session. Obviously mothers with relatively small breasts do not have large storage capacities, and those with larger breasts may vary considerably in their storage capacity depending upon the ratio of glandular to adipose tissue in their breasts. The concept of storage capacity is important to preterm mothers, as those with a small capacity to store milk in their breasts need to express more frequently to optimize their milk production than mothers with larger storage capacities.

Arterial supply

Descriptions of the blood supply to the breast have changed little since the classic dissections of lactating cadavers by Cooper in 1840.[21] Methods used to investigate the vasculature of the mammary gland in cadavers include injection of wax or size of different colours into the vessels,[21] and injection of a suspension of fine lead and subsequent radiography of the blood supply in one non-lactating woman.[26] The breast is supplied mainly by the posterior and anterior medial branches of the internal mammary artery (60%) and the lateral mammary branch of the lateral thoracic artery[27] (30%). Small sources such as the posterior intercostal arteries, the pectoral branch of the thoracoacromial artery and the subscapular artery may supply the remaining portion of blood.[17] However, there is a wide variation between women in the proportion of blood supplied by each artery[28] and there is little evidence of symmetry between breasts.[29,30]

Venous drainage

The venous drainage of the breast is divided into the deep and superficial systems[21] joined by short connecting veins. Both systems drain into the internal thoracic, axillary and cephalic veins. The deep veins are assumed to follow the corresponding mammary arteries,[29,31] while the superficial plexus consists of subareolar veins that arise radially from the nipple and drain into the periareolar vein which circles the nipple and connects the superficial and deep plexus. As with the arterial supply, symmetry of the superficial venous plexus is not apparent.[31,32]

Lymphatic drainage

Cooper carefully dissected the lymphatics of the lactating breast[21] and observed that when injections were made into these vessels the fluid always flowed away from the breast. He correctly refuted the 'extraordinary opinion' that these vessels carried chyle to the breast for formation of milk. Although a number of studies of the lymphatic anatomy of the breast have been performed since the end of the eighteenth century, it is still not fully understood. The main drainage of lymph is into the axillary nodes; however there is wide variability in the drainage pattern from any quadrant of the breast. Lymph also drains into the internal mammary nodes from both the medial and lateral portions of the breast.[33,34] Lymph may also pass through the interpectoral nodes and nodes within the breast parenchyma before reaching the axillary or internal mammary nodes.

Innervation

The lateral aspect of the breast is innervated by branches of the 4th to 6th intercostal nerves and the medial portion by branches of the 2nd to 5th intercostal nerves[17,35] while the nipple is supplied by a branch of the 4th intercostal nerve.[35] The milk ducts leading to the nipple orifices range from having an abundance of nerve fibres, to a few to none at all, while the areola and nipple are poorly innervated.[36] However, lactating women have been found to display a marked increase in areolar and nipple sensitivity within 24 h postpartum.[37] Within the glandular portion of the breast there are only a few nerves visible along the major ducts.[36,38] Some nerve fibres have been observed in the lobules nearest the major milk ducts, but otherwise the glandular tissue is free of nerve fibres and there is no evidence of any motor secretory innervation of the breast. The limited distribution of nerve fibres in the secretory tissue is supported by clinical evidence that, while the overall fullness of a distended breast can be appreciated and disease conditions can be painful, there is often no precise localization of either sensation.[14] Indeed, some women can experience the debilitating influenza-like symptoms of mastitis before they are conscious of tenderness in their breasts. These observations suggest that both the synthesis and secretion of milk are independent of neural stimulation.

BREAST GROWTH AND DEVELOPMENT

Pregnancy

In some women a heightened tenderness of their breasts even before a missed menstrual period can provide the first indication that conception has occurred. Subsequently, the superficial subcutaneous veins of the upper half of the breast become enlarged and visible and the areola usually becomes larger and more darkly pigmented. The Montgomery glands (a combination of large sebaceous glands together with rudimentary milk glands) on the areola enlarge and become more active during pregnancy. It is assumed that the secretion from these glands provides protective lubrication for the nipple and areola during lactation. These sensory and morphological changes are indicative of the major developmental changes that take place in the breast during pregnancy.

During the first half of pregnancy extension and branching of the ductal system occur, leading to extensive lobular–alveolar growth (mammogenesis) with some secretory development by mid-pregnancy. In the last trimester there is a further increase in lobular size, which is associated with hypertrophy of the cells to twice their resting size. In addition there is a further accumulation of secretion in the lumen of the alveoli. These changes usually lead to a marked increase in breast size during pregnancy. However, normal breast growth during pregnancy varies greatly between women, ranging from little or no increase to a considerable increase in size that can occur either rapidly during the first trimester or more gradually over the entire pregnancy (Fig. 4.3). Whereas Neifert et al.[39] found an association between minimal prenatal breast enlargement and insufficient lactation up to 21 days after birth, Cox et al.[40] found no such relationship. While the major increase in breast size is usually completed by week 22 of pregnancy, it is clear that for some women significant breast growth occurs during the last trimester of pregnancy (Fig. 4.3). The rate of growth of the mother's breast during pregnancy was correlated with the increase in the concentration of human placental lactogen in the mother's blood, suggesting that this hormone may stimulate breast growth in women as it does in some other mammals.[40] It is therefore likely that impaired placental function could have an impact on breast development at the time of delivery.

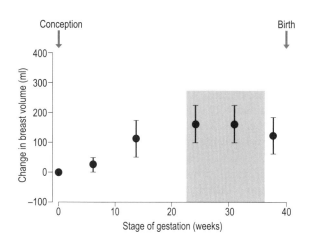

Figure 4.3 The mean (± 1 SD) increase in breast volume (ml) during pregnancy (n = 8). The shaded portion reflects the period of premature delivery. (Adapted from Cox et al.[40])

Taking these findings into consideration, it is possible that a deficiency in breast development at parturition may be more profound in very preterm mothers and mothers who have delivered intrauterine growth-restricted babies.

Lactogenesis I

Milk contains a number of components that are not produced elsewhere in the body, such as lactose, casein and α-lactalbumin. Lactogenesis I is the stage of breast development during pregnancy in which the mammary epithelial cells differentiate into lactocytes and become capable of secreting milk-specific components.[41] Lactogenesis I is identified by the detection of these milk-specific components in mammary secretion (if present), blood or urine. Since the breast secretion is not being removed by suckling, these components are resorbed into the blood through the paracellular pathway (the gaps between the lactocytes).[42] Lactose in blood is not metabolized elsewhere in the body, but is readily excreted in the urine.[43] Thus an increase in the output of lactose in urine during pregnancy is a useful indicator of lactogenesis I in women.[44]

The change in the rate of lactose excretion from preconception to delivery was related to a concomitant increase in breast size for the same period. Furthermore, the increase in the daily excretion of lactose in the urine during pregnancy was correlated with the increase in the concentration of prolactin in the blood, suggesting that prolactin may regulate the development of the synthetic capacity of the breast in pregnant women.[40] The measurement of the daily excretion of lactose in urine indicated that lactogenesis I can occur as early as 10 weeks postconception, but was highly variable between women. By week 22 of pregnancy, lactogenesis I appeared to have commenced in most, but not all, mothers (Fig. 4.4). This coincides with the time that Russo & Russo observed secretion in the lobules.[45] Therefore, it is possible that the breasts of some very preterm mothers may not have reached lactogenesis I before delivery.

Information about the hormonal regulation of breast growth and development in women during pregnancy is scanty, but the changes in the patterns of circulating hormones are now well established for women.[18] Extrapolation from animal studies suggests that the growth of the milk ducts is brought about by a combination of oestrogen, growth hormone and corticosteroids, while the proliferation of alveoli requires the further presence of progesterone and prolactin. In the absence of pituitary hormones, the ovarian steroids have either little or no mammogenic effect, but the anterior pituitary hormones may induce mammary growth in the absence of ovarian steroids. Furthermore, it appears that the high concentration of progesterone in maternal blood inhibits the secretory activity of the lactocytes during pregnancy.

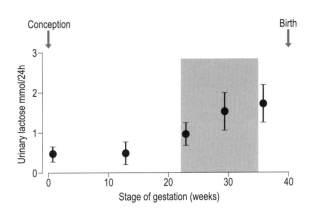

Figure 4.4 The output (mmol/24 h) of lactose in the urine (mean ± 1 SD) during pregnancy (*n* = 8). The shaded portion reflects the period of premature delivery. (Adapted from Cox et al.[40])

Current clinical practice recommends the administration of a single course of two doses of either betamethasone or dexamethasone 24 h apart to women at risk of preterm delivery.[46]

It has been suggested that progesterone and corticosteroids compete for glucocorticoid receptors in the lactocytes during pregnancy and that glucocorticoid administration during pregnancy could override the progesterone inhibition of lactogenesis II.[14] We have found that the administration of betamethasone to pregnant ewes results in precocious lactation[47] and the subsequent partial inhibition of lactogenesis II at term.[48,49] Therefore, the administration of betamethasone to women who are at risk of preterm delivery has the potential to alter normal breast development during pregnancy and parturition.

INITIATION OF LACTATION (LACTOGENESIS II) (TABLE 4.1)

Milk 'coming in' can be sensed as either a sudden feeling of fullness of the breasts or a gradual feeling of fullness occurring over a period of time. The sensation occurs between 24 and 102 h after birth, with a mean of 59–64 h,[41,50] and it has long been assumed that this was the marker of the initiation of lactation in women.[51] However, lactogenesis II, assessed by either an increase in milk production or acute changes in milk (colostrum) composition, precedes the mother sensing milk 'coming in'. Lactogenesis II is the most critical stage of the

lactation cycle as it facilitates the transition of the newborn from continuous nourishment from the umbilical cord to comparable but intermittent life support by suckling from its mother's breasts. Lactogenesis II is under hormonal control and has been shown to be triggered by the withdrawal of progesterone from the blood after birth,[52] but lactogenesis II also requires the presence of adequate levels of prolactin, insulin and adrenal corticosteroids.[53] Whereas progesterone withdrawal normally occurs just before birth in most mammals, it is delayed until after birth and the delivery of the placenta in women. Thus, irrespective of the length of gestation, little milk is produced immediately after birth. Term women produce between 39 and 169 g/day[50,54,55] in the first 48 h after birth. Therefore it is not surprising that most women are able to express only a few drops to a few millilitres of colostrum at this time. The rapid increase in milk production, lactogenesis II, normally commences between 30 and 40 h postpartum in women.[50] This has been determined objectively by test-weighing either the infant or the mother before and after each breastfeed. However, test-weighing in the immediate postnatal period is a demanding procedure[50,54] and it is possible that the baby may not consume all of the available milk (colostrum) and thus this will mask lactogenesis II.

However, lactogenesis II not only results in an increase in milk production but also results in dramatic changes in milk composition. These changes are induced by the closure of the paracellular pathway between the lactocytes,

Table 4.1 Factors that may contribute to either the inhibition or delay of lactogenesis II in preterm mothers together with potential causes and possible treatments

Factor	Cause	Treatment
Retained placental fragments	Elevated progesterone	Removal of fragments (dilatation and curettage)
Maternal type I diabetes	Unknown (possible decreased glucose uptake)	Informed support to ensure successful lactation
Maternal obesity	Unknown (possible elevated progesterone from body fat)	
Prolactin insufficiency	Prolactin switches on milk-specific genes	Domperidone, metoclopramide
Caesarean-section delivery	No labour – disturbed hormonal balance	Informed support to ensure successful lactation
Betamethasone	May induce premature lactation and subsequent partial inhibition	
Depo-Provera	Progesterone inhibition	Delay treatment until lactogenesis II is established
Anaesthetic agents	Not researched	
Breasts not emptied	Inadequate removal of milk with breast pump or engorgement – autocrine inhibition	Effective emptying of the breasts
Poor breast development	Shortened gestation	Increase frequency of pumping
Inadequate stimulation	Absence of milk ejection	Use gentle hand massage while pumping. Pump near baby. Double-pump
Drugs (alcohol, opiates)	Inhibition of milk ejection, decreased milk production, decreased milk removal by baby	Reduce or cease intake
Maternal-infant separation	Inadequate stimulation for milk ejection leading to ineffective pumping	Pump near baby and practice kangaroo mother care
Stress, fatigue	Inhibition of milk ejection	Stress management and relaxation techniques. Constant routine
Previous surgery or radiation treatment	Possible distortion or severing of ducts. Compromised innervation leading to inhibition of milk ejection	
Inadequate frequency of pumping	Milk stasis – autocrine inhibition	Increase frequency of pumping. Double-pumping
Glandular insufficiency	Unknown	

the rapid increase in the rate of milk synthesis and changes in the concentration of protective proteins in milk (e.g. secretory immunoglobulin A and lactoferrin) in a response to the increase in milk production. Thus the lipid content and concentrations of casein, lactose, calcium, phosphate, citrate and potassium increase, while the concentrations of total protein, sodium and chloride decrease at lactogenesis II.[50,56–58] These changes are normally stabilized within the first 5 days after birth.[50]

The changes in milk composition have been used as an alternative to test-weighing to assess the timing of the initiation of lactation in women.[50] The concentration of lactose in colostrum is low, < 50 mmol/l, and increases to > 150 mmol/l by day 3.[50] Lactose draws water into the Golgi apparatus[59] and leads to an increase in the volume of milk secreted. Arthur et al.[50] proposed that the time at which the lactose concentration in human milk reached 110 mmol/l was a useful objective marker of lactogenesis II. They found that this occurred at 31 h (SD 14 h) after birth. Neubauer et al.[60] proposed the use of the point of intersection of the increase in milk lactose (expressed as mmol/l) with the decrease in milk total nitrogen (expressed as g/l) as an alternative method of assessing the time of lactogenesis II. Their conclusions were similar to those of Arthur et al.[50] In addition, the increase in the concentration of citrate in the milk can be used as a metabolic marker of lactogenesis II.[50] On the other hand the decrease in the concentration of sodium in the milk reflects the closure of the paracellular pathway between the lactocytes.[61,62] Thus, together these markers demonstrate the complex coordinated changes that are required at lactogenesis II and the subsequent establishment of full lactation.

Mothers who deliver full-term babies and breastfeed on demand produce 556–705 g of milk by day 6 postpartum.[50,54,63,64] Depending on the nutritional needs of the infant, milk production at 1 month after birth ranges from 440 to 1220 g/day. This level of production is maintained from 1 to 6 months of lactation in exclusively breast-fed babies.[65,66]

Mothers who deliver preterm and express their milk appear more likely to produce less milk during the initiation of lactation than mothers who deliver full-term and breast-feed.[54,62] Mothers of babies in the special care nursery, who produced only a few drops of colostrum at each expression for the first 24–48 h after birth, showed a significant increase in milk production by 72 h after birth.[67] Milk productions of 20–550 g/day on day 5 after birth have been measured for mothers who delivered preterm (31–35 weeks' gestation) and were expressing their milk.[62]

Associated with the differences in milk production between the mothers of term and preterm infants are differences in the changes in milk composition. The concentrations of four markers of lactogenesis II (lactose, citrate, sodium and total protein) in milk collected from preterm mothers at day 5 postpartum have been measured. All these markers for the preterm mothers had much greater variation (Fig. 4.5). Furthermore, all the full-term mothers had all four markers within 3 SD of the mean for the full-term mothers, and were therefore classified as having successfully undergone lactogenesis II.[62] Only 18% of the preterm mothers had all four markers within 3 SD of the mean for the full-term mothers. The remainder of the preterm mothers had one or more of the markers greater than 3 SD from the mean concentration for full-term mothers. In addition, the preterm mothers who demonstrated one or more lactogenesis II markers outside the range for the full-term mothers had significantly lower milk productions than preterm mothers with all four markers within the range for full-term mothers. It was therefore concluded that lactogenesis II had been compromised in 82% of the preterm mothers and that mothers with more markers outside the normal range were likely to have lower milk production[62] (Fig. 4.5). The reasons for the compromised lactogenesis II are not clear but there is increasing evidence that delayed initiation could be related to maternal medications such as betamethasone given to women at risk of preterm delivery. In addition, anaesthetic agents given during childbirth have not been investigated in relation to their influence, if any, on lactogenesis II. Furthermore, other factors, such as decreased frequency of breast expression, caesarean-section delivery,[68,69] obesity[69] and type 1 diabetes[50] have been found to delay lactogenesis II in term mothers. The influence of these factors may be accentuated in mothers of very preterm babies where it is possible that lactogenesis I and breast growth are not yet complete.

However, it is of interest that given appropriate assistance it is possible for women to establish lactation in the absence of a normal pregnancy. Although the available evidence is limited, it suggests that there may be consider-

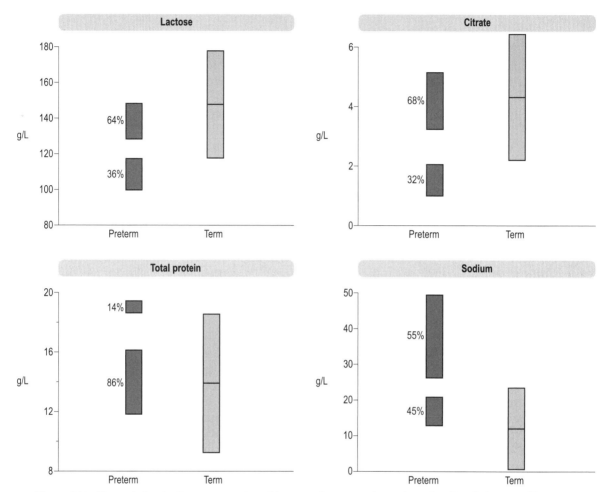

Figure 4.5 The variation in the concentration of lactose, citrate, total protein and sodium in breast milk at 5 days postpartum in preterm and term mothers. A proportion of preterm mothers had levels for lactose and citrate that were lower than the normal range for term mothers and levels of total protein and sodium that were higher than those for the normal range for term mothers. (Reproduced with permission from Cregan et al.[62])

able variation between women in their capacity to respond to these stimuli[14] (see Chapter 5). Furthermore, women who have stopped breastfeeding for up to several months can relactate and fully nourish their babies within a few days to weeks and women who have had minimal breast growth and development during pregnancy can show compensatory growth during the first month postpartum.[40]

It is recognized that for normal term mothers the early commencement of breastfeeding (within 1 h of birth) and frequent breastfeeding thereafter provide the optimum stimulation for the initiation of successful lactation. Since

breast development may be compromised by the truncation of pregnancy in preterm mothers, the timing and frequency of breast expression should be at least comparable to that recommended for term breastfeeding mothers[70,71] (see Chapter 5).

MILK COMPOSITION

Breast milk is considered the ideal nutrient for full-term infants, providing many benefits (see Chapter 1), including protecting against illness, facilitating rapid brain development and providing specific nutrients for the development of the gastrointestinal tract and a readily available source of calcium for bone development.[72–76] Feeding mother's milk to preterm babies also decreases the risk of morbidity and mortality. Numerous reports suggest that milk from mothers who delivered prematurely has a higher concentration of total protein and a lower concentration of carbohydrates than the milk from mothers who delivered at term.[77–79]

There is considerable variation in the composition of milk from term mothers within mothers, between mothers and with stage of lactation.[80] For example, at the extreme, some mothers can have twice the fat content in their breast milk from 1 to 6 months of lactation compared to other mothers.[81] Recent studies of preterm mothers have shown considerable variations in the composition of their milk during early lactation,[62] but little information is available on variation in the composition of the milk of preterm mothers in established lactation. Fortification of mother's own milk is usually based on an assumed average composition of mature human milk. If similar variation occurs in preterm mothers to that observed in term mothers, major errors may occur in matching the final composition of fortified mother's milk to the desired nutritional requirements of the preterm infant. (See Chapter 3 for a full discussion of fortification.)

Usually foremilk at the beginning of a breastfeed contains very little fat and is pale blue in appearance, whereas hindmilk at the end of a breastfeed usually contains much more fat and is dense white in appearance. Thus there is a progressive increase in the fat content of milk as it is removed from the breast, and a decrease in fat as the breast fills with milk from the end of one breastfeed to the beginning of the next breastfeed. Therefore the fat content of a sample of either fore- or hindmilk depends on the amount of milk stored in the breast at the time the sample was taken. The degree of fullness of the breast can be calculated by subtracting the minimum breast volume observed over a 24-h period from the breast volume measured at any other time. Daly et al.[25] found a close relationship between the degree of fullness of the breast and the fat content of milk; milk with low fat was associated with a full breast and that with a high fat with a breast drained of milk.

Although the physiological significance of this highly conserved feature of mammalian lactation is not known, it is of clinical importance. Either measuring the fat content or observing the opacity of the milk can provide useful information on the fullness of the mother's breasts at any point in time. The change in the fat content of milk can also be used to assess the effective removal of the available milk from the breast at either breast expression or a breastfeed.[24] It should be noted that these relationships have only been substantiated for women in established lactation; the relationships may not hold for mothers either during lactogenesis II or those with very low milk production. An innovative technique has recently been developed to enable mothers to collect expressed breast milk with a higher energy density for their preterm babies.[82,83] Mothers measure the fat content of their fore- and hindmilk by the creamatocrit technique.[84,85] They then take advantage of the progressive increase in the fat content of breast milk during expression to select the fraction of expressed milk that has a fat content (energy density) that is appropriate for their preterm baby: this has resulted in accelerated weight gain in the preterm baby.[82,83] Currently there are no simple procedures to increase the protein and micronutrients in mother's own milk for preterm babies. However adequate protein is critical for optimal growth rates in preterm infants (see Chapter 3 for information on balancing the energy and protein intake in such babies fed on predominantly hindmilk).

MILK EJECTION

Historical paintings show that it was known for thousands of years that milk letdown (milk ejection) was associated with the stimulation of either the nipple or the birth canal. But it was only in 1941 that Ely & Petersen[86] first correctly described the physiology of the milk ejection reflex in studies on dairy cows. They concluded: 'The "letting down" of milk is a conditioned reflex operated by sensory stimuli associated with milking. Afferent impulses reach the central nervous system and cause the release of oxytocin from the posterior pituitary, which in time causes a rise in milk pressure probably because of the contraction of muscular tissue, which is believed to surround the alveoli and small ducts.'[86] However, it was not until 1948 that Newton & Newton demonstrated that the milk ejection reflex was also present in lactating women.[87] They measured the amount of milk taken by a baby in timed breastfeeds when the mother was subjected to the effects of severe distractions, with and without injection of oxytocin, and concluded that the mechanism of letdown in animals held for lactating women. From these findings Newton & Newton speculated that if mothers were subjected to a stressful environment in hospital, milk ejection would be inhibited and the baby would get little milk.[87] This concern is of particular relevance to preterm mothers who are subjected to the normal hospital stresses but, in addition, have the added burden of having to express their milk for their sick babies. Thus providing an appropriate environment for the mother to express her milk is of great importance. Studies have shown that lactation is best facilitated if the mother is able to express in close proximity to her baby – providing care is taken to avoid potential stresses.[88]

It is now well established that milk ejection is critical to successful lactation in women. In most mothers only very small volumes of milk (< 5 ml) can be obtained prior to milk ejection, but some women who had large milk ducts (5–10 mm) were able to express up to 30 ml before milk ejection.[89] However, there is virtually no information available about the characteristics of milk ejection in preterm mothers. One study has shown that double-pumping is more effective at producing milk than single sequential pumping. Milk yield was higher from mothers who double-pumped.[90] A possible explanation for this finding could be related to a more efficient removal of milk during the initial milk ejection. However, more research is

required to determine the ideal conditions for the optimization of milk ejection in mothers who are expressing their milk for their preterm babies.

Although oxytocin is usually associated with stimulating uterine contractions and milk ejection, evidence is now accumulating that this hormone has a more extensive metabolic role. The stimuli that lead to the release of oxytocin from the posterior pituitary gland into the blood also cause its release from axons that pass from the paraventricular nucleus to other areas of the brain, thereby activating a series of responses that promote energy storage, calmness and socialization. Uvnas-Moberg et al. and others[91–93] have shown that buccal stimulation and cholecystokinin release associated with eating are potent stimuli, causing both the central and peripheral release of oxytocin, and result in diverse responses, including:

1. increasing energy reserves by stimulating the release of insulin
2. increasing the efficiency of food utilization by contraction of the pyloric sphincter and slowing the passage of digesta
3. promotion of calmness by lowering blood pressure, heart rate and cortisol secretion
4. modification of behaviour by promoting socialization

Although these responses are not directly related to the synthesis and secretion of milk, they are appropriate metabolic and behavioural responses for the facilitation of breastfeeding and maternal care.

ESTABLISHED LACTATION

Substrate supply and endocrine control of milk synthesis

During the 1970s it was clear that food intake was an important determinant of milk production in dairy and laboratory animals. This knowledge was extrapolated to women and it was thought that improving maternal nutrition in developing countries would increase their milk production and thereby improve the nourishment of their breast-fed babies. However, Prentice et al.[94] showed that poorly nourished women in developing counties produced as much milk as well-nourished mothers in developed countries and concluded that milk production was not particularly sensitive to food intake in women. (See Chapter 3 for further discussion of the effect of maternal diet on breast-milk composition.) At this time it was found that breast-feeding stimulated the release of prolactin and it was assumed that increasing the frequency of breastfeeding would increase the release of prolactin, which in turn would increase milk production. Subsequent studies have shown that in women, milk production was not correlated with the release of prolactin.[95] However, mothers with impaired low levels of prolactin in their blood may respond to the stimulation of prolactin secretion brought about by the administration of domperidone (Motilium)[96] (see Chapter 5).

Autocrine control of milk synthesis

Linzell & Peaker first demonstrated the autocrine control of milk synthesis (local control within each breast) in dairy goats in 1971.[59] They found that increasing the frequency of milking on one gland of a goat only increased milk production in that gland and therefore they concluded that this response was local and independent of systemic hormonal stimulation. Recently, peptides have been purified and sequenced from cow's milk that reversibly inhibit the secretion of milk through the Golgi system. Thus it appears that a local inhibitory mechanism reduces milk secretion as the mammary gland fills with milk and that the frequent removal of milk from the mammary gland will prevent this inhibition and result in increased milk production.

Studies on the rate of milk synthesis strongly suggest that a similar inhibitory control occurs in women. This autocrine inhibition explains why women with small storage capacities need either to breastfeed or express their milk more frequently than women with larger storage capacities. Indeed, the volume of milk expressed can be misleading to preterm mothers. They are

likely to express the largest volumes of milk in the early morning when the interval between breast expressions has been the greatest. However, if the volume of milk produced is divided by the number of hours from the previous breast expression, the rate of milk production (ml/h) is usually much lower when the interval between breast expressions is longer. Thus, not only is the frequency of breast expression per day important, but there should be no long intervals between breast expressions over the 24-h period if maximum milk production is to be achieved.

Thus once a preterm mother's milk supply is established, the ideal frequency of breast expression for providing milk for her baby is not absolute, but depends upon the storage capacity of her breasts. A mother with a large storage capacity who can easily drain her breasts during pumping may need to express only three or four times per day. On the other hand, a mother who has either a small storage capacity or who has difficulty draining her breasts may need to express as frequently as eight times a day. It is important that the breast expressions are spaced out over the entire 24-h period so that there are no long intervals where the amount of milk produced reaches the storage capacity and milk synthesis is downregulated. It is much easier to maintain a high supply of milk than to allow it to decline and then try to increase milk production again. Therefore, mothers should aim to produce as much milk per day for their preterm babies as would be required by a normal term baby so that an adequate milk supply is ensured when they are eventually able to breastfeed.

References

1. Jensen RJ. Handbook of milk composition. San Diego: California, USA: Academic Press; 1995:2–3.
2. Nicholas KR, Wilde CJ, Bird PH et al. Asynchronous concurrent secretion of milk proteins in the Tammar wallaby. In: Wilde CJ, Peaker M, Knight DH, eds. Intercellular signalling in the mammary gland. New York: Plenum Press; 1994:153–170.
3. Dewey KG, Peerson JM, Brown KH et al. Growth of breast-fed infants deviates from current reference data: a pooled analysis of US, Canadian, and European data sets. World Health Organization

Working Group on Infant Growth. Pediatrics 1995; 96:495–503.

4. Moyer-Mileur L, Chan GM, Gill G. Evaluation of liquid or powdered fortification of human milk on growth and bone mineralization status of preterm infants. J Pediatr Gastroenterol Nutr 1992;15:370–374.

5. Schanler RJ, Schulman RJ, Lau C et al. Feeding strategies for premature infants: randomised trial of gastrointestinal priming and tube-feeding method. Pediatrics 1999; 103:434–439.

6. Reis BB, Hall RT, Schanler RJ et al. Enhanced growth of preterm infants fed a new powdered human milk fortifier: a randomised controlled trial. Pediatrics 2000; 106:581–588.

7. Kuschel CA, Harding JE. Multicomponent fortified human milk for promoting growth in preterm infants. Cochrane Database Syst Rev 2000; 2:CD000343.

8. Yeung DL, Peters CT. Functional foods: implications of infant development and later health. Heinz Sight Infant Nutr Newslett 2001; 58:1–6.

9. Yu V, Simmer K. Enteral nutrition. In: Tsang RC, ed. Nutritional needs of the preterm infant. Philadelphia, PA: Williams & Wilkins; (in press).

10. American Academy of Pediatrics. Work group on breast-feeding. Breast-feeding and the use of human milk. Pediatrics 1997; 100:1035–1039.

11. Kavanaugh KL, Meir PP, Zimmerman B et al. The rewards outweigh the efforts: breast-feeding outcomes for mothers of preterm infants. J Hum Lact 1997; 13:15–21.

12. Meier PP, Brown LP, Hurst NM. Breast-feeding the preterm infant. In: Breast-feeding and human lactation. Boston: Jones and Bartlett; 1999:456.

13. Hartmann PE, Cregan MD. Lactogenesis and the effects of insulin-dependent diabetes mellitus and prematurity. J Nutr 2001; 131:3016S–3020S.

14. Cowie AT, Forsyth IA, Hart IC. Hormonal control of lactation. New York: Springer-Verlag; 1980:117–118; 203–204.

15. Tobon H, Salazar H. Ultrastructure of the human mammary gland. II. Postpartum lactogenesis. J Clin Endocrinol Metab 1975; 40:834–844.

16. Birkenfeld A, Kase NG. Functional anatomy and physiology of the female breast. Obstet Gynecol Clin North Am 1994; 21(3):433–445.

17. Bannister LH, Berry MM, Collins P et al., eds. Gray's anatomy, 38th edn. London: Churchill Livingstone 1995:417–424.

18. Hartmann PE. The breast and breast-feeding. In: Philipp E, Setchell M, Ginsburg M, eds. Scientific foundations of obstetrics and gynaecology, 4th edn. Oxford: Butterworth Heinemann; 1991:378–390.

19. Lawerence R. Breast-feeding: a guide for the medical profession, 4th edn. St Louis: Mosby Year Book; 1994: 53.

20. Fawcett DW. Mammary gland. In: Fawcett DW, ed. A textbook of histology. Philadelphia, PA: WB Saunders; 1986:901–912.

21. Cooper AP. The anatomy of the breast. London: Longman, Orme, Green, Browne and Longmans; 1840.

22. Ramsay DT, Kent JC, Hartmann PE. Ultrasound imaging of the anatomy of the human lactating breast. Conference proceedings. Abstract. Perinatal Society of Australia and New Zealand Christchurch, NZ; March 2002.

23. Ramsay DT, Kent JC, Hartmann PE. Breast anatomy redefined by ultrasound in the lactating breast. Conference proceedings. Australian Society for Ultrasound in Medicine. Perth, Australia. September, 2003.

24. Hartmann PE. New insights into breast physiology and breast expression and development of the symphony breastpump. In: Human lactation – the science of the art series. CD version 1.1. Baar Switzerland: Medela; Medical Technology; 2002.

25. Daly SEJ, Di Rosso A, Owens RA et al. Degree of breast emptying explains changes in the fat content, but not fatty acid composition, of human milk. Exp Physiol 1993; 78:741–755.

26. Salmon M. Arteries of gland mammaire. Ann Pathol Anat 1939; 4:481–500.

27. Vorherr H. The breast: morphology, physiology and lactation. London: Academic Press; 1974:27–30.

28. Doughty JC, McCarter DHA, Kane E et al. Anatomical basis of intra-arterial chemotherapy for patients with locally advanced breast cancer. Br J Surg 1996; 83:1128–1130.

29. Anson BJ, Wright RR, Wolfer JA. Blood supply of the mammary gland. Surg Gynecol Obstet 1939; 69:468–473.

30. Aljazaf K, Ramsay DT, Hartley B et al. Colour Doppler ultrasound imaging of the arterial blood supply of the human lactating breast. Conference proceedings. ILCA: Boca Raton, USA. July 2002.

31. Cunningham L. The anatomy of the arteries and veins of the breast. J Surg Oncol 1977; 9: 71–85.

32. Isard HJ, Ostrum BJ. Breast thermography – the mammatherm. Radiol Clin North Am 1974; 12:167–188.

33. Hultborn KA, Larsson LG, Ragnhult I. The lymph drainage from the breast to the axillary and parasternal lymph nodes, studied with the aid of colloidal Au[198]. Acta Radiol 1955; 43:52–64.

34. Turner-Warwick RT. The lymphatics of the breast. Br J Surg 1959; 46:574–582.

35. Morehead JR. Anatomy of embryology of the breast. Clin Obstet Gynecol 1982; 5:353–357.

36. Montagna W, MacPherson E. Some neglected aspects of the anatomy of human breasts. J Invest Dermatol 1974; 63:10–16.

37. Robinson JE, Short RV. Changes in breast sensitivity at puberty, during the menstrual cycle, and at parturition. Br Med J 1977; 1:1188–1191.

38. Linzell JL, Peaker M. The permeability of mammary ducts. J Physiol 1971; 216:701–716.

39. Neifert M, DeMarzo S, Seacat J et al. The influence of breast surgery, breast appearance, and pregnancy-induced breast changes on lactation sufficiency as measured by infant weight gain. Birth 1990; 17:31–38.

40. Cox DB, Kent JC, Casey TM et al. Breast growth and the urinary excretion of lactose during human pregnancy and early lactation: endocrine relationships. Exp Physiol 1999; 84:421–434.

41. Kulski JK, Hartmann PE. Changes in human milk composition during the initiation of lactation. Austr J Exp Biol Med Sci 1981; 59:101–114.

42. Arthur PG, Kent JC, Potter JM et al. Lactose in blood in nonpregnant, pregnant, and lactating women. J Pediatr Gastroenterol Nutr 1991; 3:254–259.

43. Carleton FJ, Roberts HR. Preliminary observations on the fate of intravenously administered lactose labelled with carbon-14. Nature 1959; 184:1650–1651.

44. Arthur PG, Kent JC, Hartmann PE. Metabolites of lactose synthesis in milk from women during established lactation. J Pediatr Gastroenterol 1991; 13:260–266.

45. Russo J, Russo IH. Development of the human mammary gland. In: Neville MC, Daniel CW, eds. The mammary gland: development, regulation and function. New York: Plenum; 1987:67–93.

46. National Institutes of Health Consensus Development Panel. Antenatal corticosteroids revisited: repeat courses – National Institutes of Health consensus development conference statement August 17-18 2000. Obstet Gynecol 2001; 98:144–150.

47. Hartmann PE, Cregan MD. Lactogenesis and the effects of insulin-dependent diabetes mellitus and prematurity. J Nutr 2001; 131:3016S–3020S.

48. Henderson JJ, Hartmann PE, Moss TJM et al. Maternal effects of glucocorticoid administration in the pregnant ewe: the impact on lactogenesis. Melbourne: Australian Health and Medical Research Congress, 2002.

49. Henderson JJ, Hartmann PE, Moss TJM et al. Antenatal glucocorticoids inhibit initiation of lactation in the ewe. Washington DC, Society for Gynecologic Investigation 50th Annual Meeting, March 26–30, 2003.

50. Arthur PG, Smith M, Hartmann PE. Milk lactose, citrate and glucose as markers of lactogenesis in normal and diabetic women. J Pediatr Gastroenterol 1989; 9:488–496.

51. Cadogan W. An essay upon nursing. In: Rendle-Short J, Rendle-Short M, eds. The father of child care. Life of William (1711–1797). Bristol, UK: John Wright; 1966:1–34.

52. Kulski JK, Smith M, Hartmann PE. Perinatal concentrations of progesterone, lactose and alpha-lactalbumin in the mammary secretion of women. J Endocrinol 1977; 74:509–510.

53. Forsyth IA. The endocrinology of lactation. In: Mepham TB, ed. Biochemistry of lactation. New York: Elsevier; 1983:309–349.

54. Saint L, Smith M, Hartmann PE. The yield and nutrient content of colostrum and milk in women from giving birth to one month post-partum. Br J Nutr 1984; 52:87–95.

55. Glasier A, McNeilly A. Physiology of lactation. Baillieres Clin Endocrinol Metab 1990; 4:379–395.

56. Harzer G, Haug M, Bindels JG. Biochemistry of maternal milk in early lactation. Hum Nutr Appl Nutr 1986; 40 (suppl. 1):11–18.

57. Neville MC, Allen JC, Archer PC et al. Studies in human lactation: milk volume and nutrient composition during weaning and lactogenesis. Am J Clin Nutr 1991; 54:81–92.

58. Kunz C, Lonnerdal B. Re-evaluation of the whey protein/casein ratio of human milk. Acta Paediatr 1992; 81:107–112.

59. Linzell JL, Peaker M. Mechanism of milk secretion. Physiol Rev 1971; 51:564–597.

60. Neubauer SH, Ferrus AM, Chase CG et al. Delayed lactogenesis in women with insulin-dependent diabetes mellitus. Am J Clin Nutr 1993; 58:54–60.

61. Linzell JL, Peaker M. Changes in colostrum composition and in the permeability of the mammary epithelium at about the time of parturition in the goat. J Physiol 1974; 243:129–151.

62. Cregan MD, de Mello TR, Kershaw D et al. Initiation of lactation in women after preterm delivery. Acta Obstet Gynecol Scand 2002; 81:870–877.

63. Casey CE, Hambridge KM, Neville MC. Studies in human lactation: zinc, copper, manganese and chromium in human milk in the first month of lactation. Am J Clin Nutr 1985; 41:1193–1220.

64. Hartmann PE, Sheriff J, Kent J. Maternal nutrition and the regulation of milk synthesis. Proc Nutr Soc 1995; 54:379–389.

65. Sherriff JL, Hartmann PE. Energy expenditure during lactation - a review of the literature. Austr J Nutr Diet 1995; 52:187–199.

66. Kent JC, Mitoulas LR, Cox DB et al. Breast volume and milk production during extended lactation in women. Exp Physiol 1999; 84:435–447.

67. Meier PP. Breast-feeding in the special care nursery. Prematures and infants with medical problems. Pediatr Clin North Am 2001; 48:425–442.

68. Evans KC, Evans RG, Royal R et al. Effect of caesarean section on breast milk transfer to the normal term newborn over the first week of life. Arch Dis Child Fetal Neonatal Ed 2003; 88:F380.

69. Chapman D, Perez-Escamilla R. Identification of risk factors for delayed onset of lactation. J Am Diet Assoc 1999; 99:450–454.

70. De Carvalho M, Robertson S, Friedman A et al. Effect of frequent breast-feeding in early milk production and infant weight gain. Pediatrics 1983; 72:307–311.

71. Hopkinson JM, Schanler RJ, Garza C. Milk production by mothers of premature infants. Pediatrics 1988; 81:815–820.

72. Kent JC, Arthur PG, Retallack RW et al. Calcium, phosphate and citrate in human milk at initiation of lactation. J Dairy Res 1992; 59:161–167.

73. Makrides M, Neumann MA, Byard RW et al. Fatty acid composition of brain, retina, and erythrocytes in breast- and formula-fed infants. Am J Clin Nutr 1994; 60:189–194.

74. Kelleher SL, Lonnerdal B. Immunological activities associated with milk. Adv Nutr Res 2001; 10:39–65.

75. Hartmann PE, Cregan MD, Mitoulas LR. Maternal modulation of specific and non-specific immune components of colostrum and mature milk. Adv Nutr Res 2001; 10:365–387.

76. Burrin DG, Stoll B. Key nutrients and growth factors for the neonatal gastrointestinal tract. Clin Perinatol 2002; 29:65–96.

77. Butte NF, Garza C, Johnson CA et al. Longitudinal changes in milk composition of mothers delivering preterm and term infants. Early Hum Dev 1984; 9:153–162.

78. Montagne P, Cuilliere ML, Mole C et al. Immunological and nutritional composition of human milk in relation to prematurity and mother's parity during the first 2 weeks of lactation. J Pediatr Gastroenterol Nutr 1999; 29:75–80.

79. Maas YG, Gerritsen J, Hart AA et al. Development of macronutrient composition of very preterm human milk. Br J Nutr 1998; 80:35–40.

80. Hartmann PE, Rattigan S, Saint L et al. Variation in the yield and composition of human milk. Oxford Rev Reprod Biol 1985; 7:118–167.

81. Mitoulas LR, Kent JC, Cox DB et al. Variation in fat, lactose and protein in human milk over 24 h and throughout the first year of lactation. Br J Nutr 2002; 88:29–37.

82. Valentine CJ, Hurst NM, Schanler RJ. Hindmilk improves weight gain in low-birth-weight infants fed human milk. J Pediatr Gastroenterol Nutr 1994; 18:474–477.

83. Vasan U, Meier PP, Meier WA et al. Individualizing the lipid content of own mothers' milk: effect on weight gain for extremely low birthweight infants. Pediatr Res 1998; 45:287A.

84. Griffin TL, Meier PP, Bradford LP et al. Mothers performing creamatocrit measures in the NICU: accuracy, reactions and cost. J Obstet Gynecol Neonatal Nurs 2000; 29:249–257.

85. Meier PP, Engstrom JL, Murtaugh M et al. Mothers' milk feedings in the neonatal intensive care unit: accuracy of the creamatocrit technique. J Perinatol 2002; 22:646–649.

86. Ely F, Petersen WE. Factors involved in milk ejection. J Dairy Sci 1941; 24:211–223.

87. Newton M, Newton NR. The let-down reflex in human lactation. J Pediatr 1948; 33:698–704.

88. Meier PP. Supporting lactation in mothers with very low birth weight infants. Paediatr Ann 2003; 32:317–325.

89. Kent JC, Ramsay DT, Doherty D et al. Response of breasts to different stimulation patterns of an electric breast pump. J Hum Lact 2003; 19:179–187.

90. Jones E, Dimmock PW, Spencer SA. A randomised controlled trial to compare methods of milk expression after preterm delivery. Arch Dis Child Fetal Neonatal Ed 2001; 85:F91.

91. Uvnas-Moberg K, Johansson B, Lupoli B et al. Oxytocin facilitates behavioural, metabolic and physiological adaptations during lactation. Appl Anim Behav Sci 2001; 72:225–234.

92. Nissen E, Gustavsson P, Widstrom AM et al. Oxytocin, prolactin, milk production and their relationship with personality traits in women after vaginal delivery or Cesarean section. J Psychosom Obstet Gynaecol 1998; 19:49–58.

93. Marchini G, Lagercrantz H, Winberg J et al. Fetal and maternal plasma levels of gastrin, somatostatin and oxytocin after vaginal delivery and elective cesarean section. Early Hum Dev 1988; 18:73–79.

94. Prentice A, Paul A, Prentice A et al. Cross-cultural differences in lactational performance. In: Hamosh M, ed. Human lactation 2. Maternal and environmental factors. New York: Plenum Press; 1986:13–44.

95. Cox DB, Owens RA, Hartmann PE. Blood and milk prolactin and the rate of milk synthesis in women. Exp Physiol 1996; 81:1007–1020.

96. Hale TW. Medications and mothers' milk. 10th edn. Pharmasoft Medical Publishing: Amarillo, Texas 2002; 230–232.

97. Ramsay DT, Kent JC, Hartmann RL, Hartmann PE. Anatomy of the lactating human breast redefined with ultrasound imaging Journal of Anatomy (2005) in press.

Chapter 5

Milk expression

Elizabeth Jones and Peter E Hartmann

Summary of key points

- The barriers that women encounter regarding preterm milk expression are investigated
- The principles of milk expression and the effective use of milk expression equipment are outlined and explored
- Practical guidance is given for common problems such as excessive milk, too little milk and sore nipples
- Management issues regarding relactation and induced lactation are examined

THE CHALLENGE

Human milk is an important requirement for preterm babies, promoting the establishment of enteral feeding and providing immunological protection.[1] Breastfeeding is also a key strategy to facilitate maternal–infant attachment, so often adversely affected by separation in the early postpartum period.[2] In a study carried out by Kavanaugh et al.[2] in the USA, 20 mothers were interviewed at 1 month postdischarge from a neonatal intensive care unit (NICU). All women in the study received evidence-based breastfeeding advice and support, and their comments demonstrate the value they placed on their experience. Descriptive impressions from those interviewed include:

- 'knowing that they had given their infants a good start in life'
- 'their enjoyment of the physical closeness and intimacy of breastfeeding'
- 'knowing that they were making a unique contribution to infant care'

However, it is widely acknowledged that mothers of preterm infants, especially extremely low-birth-weight neonates, experience both physiological and emotional challenges that adversely affect breastfeeding rates for this population.[3–5] The initiation of lactation may be delayed for a number of reasons (see Chapter 4.1, Table 4.1) and in addition many mothers are ill in the immediate postpartum period due to obstetric complications. Furthermore, the initiation of an expression schedule may be difficult to achieve since it may necessitate a strong commitment to a future that may seem to be very uncertain. A study carried out in the USA by Hill et al.[6] suggests that almost half of mothers of low-birth-weight infants do not express milk until 24 h after giving birth, and nearly one-quarter delay past 96 h before initiating milk expression. Even if early expression is facilitated, anxiety is a potent inhibitor of the milk ejection reflex.[7] Unless colostrum is efficiently expressed in the early period following delivery, the developmental switch needed for copious milk production is inhibited.[8] Insufficient milk volumes followed by declining production are common problems associated with preterm delivery.[9]

Whilst preterm breastfeeding rates vary worldwide, several studies suggest that mothers of preterm infants initiate and sustain breastfeeding at lower rates than mothers of term healthy babies.[10–12] These studies indicate an inverse relationship between infant gestational age and duration of breastfeeding. In a study from the USA, Furman et al.[13] sought to determine what percentage of mothers of very-low-birth-weight (VLBW) infants intended to breastfeed and how many established the practice. The results revealed that, of the 73% of mothers who intended to breastfeed, 34% continued to lactate at 40 weeks' corrected age. In a Malaysian study, the breastfeeding rate at discharge was 40% for 126 mothers of surviving VLBW infants.[14] Although these studies directly reflect the difficulties mothers encounter in sustaining milk production, they indicate that lactation can be prolonged if mothers are given encouragement and support. In recognition of the unique species-specific benefits of breastfeeding and human milk, the support and encouragement of breastfeeding are included in the *Dietary Guidelines for Australia* (see Resources).[15]

Five independent UK audits of the support given to preterm breastfeeding mothers have found that breastfeeding facilities and support in many units are far below acceptable standards.[16–20] Reasons stated by mothers encompass numerous explanations, including poor provision of milk expression equipment, lack of privacy, lactation failure, conflicting advice and rigid feeding routines. This apparently suggests that breastfeeding support programmes are not in place in many NICUs within the UK. Supporting mothers adequately is time-consuming and requires specialist knowledge and expertise. Whilst information is given regarding human lactation in UK midwifery training, considerably less is provided within the training programmes undertaken by paediatric students. This is a situation that clearly needs to be addressed as the knowledge and attitudes health professionals have about breastfeeding are crucial to the information and support mothers receive. It is imperative that all staff should receive in-service training regarding breastfeeding management and that equipment and private facilities are available for both milk expression and preterm breastfeeding. Despite the fact that breastfeeding rates are relatively high in Australia and the 'support and encouragement' of breastfeeding have been included in the *Dietary Guidelines for Australia* since 1981, there are still difficulties in providing mothers with appropriate and consistent breastfeeding and milk expression advice.[15]

Many parents find the neonatal environment intimidating and struggle to cope with the barrage of information given to them by nurses and medical staff about the care their baby is receiving. Whenever possible, it is important to discuss both the benefits of human milk and breastfeeding during the antenatal period, and it is important that this information is given in both written and verbal form.[16] Mothers with obstetric complications are often hospitalized before a decision is made to expedite delivery and are anxious about the welfare of their baby. Even mothers who do not ultimately intend to establish breastfeeding often consider expressing breast milk to be fed to their baby either by nasogastric tube or by bottle. In addition, preterm delivery often precludes the attendance at parentcraft classes so unless parents are given accurate information they will be denied an informed choice regarding infant feeding. A mother's decision to breastfeed should be documented in her nursing care plan in order to ensure that mothers who wish to initiate milk expression are given assistance to do so in the early post-partum period. The provision of research-based information and specialist advice on the benefits of breast milk to the preterm infant should be the standard of care for all mothers.

SUMMARY OF RECOMMENDATIONS

The challenge
- Discuss the benefits of breastfeeding antenatally
- Discuss the probable need for the fortification of breast milk for preterm babies
- Acknowledge emotional and physiological barriers
- Provide in-service training about breastfeeding management
- Have a breastfeeding care policy and procedures manual (clinical guidelines) for hospital staff and mothers
- Provide equipment, facilities and ongoing support

INITIATION AND ESTABLISHMENT OF LACTATION

Although few empirical data are available to provide guidance for the initiation of lactation following preterm delivery, published evidence suggests early and frequent milk expression is associated with increased breastfeeding duration. DeCarvalho et al.[9] reported that the frequency of milk expression was correlated positively with milk production in mothers of preterm infants. In another study, Hopkinson et al.[21] evaluated 32 healthy non-smoking women who gave birth to infants at 28–30 weeks' gestation and found a positive correlation between the day on which milk expression was initiated with milk volume at 2 weeks. Hill et al.[22] also reported that milk weight was positively influenced by the initiation of mechanical expression soon after birth and that there was a significant interaction between frequency and initiation. Based on these findings it appears to be imperative to minimize the time interval between delivery and initiation of milk expression.

In some cultures, colostrum is regarded as unclean and newborn infants are not put to the breast until 48–72 h following delivery. Prelacteal feeds such as boiled water, tea or diluted animal milks are given to the infant until lactation is established. There is no scientific support for these beliefs and such practices should be discouraged, particularly for preterm babies. Furthermore, Neville et al.[23] observed that a delayed removal of colostrum may result in an unsuccessful initiation of lactation. Therefore, if a mother appears reluctant to express initially it is important to ascertain if there are cultural barriers involved. When discussing the benefits of colostrum it is useful to reinforce verbal information with appropriately translated information leaflets in order to help a mother to share her decisions with her family.

Mothers should be given realistic expectations regarding initial milk volume. Many mothers who deliver preterm produce less milk during the initiation of lactation than mothers who deliver term infants and breastfeed. The amount produced can be as little as a few drops of colostrum at each expression for the first 24–48 h after birth, and there may be a significant delay before more substantial milk production begins (see Chapter 4). Hand expression can be useful initially for collecting colostrum, since colostrum is viscous and difficult to remove from a milk storage container.

There are few recommendations in the literature regarding an expression schedule (frequency) for the expressing mother using an electric breast pump. Current recommendations for mothers expressing milk for preterm infants range from 'as often as a term breastfeeding baby (8–12 times a day)'[24] to 'every three hours, with no more than a five-hour break over night'[25] to 'a minimum of five milk expressions per day and a total duration of 100 minutes per day at the breast pump'.[21] These recommendations can often be misinterpreted; for example, it may be detrimental if most of the expression periods (either by number or total time at the pump) occur during daylight hours, even though such a regime may fit the guidelines. Furthermore, these guidelines are generalized and do not take into account individual differences between mothers. It is therefore important to consider the major determinants of milk production (synthesis) and to understand how these vary between individual mothers so that recommendations relating to the individual can be developed in order to maximize milk output (see Chapter 4).

For each expressing mother to maximize her milk output, the rate of milk synthesis between expression episodes must be considered. Once milk production is established the short-term (between breast expressions) rate of milk synthesis is controlled locally within each breast and is dependent on the amount of milk stored in the breast. Previous research has shown that the greatest rates of milk synthesis occur when the breast is drained of milk, whereas the slowest rates of milk synthesis occur in the fuller breast.[26] This relationship is, however, often misrepresented, as mothers can express larger volumes of milk after long intervals between expression periods. However, when milk output is viewed in the context of volume per interval time (ml/h), the longer intervals are associated with lower overall rates of synthesis, that is, less milk is produced each hour over the longer period. Indeed, Daly et al.[27] showed that for five breastfeeding mothers and three expressing mothers, milk synthetic

rates were linear when intervals were less than 6 h but proportionally less milk was obtained for intervals greater than 6 h. Furthermore, Mitoulas (2003, personal communication) has investigated rates of milk synthesis and intervals between expression episodes in mothers expressing milk for preterm infants and found a negative relationship between rate of milk synthesis and interval between breast expressions. However, there was considerable variation between women, with the rate of milk production (ml/h) decreasing after only a 3-h interval in some women but not until up to a 7-h interval in others. At the extreme one mother was able to maintain a production of over 600 ml/day while expressing her breasts only twice per day. Thus both the duration of each expression session and the intervals between expression sessions have to be considered for an individual mother, with the object of maximizing the mother's production, but minimizing the number of minutes per day she needs to spend on milk expression. Further research is needed to identify the factors that lead to the best outcome for preterm mothers who are expressing their breast milk. However, in the absence of these data a calculation of the rate of milk production (ml/h) for a range of intervals between breast expression sessions should form the basis for advice for individual mothers.

Frequent milk expression will also help to minimize mammary engorgement, as the back-up pressure caused by mammary engorgement may make milk expression very difficult and painful. Unrelieved engorgement may also lead to milk stasis, which acts to downregulate milk volume. It is also important that women establish an abundant milk supply initially as this safeguards against either an inadequate milk supply or the decrease in milk production that often accompanies prolonged milk expression. Furthermore, frequent expression will ensure that a mother can meet the increased milk requirements of the baby as it grows.[3,6,23] Meier et al.[28] recommend that women should aim for a daily milk production of between 750 and 1000 ml/day at day 10, to ensure that they are still producing sufficient milk to facilitate infant demand at discharge. Some lactation specialists also advise that preterm mothers should imitate the growth spurt full-term healthy babies experience at approximately 2 weeks of age, by increasing the number of milk expression for several days.[29] This intervention may help to prevent the reduction in milk volume that frequently occurs 10–14 days after preterm delivery.

It is also important that the initial milk expression sessions are supervised to ensure that pump assembly and use are understood and that expression techniques are mastered. The relationship between the milk ejection reflex and milk removal should be explained.[30] It is crucial that a mother understands that when oxytocin is released, the myoepithelial cells surrounding the alveoli contract, and as milk flows into the ducts the ductal pressure rises. Oxytocin also reduces resistance to the outflow of milk from the alveoli, by shortening and widening the ducts, thus allowing removal of the milk by the vacuum applied by the breast pump. Unless the milk ejection reflex is triggered during milk expression, milk flow will be compromised, leading to a poor milk supply and declining production. If colostrum is being synthesized but not removed, this will be indicated diagnostically by the presence of lactose in maternal urine (see Chapter 4). Methods to elicit the milk ejection reflex include expressing in close proximity to the baby, breast and nipple massage, elongation of the nipple, olfactory and visual imagery and relaxation exercises.[31]

As stated, the technique of milk expression is also very important. Before positioning the milk collection set, women should be advised to sit comfortably with a straight back, and it may help to support the breast from underneath with fingers flat on the breast and the little finger at the junction of the breast and ribs. This will support the breast tissue forward into the breast shield, which should be placed with the nipple central. (When using double milk expression equipment, a mirror is useful to determine the breast shield position.) The breast shield should be held close enough to mammary tissue to obtain a patent seal, but not so firmly that the milk flow is inhibited. The milk ducts are easily compressed with light

pressure and therefore it is important not to force the rim of the breast shield into a section of the breast and obstruct drainage from the area.[30] Mothers should also be informed that it is essential to continue to express until milk flow ceases. The last few drops of milk are high in fat and contribute substantially to the energy value of milk. When a mother is not committed to long-term milk expression and does not wish to establish breastfeeding, the expression frequency should be tailored directly to the length of time she wishes to provide breast milk. It is important to warn against abruptly discontinuing milk expression since the preceding engorgement may precipitate mastitis. Furthermore, mothers should be advised against abruptly discontinuing milk expression if either mammary inflammation or pain develops, since frequent milk removal is crucial to the healing process.

Clinically, the fat and energy content of expressed milk can be estimated by a simple method referred to as a creamatocrit, which involves collecting a well-mixed sample of expressed breast milk in a capillary tube and spinning it in a centrifuge.[32,33] Using a published regression graph an estimate can be found of caloric content[32,33] (see Chapter 3: Table 3.4). If the caloric value is low it may be helpful to determine if the mother is restricting the length of time she is expressing. It is important to empty the breast completely to obtain both fore- and hindmilk.[34] Mothers should aim to achieve a creamatocrit between 6 and 8%. Women should be reassured that this is not a surveillance procedure, but simply a method to enable staff to pick up problems early and find solutions.

SUMMARY OF RECOMMENDATIONS

- Give realistic advice
- Minimize the time between delivery and first expression
- Demonstrate the principles and techniques of milk expression
- Teach pump assembly and use

> **Box 5.1 Case study – lacto-engineering**
>
> Case study
> Baby X was born at 28 weeks' gestation and received his mother's own expressed fresh breast milk from birth. Although the breast milk he received was fortified at 14 days, subsequent weight gain and growth were poor. His mother's milk yield was copious, and she was producing 500 ml/breast per expression. He was fed 3-hourly and his fluid requirements were 22 ml per feed. A sample was taken of fore-, mid- and hindmilk (at the beginning of a milk expression, after 200 ml had been expressed and from the last bottle expressed from each breast). The foremilk contained only 1.7 g/100 ml of fat (49 kcal/100 ml). A combination of mid- and hindmilk brought the value of fat up to 5.6 g/100 ml (89 kcal/100 ml). The volume fed to the baby was increased from 150 to 200 ml/kg. We continued to fortify the milk with breast-milk fortifier. His weight and growth improved dramatically and catch-up growth was achieved. His mother was very pleased that, with a simple nutritional intervention, her baby began to thrive on her milk.

- Maximize production (frequent pumping)
- Tailor long-term expression frequency to mammary storage capacity
- Carry out creamatocrit testing for quality control

KANGAROO MOTHER CARE

Neonatal units worldwide have been implementing kangaroo mother care (KMC).[35] In the UK, the term 'skin-to-skin holding' is more commonly used. Bergman & Jurisoo[35] argue that the worst-case scenario for any infant is separation from its mother. Infants commonly exhibit a 'protest despair' behavioural response, which can be demonstrated by a rise in glucocorticoids. KMC has been shown to reduce these levels markedly. During KMC the infant is clad only in a nappy and hat and is placed vertically on the skin between the breasts of the mother (Fig. 5.1). The infant is covered with a blanket and kept in this position for an extended period of time, usually no less than 30 min and sometimes for numerous hours.[35] A series of studies have been conducted in many countries demonstrating both the safety of KMC and its effectiveness in promoting physiological stability in preterm infants.[35–39]

Although the relationship between KMC and lactational outcome has not been studied as rigorously, breastfeeding duration appears

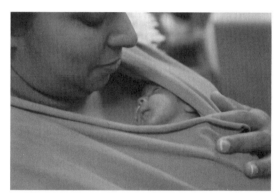

Figure 5.1   Kangaroo mother care (KMC).

to be longer for the KMC group than the controls.[36,37,40,41] Hurst et al.[37] evaluated the effects of skin-to-skin contact on maternal 24-h milk volume in mothers of preterm infants. Results showed that the average volume for the 24-h period was 499 ml in the experimental group, compared with 218 ml in the control group. For 2 weeks, the study group had a strong linear increase in milk volume, in contrast to no substantial change in the control group. The number of mothers who discontinued milk expression was similar in both groups. However, of the six who dropped out of the control group, all had low milk volumes (range 90–360 ml/day) at the time they stopped expressing. In contrast, the three mothers who dropped out of the KMC group had been able to provide their infants totally with expressed breast milk throughout their hospital stay. The results of this study should be replicated with a larger sample size, since the intervention is easy to achieve and inexpensive to implement.

A review of prospectively collected data on morbidity and diet in premature infants in Houston, Texas, showed that infants fed exclusively on fortified human milk had a significantly lower incidence of necrotizing enterocolitis (NEC), and sepsis, and fewer positive blood cultures than infants fed preterm formula or a mixture of fortified human milk and preterm formula.[42] The infants in the exclusively fortified human milk group had more episodes of KMC with their mothers than those fed preterm formula. Since one of the important protective effects of human milk on the recipient infant operates via the enteromammary immune system, KMC may be particularly important since mothers can be induced to make specific antibodies against the nosocomial pathogens in the neonatal environment. The researchers argue that the lower incidence of infection in the exclusively human milk group strongly suggests that KMC may be a means of providing species-specific antimicrobial protection for both term and premature infants. However, there is a need for a randomized controlled trial to assist in the development of a proper evidence base to test this assumption.

SUMMARY OF RECOMMENDATIONS

- The use of KMC will promote intimate skin-to-skin contact between infant and mother
- Encourage KMC to stimulate milk production
- Frequent KMC may trigger mammary antibody production

PROBLEMS

Too little milk

As discussed earlier, an insufficient milk supply can be an insurmountable problem for mothers dependent on milk expression to sustain lactation. When counselling a mother with lactation problems it is imperative to take a complete lactation history. It is important to try to persuade mothers not to focus solely on the volume of milk they express as this may lead to anxiety. Another angle is to encourage mothers to try to incorporate a wide range of strategies to elicit the milk ejection reflex such as instigating more frequent KMC and promoting expression in close proximity to the baby's cot. It is important to provide privacy when a mother expresses in an intensive care room, by the use of screens or positioning a mother so that she is facing the wall to ensure that she is not in full view of other parents and staff. Such interventions will sometimes work quickly: for example, the type of breast pump a mother uses can also determine how successfully milk is removed.

There are currently no published studies available to address the phenomenon of long-term expression for the mothers of preterm infants, and this is an area that urgently needs to be addressed. The clinical strategies that are currently in place focus primarily on the pharmacological enhancement of prolactin secretion. Prolactin is an important hormone for both the development of secretory alveoli and for the synthesis of milk proteins by the alveolar cells. Both metoclopramide and domperidone exert their pharmacologic effects through interactions with dopamine receptors, resulting in increased prolactin levels. Seema et al.[43] conducted a randomized controlled trial in which 50 mothers with partial or complete lactation failure were randomly assigned to two groups. Relactation was attempted in both the groups, with clinical support and repeated suckling. In addition group 1 mothers were given metoclopramide. The time of the first appearance of milk secretion and time of partial and complete relactation were comparable in both groups. Maternal factors such as nutrition, parity, feeding practices in previous babies, lactation gap and infants' initial refusal to suck at the breast did not influence the outcome as long as repeated suckling was ensured. It was concluded that galactagogues were not shown to offer any benefit.[43] This study was not placebo-controlled.

A randomized, double-blind, placebo-controlled trial was performed by da Silva et al.[44] to investigate the efficacy of domperidone in augmenting milk production in mothers of premature infants. Unlike metoclopramide, domperidone does not cross the blood-brain barrier and therefore does not have central nervous system side-effects.[45] Twenty patients were randomly assigned to receive either domperidone or placebo for 7 days. Breast milk was collected using a simultaneous (double) breast pump. Data from 16 patients were available for analysis. When compared with baseline values, the mean increase in milk volume represented 44.5% in the domperidone group and 16.6% in the placebo group. The serum prolactin levels were similar in both groups at baseline but by day 5 they were significantly higher in the domperidone group. Prolactin levels returned to baseline levels in both groups 3 days after the last dose of medication. The authors were unable to determine whether the increase in milk volume was sustained. However, the proportion of mothers discharged from hospital breastfeeding did not differ between the two groups. It was concluded that in the short term domperidone increases milk production in women with a low milk supply.[44]

Evidence based on clinical experience suggests that intervention with domperidone or metoclopramide is particularly effective in arresting the decline in milk production that can occur at days 10–14 postpartum in preterm mothers. Although the reasons for a diminishing milk supply are not clear, it is possible that some women may have abnormally low prolactin levels in the postpartum period and that stimulation of prolactin secretion may facilitate the initiation and establishment of lactation in these mothers.

There are several practical problems involving the use of both metoclopramide and domperidone. Currently, these medications are not licensed to augment lactation or for relactation (in the UK) and domperidone does not have approval from the US Food and Drug Administration for augmenting lactation. Another barrier is that an evidence-based protocol for drug timing and dosage in respect to metoclopramide has yet to be developed. Furthermore, most interventions for the stimulation of prolactin have been carried out without first assessing the mother's prolactin status. Measuring serum prolactin just before milk expression (basal prolactin level) and again 45 min after the commencement of breast expression (stimulated prolactin level) can determine if the mother's prolactin is in the normal range.[46] Intervention would only be expected to be beneficial if the mother has abnormal lactational prolactin levels before a galactagogue is prescribed.

However, the most contentious issue is that the role of prolactin in lactogenesis II is currently far from defined.[47] Since postpartum levels are similar in both breastfeeding and non-breastfeeding women, some mammary physiologists speculate that ineffective breast emptying in the immediate postpartum period may lead to high sodium concentrations in breast milk which may impede the cascade of physiological changes that bring about lactogenesis II.[47] The identification of chemical markers that appear to provide a new index for predicting which women are likely to have problems initiating lactogenesis II, is a breakthrough for the management of lactation following preterm delivery (see Chapter 4). The results of this study will help practitioners to identify which women are most at risk of lactation failure and to intervene early in their lactation management to maximize milk production.

Too much milk

Some mothers produce a vast quantity of milk, so much so that storage can sometimes create quite a dilemma. Mothers with an abundant supply must be encouraged to drain their breasts since they are particularly vulnerable to milk stasis and it is extremely important to warn mothers to observe for signs of mastitis such as tenderness and inflammation of the breast as well as flu-like systemic symptoms. Mothers with mastitis should be encouraged to carry on expressing on a regular basis, since the discontinuation of the removal of milk from the breast will only make the situation worse. During the early period of establishing breastfeeding, mothers may need to 'wean their milk supply down', so they do not remain dependent on milk expression in the postdischarge period. They can do this by decreasing the frequency of expression slowly. During this period it is essential to prevent unrelieved engorgement. Hand expression is useful to soften the breasts gently.

During the early period of introducing enteral feeds staff must be vigilant, particularly if mothers are utilizing multiple bottles to store milk in each expression session, since an infant could be fed exclusively on foremilk. As milk is removed from the breast the fat content increases so that the first milk removed has a low fat content and the milk removed when the breast is almost drained has a high fat content. The creamatocrit technique can also be very useful to determine breast emptying. Pale blue milk has a low fat content and indicates a full breast, whereas dense white milk has a high fat content and indicates that the breast has been drained of milk[48] (Fig. 5.2). Therefore, feeding foremilk is detrimental to the caloric value of the feed and will lead to poor infant growth (Box 5.1). Mothers with too much milk are perfect candidates for a hindmilk policy (see Chapter 3).

When a baby is establishing breastfeeding the issues of fore- and hindmilk become much less easily defined. Babies, when regulating their own intake, do not receive either fore- or hindmilk but a mixture between the two spectrums. Milk that has not been taken in one feed will remain in the mammary gland. Therefore, the feed may start with hindmilk rather than foremilk.[49] A poor understanding of the physiology of lactation has led to the terminology of 'foremilk and hindmilk' being used inappropriately when advising mothers of term healthy babies about relatively basic management problems. This is a problem that needs to be addressed. In particular, the variation in the composition of breast milk within and between mothers must be recognized and the fortification of breast milk for preterm babies should be evidence-based, that is, based on the measurement of the composition of the mother's breast milk (see Chapter 3).

Sore nipples

The primary culprit for sore nipples during milk expression is the use of a collection funnel (i.e. breast shield) that is too small. Milk collection sets should be measured to the size and shape of individual mothers, since women with either large or wide nipples may have difficulty with a set that has either a small opening or narrow slope[50] (Fig. 5.3). The ideal range is 68–82 mm outer diameter and 35–40 mm depth of flare.[50] Unless a collection set is used that fits the anatomical configuration of the breast, nipple tissue will rub against the sides of the tunnel, causing friction, leading to severe nipple excoriation and predisposing a mother to a risk of mastitis through bacterial invasion. Milk drainage may also be compromised, leading to maternal engorgement and a decrease in milk production.

Fore ←———————— ————————→ Hind

Full Breast   **Drained Breast**

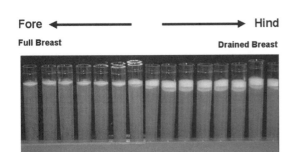

Figure 5.2   Increase in the fat content of breast milk in milk samples collected every 60 s during a 15-min breast expression with an electric breast pump.

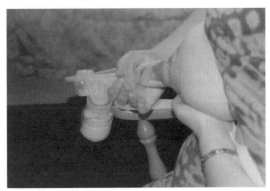

Figure 5.3   Large glass breast shield.

Another common cause of sore nipples is the use of excessive vacuum. Therefore, mothers should be advised to increase the vacuum slowly until the suction becomes slightly uncomfortable and then to decrease the vacuum by 10%. This will not affect milk output with hospital-grade breast pumps. Sometimes a mother using an electric breast pump that does not have a valve between the shield and the collection bottle will report that her nipples feel comfortable when she begins to express but start to feel painful as the session progresses. This is because the amount of negative pressure increases as the bottle fills with milk and thus adjustment of the vacuum during milk expression is required. When using an electric breast pump a mother should be advised to turn off the pump to release the vacuum before she removes the funnel from her breast. If nipple tissue is severely traumatized, it may be beneficial to encourage hand expression until healing occurs.

SUMMARY OF RECOMMENDATIONS

Too little milk
- Take a history to inform treatment
- Determine expression technique
- Check milk expression equipment
- Encourage techniques to elicit the milk ejection reflex
- Promote skin-to-skin contact
- Reassure, when possible
- Measure serum prolactin levels before prescribing galactagogues

Too much milk
- Relieve engorgement
- Encourage breast emptying
- Have a hindmilk policy (if appropriate) with creamatocrit monitoring

Sore nipples
- Match breast shield tunnel diameter to maternal nipple size and breast shape
- Centre nipple in breast shield
- Increase vacuum slowly until it feels uncomfortable and then decrease the suction by 10%

- Stop pump before removing the shield
- If trauma occurs, hand expression is helpful until healing occurs

METHODS

Hand expression

Mothers who are expressing their milk should be offered the opportunity to learn how to hand-express (Fig. 5.4). It is important to stimulate the milk ejection reflex before beginning to express by applying a warm flannel (washcloth) to the breasts and gentle breast and nipple massage.

The UK Royal College of Midwives[51] recommends the following method:

1. Advise the mother to adopt a comfortable upright position
2. Suggest that she places her little finger at the base of her breast, against her ribs, and spreads her other fingers slightly to support her breast. Her thumb will be on top
3. It is helpful to ensure that her first finger and thumb are opposite each other, making a C-shape around her breast
4. Suggest that she squeeze her thumb and first finger gently together, and hold the squeeze for a count of three, then release
5. She should keep her finger and thumb in the same position and continue to squeeze and release until she see drops of milk appearing at the nipple. It can take several minutes before this occurs
6. Sometimes it can be more effective to press the whole hand back and in towards the breast, just before applying pressure by squeezing

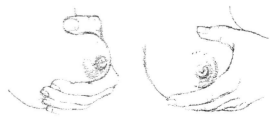

Figure 5.4   Hand expression. (Adapted from Royal College of Midwives.[51])

7. It is important to avoid sliding the thumb over the surface of the breast as any friction may damage the skin

8. When milk flow slows, the woman should rotate her hand slightly in order to drain a different section of the breast

9. When her fingers get tired, suggest that she change hands or breasts

10. Milk should be collected in a sterile, wide-mouthed container

Hand pumps

Manual breast pumps are those that are not automated in any way. There are currently three types on the market: bulb pumps (Fig. 5.5), cylinder pumps (Fig. 5.6) and trigger pumps (Fig. 5.7). A manual pump operated by a suction-creating bulb at one end should *never* be used for milk collection, as the bulb is not amenable to proper sterilization. Milk can enter the bulb during pumping and become contaminated with bacteria. This milk is not suitable for infant feeding.

Trigger pumps create a vacuum by using the trigger handle. Cylinder pumps consist of two cylinders and they create a vacuum when the mother pulls the outer cylinder down. Hand pumps produce less suction than automated pumps and can be useful to relieve engorgement and in cases where a mother needs to express infrequently. They should not be recommended for prolonged milk expression or if a mother has a history of repetitive strain injury. It is important that the vacuum applied

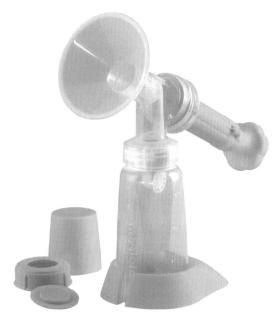

Figure 5.6   Cylinder pump.

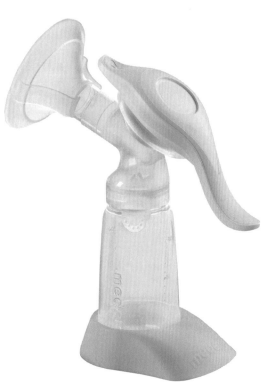

Figure 5.7   Trigger pump.

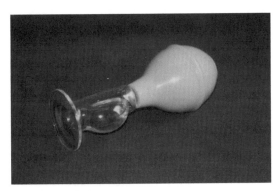

Figure 5.5   Bulb pump.

to the breast is released every 1–2 s, rather than waiting for a decrease in milk flow, as holding the vacuum for excessive periods of time will cause bruising of the breast tissue.

Electric pumps

The Human Milk Banking Association of North America[52] recommends that mothers use an electric breast pump when milk expression is required over a long period of time. In selecting an electric breast pump the following criteria should be met:

1. The pump must be easy to assemble
2. The pump should be fully automatic, with a cyclic suction rhythm that mimics infant suckling
3. Vacuum strength should not exceed 250 mmHg, and should be easily regulated
4. The drive and sucking system should be separate to ensure that no contamination from milk spillage can enter the pump
5. The pump selected should provide a system of collection that enables milk to be pumped directly into any storage container that utilizes a universal thread. This avoids the need to transfer collections from one container to another
6. All parts should be easy to wash by hand or in a dishwasher. The parts should be made of materials that will withstand cold sterilization methods, boiling and autoclaving

The principles regarding milk expression technique are the same, regardless of which breast pump is selected. Before use, women should be familiar with the manufacturers' instructions regarding assembly, cleaning and storage. Equipment must be sterilized before it is used to collect milk.

There is now considerable evidence to show that the use of an electric breast pump results in greater milk yield than other expression methods such as either hand expression or a manual breast pump,[53,54] and it is therefore the recommended method of milk expression.[24,25] Mitoulas et al.[55] found that the volume of milk removed over the first 5 min after milk ejection using a hospital-grade breast pump was not significantly different from the mean daily volume of milk consumed by the baby at a breastfeed from the same breast. Jones et al.[56] conducted a randomized controlled trial to compare sequential (single) and simultaneous (double) breast pumping on the volume of milk expressed and its energy content (Fig. 5.8). The secondary objective was to measure the effectiveness of breast massage on milk volume and fat content. The results were unequivocal and showed that simultaneous pumping (expressing both breasts simultaneously, i.e. double-pumping) was significantly more effective than sequential pumping and massaging before expressing was significantly more effective than non-massage in terms of the total milk volume obtained and the total fat in grams. Several studies have observed that double-pumping also reduces expression time and avoids milk loss from leakage from the other breast, which frequently occurs when only one breast is being pumped.[56–58] Double-pumping also elicits a greater prolactin response.[59]

Double-pumping can be difficult for mothers, since both hands are needed to hold the breast shields. This is particularly frustrating for a mother who is dependent on long-term exclusive expressing (such as a mother of a baby with Pierre Robin syndrome), since she will be unable to do anything else while she is expressing. A tailor-made halterneck bra that holds the breast shields in place will allow her to eat and drink or talk on the phone while she is expressing (Fig. 5.9). Many mothers have reported that they felt more relaxed while they

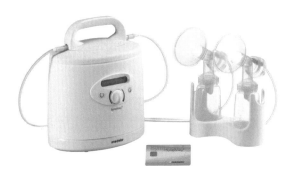

Figure 5.8   Double breast pump.

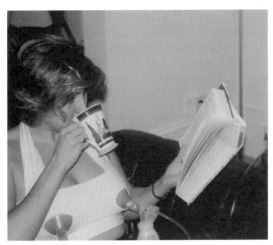

Figure 5.9   Double-pumping bra.

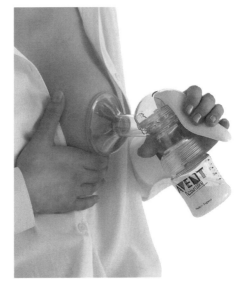

Figure 5.10   Study (manual) pump.

were expressing after utilizing the bra and that their milk supply increased (E Jones, personal communication 2004; see Resources). One mother reported that she was able to produce more milk than her son needed and could donate milk to her local milk bank.

Fewtrell et al.[60] compared the efficacy of expressing a single breast with either a standard electric pump or a manual pump (Fig. 5.10) during early lactation in preterm mothers, and reported that milk removal was more efficient with the manual pump. However, the average milk production in this study was about 200 ml/24 h and the mothers only pumped four times per 24 h. Thus, for mothers with higher milk productions, double pumping 6–8 times per 24 h using an electric breast pump offers considerable savings in the amount of time that mothers need to spend pumping each day.

It is of interest that Mitoulas et al.[61] used an experimental software-controlled electric breast pump to generate six different vacuum patterns varying from 20 to 55 cycles/min. The researchers found that the volume of milk removed from the breast over a 5-min pumping period varied between the patterns. In addition, differences in the profile of the vacuum curve resulted in significant differences in the comfort of breast expression. Since various models of electric breast pumps have different vacuum patterns, if a pump feels uncomfort-able, a mother should be encouraged to try an alternative pattern, as it may be more suitable for her. However, further research is required to maximize the efficiency of electric and manual breast pumps, particularly during the initiation of lactation in preterm mothers.

SUMMARY OF RECOMMENDATIONS

Hand expression
- All mothers should be taught hand expression

Hand pumps
- Bulb pumps should never be used for milk collection
- Hand pumps produce less suction than automated pumps
- Hand pumps should not be used on a long-term basis for mothers with a history of repetitive strain injury or for prolonged pumping
- Vacuum should be released every few seconds to prevent bruising of the breast tissue

Electric pumps
- Mothers dependent on long-term expression should use an electric breast pump

- Simultaneous (double) pumping reduces expression time
- Simultaneous pumping combined with breast massage improves milk volume and fat yield
- Differences in the vacuum pattern have resulted in significant differences in the comfort of breast expression

RELACTATION/INDUCED LACTATION

Even when mothers receive clinical support to sustain lactation following preterm delivery, some women find it very difficult to sustain a milk supply. However, breastfeeding can be re-established with maternal determination. The resumption of the production of breast milk without a further pregnancy is called 'relactation'.[62] There is evidence to suggest that many women who relactate can eventually produce enough milk to breastfeed an infant exclusively. 'Induced lactation' is defined as the means of establishing a milk supply in a mother who has never been pregnant.[62] The amount of milk produced is often inadequate for exclusive breastfeeding.

There are several important factors directly related to the infant and the mother which affect the success of relactation. One of the primary requirements is that the infant should suckle. The baby's willingness to suck is re-lated to infant age at the time of relactation, the time that has elapsed since the infant stopped breastfeeding and the infant's feeding experi-ence during the gap.[63,64] If the baby is of low birth weight, the length of time before the breast can be introduced also affects infant respon-siveness.[64] Seema et al.[43] found that if breastfeeding had been completely discontinued 74% of babies refused to suckle initially, mostly because of difficulties in correctly attaching to the breast. The use of a supplementary nursing system can be very helpful during this process to entice an infant to continue to suckle at the breast (see Chapter 10, Fig. 10.10). The pro-vision of skilled support and encouragement also appears to be a key prerequisite.

The key factors relating to maternal success are the mother's motivation and her lactation gap. Bose et al.[64] postulate that the likelihood of successful relactation and the rapidity of the onset of lactation correlate positively with a shorter postpartum interval. Mothers reached their maximum potential for milk production in varying periods of time (8–58 days). Auerbach & Avery[65] argue that if the production of milk is the sole goal for relactation, mothers are more likely to find difficulty in re-establishing an exclusive milk supply than if the primary importance of re-establishing breastfeeding is based on the mother-infant relationship. While exclusive breastfeeding is the ultimate goal, it is important to inform mothers that for babies some breast milk is better than no breast milk and that partial breastfeeding is a very worth-while outcome.[66]

The World Health Organization offers clear guidance for practice:[62]

- Provide counselling for the mother or adop-tive mother
- Assess the reason for the difficulty
- Stimulate the nipple by infant suckling, milk expression or KMC
- Provide a nutritional supplement (without using bottles)
- Observe changes in infant stooling (texture: soft, colour: yellow)[54]

After relactation has started:

- Put the infant to the breast 8–12 times in 24 h
- Encourage the infant to suckle on both breasts (for at least 10–15 min)
- Ensure attachment and positioning are correct
- Offer dietary supplements by cup

In cases where mothers have never previously lactated (adoption/surrogate mothers), prepara-tions of oestrogen, progesterone or hormonal contraceptives are sometimes used to mimic pregnancy and to stimulate breast development (induced lactation).[67,68] Milk production is ex-pected to start several days after the hormones are discontinued. Doses of chlorpromazine or metoclopramide or preferably domperidone are also given to act as prolactin enhancers. However no controlled studies have been ident-ified to guide this practice. Furthermore, it is unclear how effective the medications are on the initiation of lactation since infant suckling is actively encouraged.

Antipsychotics such as sulpiride have been evaluated, but significant amounts of the drug are secreted in milk, with possible adverse effects on the infant.[62] A variety of galactogogues such as brewer's yeast, herbal teas and warm cereal drinks have been used by relactating mothers. Few have been evaluated scientifically. Alcohol, particularly beer, is also recommended for increasing milk production by raising prolactin levels. However, one trial has shown that consumption of alcohol reduced the infant's intake of breast milk at the following feed.[69] Finally, another natural product, fenugreek, has been purported to be effective in anecdotal reports. Gaby[70] suggests that the use of this agent may be warranted after considering risks versus benefits.

In conclusion, Biancuzzo[71] suggests that the closeness of the mother–infant relationship is, in itself, a measure of success for either relactation or induced lactation. However, she argues that some physiologic outcomes are also important. She warns that is important to be aware that the extent to which women can either completely or partially lactate varies considerably, and that infant dehydration and failure to thrive are very real possibilities.[71] Despite strong maternal motivation and a good support network, it is unwise to assume that all babies will receive adequate nutrition without supplementation. There are currently few studies to address breastfeeding problems such as insufficient milk, relactation and in-duced lactation. The studies that currently exist are small and some have serious methodological flaws. A co-ordinated programme of work is urgently needed to address the inter-related physical, psychological, professional, social and cultural issues that encompass this issue.[72] Until this can be undertaken there is very little robust evidence to guide practice.

SUMMARY OF RECOMMENDATIONS

Commencing relactation
- Take a history
- Provide counselling and ongoing skilled support
- Stimulate of the nipple by infant suckling, milk expression and skin-to-skin contact
- Ensure attachment and positioning are correct
- Use a supplementary nursing system to encourage the baby to suckle for longer periods at the mother's breast
- Provide a nutritional supplement, if necessary, after a breastfeed (without using bottles)
- Observe changes in infant stooling (texture and colour)

After relactation has started
- Put infant to the breast 8–12 times in 24 h
- Encourage the infant to suckle on both breasts (for at least 10–15 min)
- Ensure attachment and positioning are correct
- Offer dietary supplements by cup
- Monitor weight, length and head circumference

References

1. Mathur NB, Dwarkadas AM, Sharma VK et al. Anti-infective factors in preterm human colostrum. Acta Paediatr Scand 1990; 79:1039–1044.
2. Kavanaugh K, Meier P, Zimmermann B et al. The rewards outweigh the efforts: breastfeeding outcomes for mothers of preterm infants. J Hum Lact 1997;13:15–21.
3. Neifert M, Seacat J. Practical aspects of breastfeeding the premature infant. Perin Neonatol 1988; 12: 24–30.
4. Meier P, Brown L. State of the science: breastfeeding for mothers and low birth weight infants. Nurs Clin North Am 1996; 31:351–365.
5. Cregan M, De Mello T, Hartmann PE. Initiation of lactation in women after preterm delivery. Acta Obstet Gynecol Scand 2002; 81:870–877.
6. Hill P, Brown L, Harker T. Initiation and frequency of breast expression in breastfeeding mothers of LBW and VLBW infants. Nurs Res 1995; 44:352–355.
7. Newton M, Newton NR. The let-down reflex in human lactation. J Pediatr 1945; 33:698–704.
8. Kulski JK, Hartmann PE, Martin JD et al. Effects of bromocriptine mesylate on the composition of the mammary secretion in non-breastfeeding women. Obstet Gynaecol 1978; 52:38–42.

9. DeCarvalho M, Robertson S, Merkatz R et al. Milk intake and frequency of feeding in breast fed infants. Early Hum Dev 1982; 72:155–163.

10. Kaufman K, Hall L. Influences of the social network on choice and duration of breastfeeding in mothers of preterm infants. Res Nurs Health 1989; 12:149–159.

11. Hill PD, Ledbetter RJ, Kavanaugh KL. breastfeeding patterns of low birthweight infants after hospital discharge. J Obstet Gynecol Neonatal Nurs 1997; 26:189–197.

12. Nyqvist KH, Ewaald U. Successful breastfeeding in spite of early mother-baby separation for neonatal care. Midwifery 1997; 13:24–31.

13. Furman L, Minich N, Hack M. Correlates of lactation in mothers of very low birth weight infants. Pediatrics 2002;109:e57.

14. Boo NY, Goh ES. Predictors of breastfeeding in very low birth weight infants at the time of discharge from hospital. J Trop Ped 1999; 45:195–201.

15. http://www.nhmrc.gov.au/publications/synopses/dietsyn.htm. (Australian Government National Health & Research Council)

16. Pantazi M, Jaeger M, Lawson M. Staff support for mothers to provide breast milk in pediatric hospital and neonatal units. J Hum Lact 1998; 14:291–296.

17. Garcia J, Redshaw M, Fitzsimmons B et al. First class delivery: a national survey of women's views of maternity care. London: Audit Commission; 1998.

18. Dodds R. Supporting breastfeeding of babies in neonatal units. Pract Midwife 1999; 2:23–27.

19. Gready M, Newburn M, Dodds R et al. Birth choices – women's expectations and experiences. London: National Childbirth Trust; 1995.

20. Ingram J, Redshaw M, Harris A. breastfeeding in neonatal care. Br J Midwifery 1994; 2:412–418.

21. Hopkinson J, Schanler M, Garza C. Milk production by mothers of premature infants. Pediatrivs 1988; 81:815–820.

22. Hill P, Aldag J, Chatterton R. Initiation and frequency of pumping and milk production in mothers of non-nursing preterm infants. J Hum Lact 2001; 17:9–13.

23. Neville M, Morton J, Umemura S. Lactogenesis. The transition from pregnancy to lactation. Pediatr Clin North Am 2001; 48:35–52.

24. Meier PP, Engstrom JL, Mangurten HH et al. breastfeeding support services in a neonatal intensive care unit. J Obstet Gynecol Neonatal Nurs 1993; 22:338–347.

25. Schanler RJ, Hurst NM, Lau C. The use of human milk and breastfeeding in premature infants. Clin Perinatol 1999; 26:379–398.

26. Daly SEG, Owens RA, Hartmann PE. The short-term synthesis and infant-regulated removal of milk in lactating women. Exp Physiol 1993; 78:209–220.

27. Daly SE, Kent JC, Huyuh DQ et al. The determination of short-term breast volume changes and the rate of synthesis of human milk using a computerized breast measurement. Exp Physiol 1992; 77:79–87.

28. Meier P, Brown L, Hurst N. breastfeeding the preterm infant. In: Riordan J, Auerbach K, eds. breastfeeding and human lactation, 2nd edn. Boston, MA: Jones and Bartlett; 1998:449–481.

29. La Leche League International. Prematurity. In: La Leche, the breastfeeding answer book, 3rd edn. Schaumburg; IL: 2002:279–326.

30. Ramsay DR, Kent JC, Owen RA et al. Ultrasound imaging of milk ejection in the breast of lactating women. Pediatrics 2003; 113:361–367.

31. Biancuzzo M. breastfeeding the newborn. Clinical strategies for nurses, 2nd edn. St Louis, MO: Mosby; 2003:169.

32. Lucas A, Gibbs JA, Lyster RL. Creamatocrit: simple technique for estimating fat concentration and energy value in milk. Br Med J 1978; 1:1018.

33. Lemons JA, Schreiner RL, Gresham EL. Simple method for determining the caloric and fat content of human milk. Pediatrics 1980; 66:626.

34. Griffin TL, Meier PP, Bradford LP et al. Mothers performing creamatocrit measures in the NICU: accuracy, reactions and cost. J Obstet Neonatal Nurs 2000; 29:249–257.

35. Bergman NJ, Jurisoo LA. The 'kangaroo method' for treating low birth weight babies in a developing country. Trop Doc 1994; 24:57–60.

36. Charpak N, Ruiz-Pelaez JG, Figueroa de CZ et al. A randomized, controlled trial of kangaroo mother care: results of follow-up at 1 year of corrected age. Pediatrics 2001;108:1072–1079.

37. Hurst NM, Valentine CJ, Renfro L et al. Skin-to-skin holding in the neonatal intensive care unit influences maternal milk volume. J Perinatol 1997; 17:213–217.

38. Hofer MA. Early relationships as regulators of infant physiology and behaviour. Acta Paediatr 1994; 397 (suppl.):47–56.

39. Whitelaw A, Heisterkamp G, Sleath K et al. Skin to skin contact for very low birth-weight infants and their mothers. Arch Dis Child 1988; 63;1377–1380.

40. Anderson GC. Current knowledge about skin-to-skin (kangaroo) care for preterm infants. J Perinatol 1991; 11:216-226.

41. Ludhington-Hoe S, Swinth JY. Developmental aspects of kangaroo care. J Obstet Gynecol Neonatal Nurs 1997; 25:691–703.

42. Schanler RJ, Oh W. Fortified human milk improves the health of the premature infant. Pediatr Res 1996; 40:551A.

43. Seema, Patwari AK, Satyanarayana L. Relactation: an effective intervention to promote exclusive breastfeeding. J Trop Pediatr 1997; 43:213–216.

44. da Silva OP, Knoppert DC, Angelini MM et al. Effect of domperidone on milk production in mothers of premature newborns: a randomized, double-blind placebo-controlled trial. Canadian Med Ass J 2001; 164:17–21.

45 Hales TW. Medication and mother's milk, 10th edn. Amarillo, TX: Pharmasoft; 2002:230–232.

46. Cox DB, Owens RA, Hartmann PE. Blood and milk prolactin and the rate of milk synthesis in women. Exp Physiol 1996; 81:1007–1020.

47. Neville M, Morton J, Umemura S. The transition from pregnancy to lactation. Pediatr Clin North Am 2001; 48:35–52.

48. Daly EEJ, Di Rosso A, Owens RA et al. Degree of breast emptying explains changes in fat content, but not fatty acid composition of human milk. Exp Physiol 1993; 78:741–755.

49. Gunther M. Infant feeding. London: Methuen; 1970:98.

50. Johnson CA. An evaluation of breast pumps currently available on the American market. Clin Pediatr (Phila) 1983; 22:40 45.

51. Royal College of Midwives. Successful breastfeeding, 3rd edn. Edinburgh: Churchill Livingstone; 2002:102–103.

52. Arnold L. Recommendations for collection, storage and handling of a mother's milk for her own infant in a hospital setting, 3rd edn. Sandwich, MA: Human Milk Banking Association of North America; 1999.

53. Garza C, Johnson CA, Harrist R et al. Effects of methods of collection and storage on nutrients in human milk. Early Hum Dev 1982; 6:295–303.

54. Paul VK, Singh M, Deorari AK et al. Manual and pump methods of expression of breast milk. Ind J Pediatr 1996; 63:87–92.

55. Mitoulas LR, Lai CT, Gurrin LC et al. Efficacy of breast milk expression using an electric breast pump. J Hum Lact 2002; 18:344–352.

56. Jones E, Dimmock PW, Spencer SA. A randomised controlled trial to compare methods of milk expression following preterm delivery. Arch Dis Child Fetal Neonatal 2001; 85:F91–F95.

57. Hill PD, Aldag JC, Chatterton RT. Effects of pumping style on milk production of mothers of non-nursing preterm infants. J Hum Lact 1999; 15:209–216.

58. Auerbach KG. Sequential and simultaneous breast pumping: a comparison. Int J Nurs Stud 1990; 27:257–265.

59. Zinaman MJ, Hughes V, Queenan JT. Acute prolactin and oxytocin responses and milk yield to infant suckling and artificial methods of expression in lactating women. Pediatrics 1992; 89:437–440.

60. Fewtrell MS, Lucas P, Collier S et al. Randomized trial comparing the efficacy of a novel manual breast pump with a standard electric breast pump in mothers who delivered preterm infants. Pediatrics 2001; 107:1291–1297.

61. Mitoulas LR, Lai CT, Gurrin LC et al. Effect of vacuum profile on breast milk expression using an electric breast pump. J Hum Lact 2002; 18:353–360.

62. Relactation: a review of experience and recommendations for practice. Geneva: World Health Organization; 1998.

63. Auerbach KG, Avery JL. Induced lactation. A study of adoptive nursing by 240 women. Am J Dis Child 1981; 135:340–343.

64. Bose CL, D'Ercole AJ, Lester AG et al. Relactation by mothers of sick and premature infants. Pediatrics 1981; 67:565–569.

65. Auerbach KG, Avery JL. Relactation: a study of 366 cases. Paediatrics 1980; 65:236–242.

66. Howie PW, Forsyth JS, Ogston SA et al. Protective effect of breastfeeding against infection. Br Med J 1990; 300:11–16.

67. Nemba K. Induced lactation: a study of 37 non-puerperal mothers. J Trop Pediatr 1994; 40:240–242.

68. Adoptive Nursing Resource Website. Available online at: http://www.fourfriends.com.abrw/.

69. Menella JA, Beauchamp GK. The transfer of alcohol to human milk. N Engl J Med 1991; 325:981–985.

70. Gaby MP. Galactogogues: medications that induce lactation. J Hum Lact 2002; 18:274–279.

71. Biancuzzo M. Successful milk production and transfer. In: Biancuzzo M, ed. breastfeeding the newborn: clinical strategies for nurses, 2nd edn. St Louis, MO: Mosby; 2003 :175–177.

72. Renfrew M, Woolridge M, Ross McGill H. Enabling women to breastfeed. London: Stationery Office; 2000:72.

Chapter 6

Human milk banking

Gillian Weaver

A human milk bank collects, screens, stores, processes and distributes donated breast milk.

INTRODUCTION

For a variety of reasons, not all babies on a neonatal unit (NNU) are able to receive their own mother's expressed breast milk. This may be because of the mother's own health problems, the location, if separated geographically from her baby or her inability to establish or maintain lactation for reasons of stress or anxiety.

When the mother's own breast milk (maternal expressed breast milk or MEBM) is unavailable, the clinicians are faced with the choice of delaying or stopping enteral feeds, using formula milk or offering donor breast milk (DEBM). If DEBM is the enteral feed of choice, it should always be obtained from a human milk bank that is known to adhere to nationally accepted and accredited guidelines.

HISTORY

Milk banking began in a formalized way in Vienna in 1909 with the opening of the first human milk bank. Ten years later a second bank opened in Boston, Massachusetts, USA and this became the model for milk banks in other American cities, including Chicago, New York and Los Angeles. The Dionne quintuplets, born in Quebec, Canada, in the 1930s, received almost 250 litres of breast milk from donors in North America and Canada.[1]

The first milk bank in the UK was established at Queen Charlotte's Hospital in West London following the use of DEBM to feed a set of quadruplets. The St Neot's quads, born in 1935, became the first set of quads to survive in the UK and this in turn led to charitable funds being used to develop a milk-banking facility that could provide DEBM for other infants. The Queen Charlotte's Hospital Milk Bureau was officially opened in 1939, after which DEBM was regularly sent to London from Cardiff and other centres and the processed milk was used to feed babies as far afield as Edinburgh. The methods of heat treatment and standards adopted were similar to those used in the milk bank in Boston in the USA.[2]

Following the Second World War, several hospitals followed the lead of Queen Charlotte's and breast milk banks were established in other centres in the UK, starting with Cardiff and followed by Birmingham and Bristol. The subsequent decades saw the popularity of milk banking follow the patterns of breastfeeding, with the largest growth in numbers during the 1970s and early 1980s. However in the mid 1980s the discovery that human immunodeficiency virus (HIV) could be transmitted via breast milk brought milk banks under threat of closure. The Department of Health and Social Security, in two letters sent to all doctors and nursing officers in England in 1988[3] and 1989,[4] decreed that all donors should be screened for HIV and all DEBM should be pasteurized. At the time, not every milk bank routinely pasteurized all donor milk and it was also felt that women would be reluctant to volunteer to be tested for HIV infection. In addition, new artificial milks designed for feeding preterm infants were being increasingly used on NNUs, substantially reducing the demand for DEBM. The net result was a dramatic drop in the numbers of milk banks in the UK from approximately 70 in the early 1980s to six by 1990. This trend was mirrored throughout Europe and North America. However, since then, numbers in the UK have increased steadily. This has been due to the ready acceptance of serology tests by prospec-

tive donors, the publication of research providing evidence for the benefits of human milk for preterm infants[5] and the support available from the UK Association for Milk Banking (UKAMB).[6] The UKAMB is a charity, formed in 1997, to promote milk banking as well as to set standards and to review guidelines regularly.

LOCATION OF MILK BANKS

The UK

There are 17 established milk banks in the UK, with several others in the planning stage (see Fig. 6.1). However there are still large areas with none, including the whole of Wales, the south-west of England and much of the northeast and Scotland. Furthermore, most milk banks in the UK are funded to supply the NNU in their own hospital or NHS trust and are only able to offer donor milk to other hospitals if they have a surplus. Staffing and budget limitations preclude some milk banks from routinely providing milk to other units. In response to this and the growing awareness of the benefits of donor milk, hospitals are once again starting their own milk banks.

The milk bank in Irvinestown in Northern Ireland came about in part as the result of the inability of a paediatrician to obtain DEBM for a sick baby from milk banks in England. Subsequently the recognition of the need for a milk bank in the province was incorporated into a document published by the Breast-feeding Strategy Group for Northern Ireland.[7] Within 2 years the milk bank was operating to a very high level of effectiveness and supplying DEBM to hospitals throughout Northern Ireland as well as to some south of the border. Very importantly, every hospital with an NNU in Northern Ireland is able to accept donations of milk for the bank.

The existence of satellite milk banks is also on the increase on the UK mainland. Satellite banks are able to recruit donors and store the frozen donations. The milk is then transported to the main centre for processing. Formalized arrangements for this are in their infancy but it

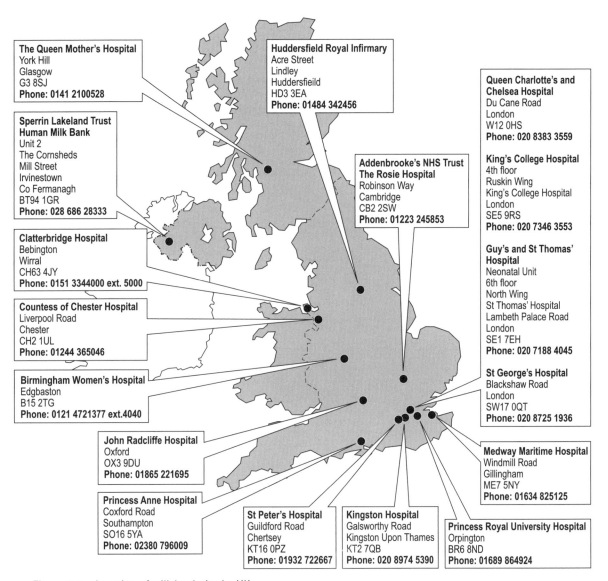

The Queen Mother's Hospital
York Hill
Glasgow
G3 8SJ
Phone: 0141 2100528

Huddersfield Royal Infirmary
Acre Street
Lindley
Huddersfield
HD3 3EA
Phone: 01484 342456

Queen Charlotte's and Chelsea Hospital
Du Cane Road
London
W12 0HS
Phone: 020 8383 3559

Sperrin Lakeland Trust Human Milk Bank
Unit 2
The Cornsheds
Mill Street
Irvinestown
Co Fermanagh
BT94 1GR
Phone: 028 686 28333

Addenbrooke's NHS Trust The Rosie Hospital
Robinson Way
Cambridge
CB2 2SW
Phone: 01223 245853

King's College Hospital
4th floor
Ruskin Wing
King's College Hospital
London
SE5 9RS
Phone: 020 7346 3553

Clatterbridge Hospital
Bebington
Wirral
CH63 4JY
Phone: 0151 3344000 ext. 5000

Guy's and St Thomas' Hospital
Neonatal Unit
6th floor
North Wing
St Thomas' Hospital
Lambeth Palace Road
London
SE1 7EH
Phone: 020 7188 4045

Countess of Chester Hospital
Liverpool Road
Chester
CH2 1UL
Phone: 01244 365046

Birmingham Women's Hospital
Edgbaston
B15 2TG
Phone: 0121 4721377 ext.4040

St George's Hospital
Blackshaw Road
London
SW17 0QT
Phone: 020 8725 1936

John Radcliffe Hospital
Oxford
OX3 9DU
Phone: 01865 221695

Medway Maritime Hospital
Windmill Road
Gillingham
ME7 5NY
Phone: 01634 825125

Princess Anne Hospital
Coxford Road
Southampton
SO16 5YA
Phone: 02380 796009

St Peter's Hospital
Guildford Road
Chertsey
KT16 0PZ
Phone: 01932 722667

Kingston Hospital
Galsworthy Road
Kingston Upon Thames
KT2 7QB
Phone: 020 8974 5390

Princess Royal University Hospital
Orpington
BR6 8ND
Phone: 01689 864924

Figure 6.1   Location of milk banks in the UK.

is a step towards the establishment of regional centres. The overall picture remains one in which there exists a widespread inequality of access to DEBM that is not reflected elsewhere within the provision of the UK's nationalized health services.

North America

In North America, the number of milk banks has remained comparatively low and static since the late 1980s, although some of the US banks collect, process and supply very large volumes of milk. The Mothers' Milk Bank in Denver, Colorado, regularly processes over 3000 litres of DEBM per year. This is 6–8 times the volumes processed in the largest UK milk banks and as much as all the UK banks combined. Currently there are six milk banks in the USA and one in Canada (see Fig. 6.2).

In the USA, whilst there are many similarities, most milk banks operate on a fundamentally

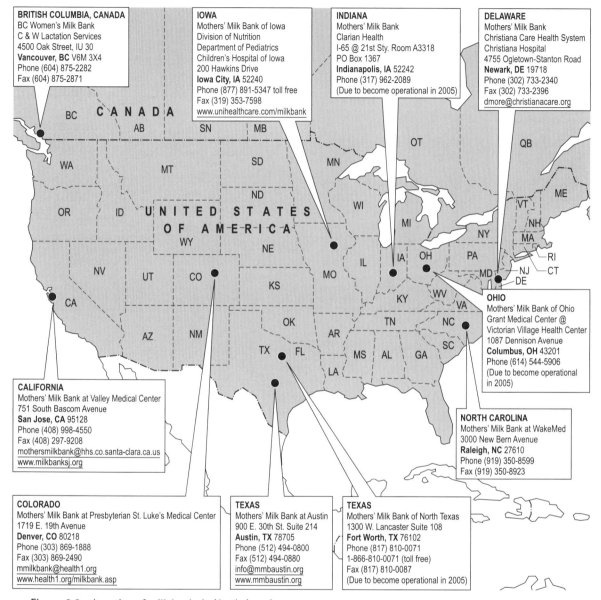

BRITISH COLUMBIA, CANADA
BC Women's Milk Bank
C & W Lactation Services
4500 Oak Street, IU 30
Vancouver, BC V6M 3X4
Phone (604) 875-2282
Fax (604) 875-2871

IOWA
Mothers' Milk Bank of Iowa
Division of Nutrition
Department of Pediatrics
Children's Hospital of Iowa
200 Hawkins Drive
Iowa City, IA 52240
Phone (877) 891-5347 toll free
Fax (319) 353-7598
www.unihealthcare.com/milkbank

INDIANA
Mothers' Milk Bank
Clarian Health
I-65 @ 21st Sty. Room A3318
PO Box 1367
Indianapolis, IA 52242
Phone (317) 962-2089
(Due to become operational in 2005)

DELAWARE
Mothers' Milk Bank
Christiana Care Health System
Christiana Hospital
4755 Ogletown-Stanton Road
Newark, DE 19718
Phone (302) 733-2340
Fax (302) 733-2396
dmore@christianacare.org

OHIO
Mothers' Milk Bank of Ohio
Grant Medical Center @
Victorian Village Health Center
1087 Dennison Avenue
Columbus, OH 43201
Phone (614) 544-5906
(Due to become operational in 2005)

CALIFORNIA
Mothers' Milk Bank at Valley Medical Center
751 South Bascom Avenue
San Jose, CA 95128
Phone (408) 998-4550
Fax (408) 297-9208
mothersmilkbank@hhs.co.santa-clara.ca.us
www.milkbanksj.org

NORTH CAROLINA
Mothers' Milk Bank at WakeMed
3000 New Bern Avenue
Raleigh, NC 27610
Phone (919) 350-8599
Fax (919) 350-8923

COLORADO
Mothers' Milk Bank at Presbyterian St. Luke's Medical Center
1719 E. 19th Avenue
Denver, CO 80218
Phone (303) 869-1888
Fax (303) 869-2490
mmilkbank@health1.org
www.health1.org/milkbank.asp

TEXAS
Mothers' Milk Bank at Austin
900 E. 30th St. Suite 214
Austin, TX 78705
Phone (512) 494-0800
Fax (512) 494-0880
info@mmbaustin.org
www.mmbaustin.org

TEXAS
Mothers' Milk Bank of North Texas
1300 W. Lancaster Suite 108
Fort Worth, TX 76102
Phone (817) 810-0071
1-866-810-0071 (toll free)
Fax (817) 810-0087
(Due to become operational in 2005)

Figure 6.2   Location of milk banks in North America.

different basis from those in the UK. Far from being a local service, most of the US banks recruit donors from a much larger geographical area (often over several states) and supply DEBM irrespective of the location of the recipient. Older babies and those with formula intolerance are more likely to be fed donor milk than in the UK. Health insurance companies in the USA usually pay for the DEBM.

A global perspective

Overall, on a global basis, milk banking is increasing. In recent years, some countries have established their first milk banks (Spain, South Africa), some are increasing the numbers of milk banks annually (UK, Brazil), some continue to work towards their first milk bank (Australia) but a few have struggled to maintain the milk banks they have (Canada, France). The country with the most milk banks is Brazil where a national association underpins a flourishing system of staff training and uniformity of practice. Other South American countries have used the Brazilian model when starting up their own milk banks.

Most European countries have milk banks, although the numbers vary considerably, with Scandinavia, France and Germany having far more than Spain and Italy. Milk banks are also well established in India and China. Protocols vary between countries and as yet there are no international moves to standardize practices.

THE SCALE OF HUMAN MILK BANKING

The size of milk banks both in the UK and overseas differs widely in terms of staffing levels, number of donors recruited and volume of milk processed and supplied. There is no such thing as the average milk bank and no individual model for their organization and operation. However the overall picture seems to be one of growth.

As shown in Figures 6.3 and 6.4, both the number of donors and the volume of DEBM have increased in recent years in the UK.

In part, the rise is accounted for by the greater number of banks; however some individual milk banks have also seen growth in the numbers of donors recruited and subsequent volumes of milk donated.

WHY USE DONOR BREAST MILK? (SEE CHAPTERS 1 AND 3)

There are several established short-term benefits and some long-term benefits associated with the use of donor milk. The short-term benefits include the earlier tolerance of enteral feeds[8] and

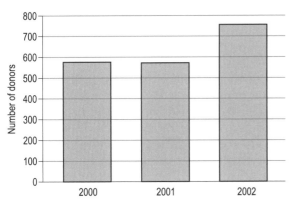

Figure 6.3 Numbers of donors to UK milk banks, 2000–2002.

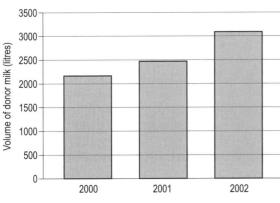

Figure 6.4 Volumes of donor breast milk collected (litres) 2000–2002.

the reduced risk of infection[9] and necrotizing enterocolitis (NEC).[10] In the longer term, lower diastolic blood pressure[11] and a reduced risk of insulin resistance in later childhood[12] have been suggested.

However the published evidence for these benefits is sometimes sparse; it rarely reflects current practice in milk banks and on NNUs or it is not universally accepted as being relevant to the developed world. Widely divergent opinions are held within paediatric circles and attitudes to the use of DEBM reflect this. Comments like: 'I do not believe there is any place for donor milk in developed countries' and 'DEBM is an invaluable resource for NNUs, enabling the early introduction of enteral nutrition and conveying immunological benefits in the absence of the mother's breast milk' demonstrate the polarization of opinion.

In practice in the UK, DEBM is most commonly provided for preterm infants in NNUs in the absence of the mother's own breast milk. Those weighing less than 1800 g, particularly with a history of intrauterine growth restriction, are likely to be prioritized. An antenatal history that has included a consistently absent or reversed end-diastolic flow will also ensure high priority for DEBM as these infants are at increased risk of developing NEC. A meta-analysis[13] published in 2003 concluded that feeding DEBM rather than preterm formula may reduce the risk of NEC. Donor milk is also often the enteral feed of choice where a diagnosis of NEC has been previously made, particularly if surgical intervention was required, and requests to the Queen Charlotte's Hospital Milk Bank from other hospitals reflect this.

The cost benefits inherent in the use of DEBM are largely hidden because of its protective nature. Bisquera et al.,[14] working in the USA, calculated the additional length of hospital stay involved when an infant develops NEC. When translated into costs to the UK health service, these figures can easily amount to £40 000 per baby. If the benefits of DEBM were only measured in respect to the incidence of NEC, its provision would still prove to be cost-effective. Similarly, there are major cost benefits associated with the earlier tolerance of

enteral feeds as this is directly associated with length of stay on the NNU.

As previously discussed, the birth of a preterm baby is a stressful experience for the mother. When twins, triplets and higher-order multiples are born in hospitals with milk banks, they are often the recipients of DEBM. Not only does the mother have several babies to worry about, they will also need two or three times the daily volume compared to a singleton.

DEBM is not widely used for feeding infants following gut surgery; however, where there is insufficient MEBM it is likely to be the enteral feed of choice on units with regular and easy access to donor milk. Published evidence for the benefits of donor milk in these situations is lacking and randomized trials have not been undertaken.

Undoubtedly, a paradox exists when looking for clinical justification for the provision of DEBM. Evidence-based recommendations derived from systematic reviews of the research literature are seemingly required to justify the establishment of regional milk banks capable of supplying all infants who might benefit from DEBM. However, without a network of well-established banks it would be difficult to supply the volumes of donor milk that would be required for such trials. It would also raise ethical concerns if infants were to be randomized to receive DEBM or a formula milk on NNUs where DEBM was currently the preferred enteral feed choice in the absence of the mother's own milk. Anecdotal evidence abounds and there is no shortage of unpublished case histories that provide testimony to the benefits – and in some cases life-saving attributes – of DEBM. There is still little published work providing statistically significant evidence in favour of the use of DEBM. However, the non-significance of the results of trials undertaken without the dual benefits of modern pasteurization equipment and the improved suitability of DEBM as currently available from most milk banks should not be interpreted as providing evidence of a lack of benefit. Absence of evidence is not evidence of absence. DEBM is mostly used as the means to initiate enteral feeds and it is often used in addition to a mother's own milk. It rarely provides the sole source of enteral nutrition. Only occasionally is DEBM the single long-term source of enteral nutrition and so it does not easily lend itself to studies that would require randomization to either DEBM or preterm formula.

Despite a similar lack of evidence in favour of the use of DEBM for older children and for adults, a wide range of uses of donor milk has been recorded from some UK and US milk banks (Boxes 6.1 and 6.2).

When the numbers of babies receiving DEBM from the Queen Charlotte's Hospital Milk Bank were analysed in terms of the total days that infants received DEBM, 43% of the recipients received it for 3 days or less, with 27% receiving it for more than 1 week. DEBM is primarily used during the establishment of enteral feeds and is often no longer required once the mother's own milk comes in at around day 3 or 4. The babies that received the DEBM long-term were largely infants that were recovering from NEC and whose own mothers had been unsuccessful in maintaining their lactation for more than a few weeks.

In some countries, for example Denmark and Brazil, babies born to HIV-positive mothers are fed with DEBM. In Durban, South Africa, a milk bank has been set up to provide donor milk for babies who have been orphaned or abandoned as a result of HIV and acquired immunodeficiency syndrome (AIDS). The establishment of the milk bank was the idea of Professor Anna Coutsoudis and was partly funded by the United Nations Children's Emergency Fund (UNICEF). The Ithembalethu Milk Bank (translates to 'I have a destiny') has quickly led to plans for other similar milk banks in Cape Town and Johannesburg.

Box 6.1   Additional recorded uses for donor breast milk in the UK

- Hirschsprung's disease
- Baby born to ventilated mother or mother too ill to express
- Term babies with renal problems
- Term babies where there is a temporary need (e.g. phototherapy)
- Term babies of diabetic mothers establishing feeds
- Short gut syndrome
- Gastroschisis
- Ulcerative colitis (adult)

Box 6.2   Additional recorded uses for donor breast milk in the USA

- Allergies
- Feeding/formula intolerance
- Immunologic deficiencies
- Postoperative nutrition
- Infectious diseases
- Inborn errors of metabolism
- Liver transplant (adult)
- Cancer (adults)
- Adoptees
- Surrogate infants

GUIDELINES

Comprehensive, authoritative donor milk-banking guidelines have been available in the UK since 1994.[15–17] The first and second editions were published by the Royal College of Paediatrics and Child Health (RCPCH) or its predecessor, the British Paediatric Association. The third edition is evidence-based and the evidence is graded in accordance with the Scottish Intercollegiate Guideline Network (SIGN). It was published in September 2003 by the UKAMB and has been endorsed by the RCPCH. This latest edition[17] includes a section on the justification for the use of DEBM together with recommendations for donor recruitment and selection, donor serology screening, microbiological testing (both pre- and postpasteurization), heat treatment of the milk and record-keeping.

In the USA, the Human Milk Banking Association of North America (HMBANA)[1] publishes *Guidelines for the Establishment and*

Operation of a Donor Human Milk Bank, a document that is reviewed annually.

DONOR RECRUITMENT, SELECTION AND SCREENING

There are two main groups of potential breast milk donors. The first group includes any healthy breast-feeding mother whose baby is thriving and who is willing to express milk for the milk bank on a regular basis. The second group contains those mothers who have already stored their own milk at home or in a hospital freezer for their baby. Every woman who is donating breast milk to the bank is carefully screened and must meet the strict selection criteria laid down in the local or national guidelines. Mothers are recruited from both groups as a result of local information (hospital literature or verbally from hospital or community staff) or from magazines, newspapers or journals containing articles about milk banks and the uses of donor milk.

Once screened and recruited, mothers of healthy babies usually express daily at home for the bank, although some choose to do so less frequently. They use their own pump or one supplied by the milk bank and store the breast milk frozen in sterile containers, again supplied by the milk bank. Donors from the second group (hospitalized infants) will mostly have stored their milk frozen whilst establishing or maintaining their milk supply because their baby has been born prematurely or has been cared for on a neonatal or paediatric unit. Some mothers in this situation express for many weeks before their baby is able to tolerate any or appreciable volumes of milk. Others have simply found that their daily supply exceeds their baby's needs and the extra provides a gradually increasing store. In some cases both sets of mothers may build up a store comprising many litres of frozen breast milk. If offered as a donation, milk bank staff will want to make sure that the milk will not be needed for the mother's own baby before going ahead with recruitment procedures. This usually means waiting until the baby is about to be discharged,

fully breastfeeding. It is not uncommon for women who were once producing amounts of milk in excess of their baby's requirements to find that their supply dwindles with time. Some of these mothers do need to draw on their frozen stocks before establishing breastfeeding; others end up using all of the stored breast milk.

Although selection criteria vary between countries, most donors fit the following criteria:

- healthy
- not using any drugs
- non-smokers
- not taking routine medication (see exceptions below)
- drinking fewer than 2 units of alcohol per day
- willing to undergo a blood test for infections transmitted via breast milk, including HIV

Most routine medications prohibit a woman from becoming a donor; however there are some exceptions, including asthma inhalers, eye and nasal drops, thyroxine, insulin and the progesterone-only contraceptive pill.

UK guidelines (3rd edition)[17] also specify a low caffeine intake (three or fewer caffeinated drinks per day) and exclude mothers who are in the process of weaning their baby at the time they wish to become a donor. In addition the volunteer donor will be asked if she has dietary restrictions, about any exposure to tuberculosis and if she has received a blood transfusion. Questions are also asked that are designed to highlight if a prospective donor is at greater than average risk of incubating Creutzfeldt–Jakob disease (CJD). This last question is precautionary. There is no evidence that CJD, and in particular variant CJD, is transmitted via breast milk, but that does not totally rule out the possibility. In the absence of a test for CJD, everything possible must be done to identify prospective donors who might be at higher risk of contracting the disease. UK milk-banking guidelines[17] have drawn upon the UK Department of Health in listing exclusion criteria.[18] In North America, as with blood donation, women are not able to donate their breast milk if they have lived in the UK.

In the UK, most other European countries, North America and Brazil, donations are provided without any form of payment. This is a most important safeguard, helping to ensure that the donor is motivated by altruism and the desire to help sick babies rather than from any pecuniary need.[19] The phrase 'the milk of human kindness' is therefore truly appropriate in these circumstances. In the early days of milk banking in the UK, when mothers were paid, DEBM was routinely tested for the presence of cow's milk to ensure milk banks were getting what they were paying for. Some European countries continue to maintain their tradition of paying mothers for their milk – a prolific donor to a milk bank in Norway was widely reported in the UK to have purchased a new car with the proceeds of her sales of breast milk, having received £11 per litre. Similar publicity has been given to women in other countries who benefited well financially from their breast milk going to milk banks. However, on the whole, even in poorer countries where the alternatives to DEBM are less safe and relatively more costly, breast milk, in common with other tissues, is donated and not sold.

Prospective donors are provided with leaflets that explain the selection procedures. UKAMB publishes a series of leaflets covering all aspects of donor selection.[20] During recruitment, milk bank staff explain to donors the reasons for all the selection criteria, take their medical history and answer any questions. In the USA, where, because of the distances involved, face-to-face meetings with the donors are less likely, the donor's family physician is also consulted.

The discussion with donors will include the blood tests. According to the document *Guidelines for Pretest Discussion on HIV Testing*,[21] pre-(HIV) test counselling of prospective donors is not necessary because the blood test is part of a routine screening procedure. However pretest discussion of the issues involved is recommended. Such issues might include reference to the position regarding life insurance. Importantly, in the UK and elsewhere, being tested for HIV as part of a screening procedure for milk banks will not affect a donor's ability to obtain or renew life insurance as long as the result is negative. In recent years the experience within UK milk banks has been that many donors have already been screened for HIV as part of their routine antenatal tests. However current guidelines recommend that serology testing must take place again at the time the donor is recruited. Additional safeguards have been incorporated into the third edition of the UK guidelines with the inclusion of two new recommendations. These are to repeat blood tests at 2-monthly intervals and quarantine milk during that period or to retest donors 3 months after the final donation of milk (with the milk having been used in the meantime). Both these practices are designed to identify any donor who seroconverts after the initial blood test. A donor's written consent to the blood tests is taken. It should be noted that in Norway and Germany, where some raw donor milk is used, repeat blood tests are also routinely undertaken.

The written information provided for donors also requests that they provide the milk bank with any relevant information if their circumstances change (for example, requiring a course of medication such as antibiotics would temporarily exclude them as a donor, as would some vaccinations). Similarly, if their risk status for becoming infected with blood-borne viruses changes, they must no longer donate their milk.

Suitable arrangements are made to collect the donor milk unless, as is the case in some milk banks, donors are required to deliver the milk themselves. In parts of Brazil, firefighters spend their quiet periods collecting DEBM on behalf of milk banks – a system that works very well but which has so far not been replicated elsewhere. Frozen donor milk is couriered around the USA from donor to milk bank as well as from milk bank to the recipient's hospital or home. Some milk banks depend upon the services of volunteers; others restrict the recruitment of donors to within a specific geographical area to ensure that milk bank staff are able to collect their donations. The use of designated freezers in local pharmacy stores, health centres and, in a few cases, the homes of volunteers all contribute to the means by which DEBM reaches the milk bank from the donors' homes.

Screening

All prospective donors should be screened via a blood test. A negative test result for antibodies to the following viruses:

- HIV1 and 2
- HTLV1 and 2 (human T lymphotrophic viruses)
- hepatitis B
- hepatitis C

and to the bacterium of syphilis will be required prior to acceptance of a donor.

Many donors return following the birth of subsequent babies and any mother who is being recruited again following a second pregnancy should be rescreened.

It is important to note that any prescriber of DEBM should ascertain which blood tests have been performed on donors (together with confirmation that other recommendations are being followed). Blood tests vary between countries and between individual banks.

In the UK, it is recommended that the tests take place in a location convenient to the donor but that results are always given in person and that every milk bank has a designated expert available in the case of a positive or equivocal result. Encouraging prospective donors to self-exclude themselves if they have risk factors for any of the infections has thus far proved successful and there have been no positive test results for HIV since screening began in the UK in the late 1980s. However, whilst it is acknowledged that donors are generally from a low-risk population, milk banks cannot be complacent and should be prepared for the possibility of a positive test result and be able to share that information with the donor in as sensitive and helpful a way as possible, with immediate access to appropriate counselling and medical advice.

MICROBIOLOGY

Expressed breast milk may contain bacteria and viruses that are there by virtue of underlying infections of the mother or contamination during the collection and handling of the milk.

Screening via blood tests helps to rule out viruses that are of significance. Cytomegalovirus (CMV) is inactivated by the freezing and heat treatment that are standard in UK and US milk banks[22] and so screening by blood test is not required. In countries such as Germany and Norway, where some DEBM is used raw, the donor is screened and only breast milk from CMV-negative mothers is accepted for feeding raw.

Donors are provided with information to ensure they collect their milk safely. This includes details about how to sterilize equipment and the need for good hand-washing before expressing. Nevertheless, some bacterial contamination of breast milk is usual. Bacteriological testing of DEBM differs between countries. In the UK, guidelines state that before pasteurization, milk containing any pathogens or contamination by non-pathogenic organisms above an acceptable limit (higher than 10^5 colony-forming units per ml) should not be issued from the milk bank. Elsewhere, reliance on postpasteurization testing may be commonplace but, in all cases, once pasteurized, the milk must show no bacterial growth after 48 hours.

POOLING OF DONOR BREAST MILK

The 2003 third edition of the UK guidelines[17] recommend that DEBM should *not* be pooled between donors. This is to minimize any risk of transmission of infection by minimizing the number of donors per recipient and this has been adopted largely as a result of questionmarks over the possible transmission of CJD via breast milk (see above). Before the 2003 edition, milk banks were encouraged to pool samples of breast milk from between four and six donors. The rationale for this was to provide a final product that would maintain a more consistent composition, given the variable nature of breast milk. Donors are at different stages of lactation, the milk is expressed at varying times of the day and donations contain more or less foremilk or hindmilk as well as the purely individual variations that are known to exist (see Chapter 3). Milk banks may still pool donations of milk from the same donor. North American milk banks continue to pool DEBM.

Where the DEBM has been donated by the mother of a preterm baby, particularly if expressed early in her lactation, the resultant milk is likely to be particularly valuable for feeding to other preterm infants as it is higher in protein and may contain more immunoglobulin A (see Chapter 1).

NUTRITIONAL ANALYSIS

It is unusual for UK milk banks to provide nutritional analyses of the DEBM. It is only feasible where the milk is pooled and has always required specialist instrumentation that is expensive and labour-intensive. A recent survey of UK milk banks showed that only two of the 16 milk banks routinely analyses the donor milk.[23] However, recently published work,[24] supported by the Irvinestown Milk Bank in Northern Ireland, concludes that routinely used equipment can provide practical, quick and reliable protein and triglyceride assays. Knowledge of the protein and fat content of DEBM will aid clinicians when faced with a baby whose rate of growth gives cause for concern.

HEAT PROCESSING

In the early days of milk banking, the temperature and time combination for the heat treatment of DEBM were directly derived from the pasteurization of cow's milk. Known as Holder pasteurization, this was a method that ensured the bacterium responsible for tuberculosis in cattle was destroyed, preventing its transmission to humans via the milk. Holder pasteurization of breast milk involves raising the temperature of the milk to 62.5°C and maintaining it there for 30 min, after which it is quickly cooled. The rapid cooling helps to minimize losses of heat-labile components of the milk. This temperature–time combination is once again recommended for UK milk banks. However in other countries (and in the UK before the recent edition of the guidelines), lower temperatures are acceptable.

The minimum temperature for the heat treatment arose from the determination that heat-treating breast milk at 56°C for 30 min inactivated HIV.[25] As a result of this work, the option of heating breast milk to a chosen temperature between 57 and 63°C was offered. The upper limit of 63°C reflects the higher losses of beneficial constituents of the milk at temperatures above this. The lower temperatures provide the advantage of increased retention of anti-infective components of the milk, and in particular the immunoglobulin that is largely present in breast milk (secretory immunoglobulin A), lactoferrin and lysozyme. However in the light of the growing incidence of tuberculosis in the UK and the overriding precautionary principle when making recommendations for human milk banking, the UK guidelines stipulate heat treatment at 62.5°C for 30 min.

The method by which the required heat treatment is carried out varies from country to country. Some use laboratory water baths to provide the heat treatment and then transfer the containers of milk to an ice bath to bring about the rapid fall in temperature. In the UK and Europe, specialized equipment that both heats and cools the milk is readily available. The human milk pasteurizers operate automatically throughout the whole cycle and are computerized to ensure they are easy to use. A permanent record of the heat treatment is provided and this should be maintained as part of the milk bank records.

HANDLING AND STORAGE OF DONOR BREAST MILK

Breast milk should be handled aseptically at all times in the milk bank. Sterile containers, jugs and other equipment are used and raw breast milk is clearly differentiated from pasteurized by means of different containers or colour-coded lids. The use of laminar flow cabinets, although uncommon in milk banks, does help to prevent contamination of the DEBM whilst being tested and handled in the milk bank.

The organization of the storage of the DEBM is designed to keep milk in different stages of the milk-banking process separate. Hence raw and pasteurized breast milk should not be stored together and all freezers should be clearly labelled. Once issued from the milk bank, the responsibility for the handling of the pasteurized DEBM will no longer lie with the milk bank. All users of donor milk should be clear about its subsequent storage, thawing and use.

Frozen, pasteurized DEBM should be thawed in a refrigerator but if needed at short notice the container may be held under running cool water, avoiding the cap area, until sufficient milk has defrosted. Once thawed, pasteurized DEBM may be stored for up to 24 h at 4°C.

RECORD-KEEPING

The importance of comprehensive and accurate record-keeping is well recognized and a suitable audit trail should be established. Details to be recorded include all relevant health and lifestyle donor information together with copies of consent forms and blood-test results. Donor identification numbers should be allocated to ensure confidentiality. Every sample of milk must be traceable from donor to recipient and vice versa, including details of any pooling where relevant. Pasteurization records should be maintained, preferably attached to the documentation referring to each batch of milk undergoing processing. All microbiological results should also be attached. Where bottles of DEBM are sent to other hospitals for unspecified infants, donor milk record cards that are returned to the milk bank help to ensure accurate record-keeping. Milk bank records should be maintained for at least 10 years. In addition, a proposed innovation is also to archive samples of milk and blood from each donor for 10 years. Figure 6.5 is a flow diagram of the main procedures, with suggestions for points of audit.

OPENING A NEW MILK BANK

Careful consideration needs to be given to the suitability of the premises. Little specialized equipment is needed to operate a milk bank except for the means to pasteurize the breast milk. However a dedicated refrigerator and freezers will be needed. The freezers and fridges should incorporate an acceptable temperature range with associated alarms (preferably linked to a switchboard or hospital security), externally visible temperature monitors and a lock. Domestic fridges and freezers are not suitable.

Containers and other equipment to store, pool and mix the milk will be required and should be disposable or autoclavable. The dangers of glass chipping are worth noting and glass should never be reused unless manufactured for that purpose. Most milk banks obtain containers specifically designed for the storage of breast milk. Tamper evidence is an important consideration when milk is being transported or stored in areas without constant supervision.

Most donors have their own breast pump, either a hand or small electric type; however it is usual for milk banks to supply these if required. Donors should also be provided with the means of clearly labelling their milk.

Any group considering opening a new milk bank in the UK should approach UKAMB for advice and support. Milk banks operate under the guidance of a management committee and/or a medical director. They are not suitable initiatives for a group of interested individuals but should be part of a medical establishment. It is also worthwhile for anyone initiating the development of a new milk bank to contact all hospitals in the region to discern if the demand for DEBM will best be met by establishing a regional bank.

TRAINING

Anyone working in a milk bank should participate in specialized training. This includes basic food hygiene as well as becoming familiar with all the procedures involved in the recruitment and selection of donors, the testing and processing of the milk and an overview of milk banking. There is no UK provision of

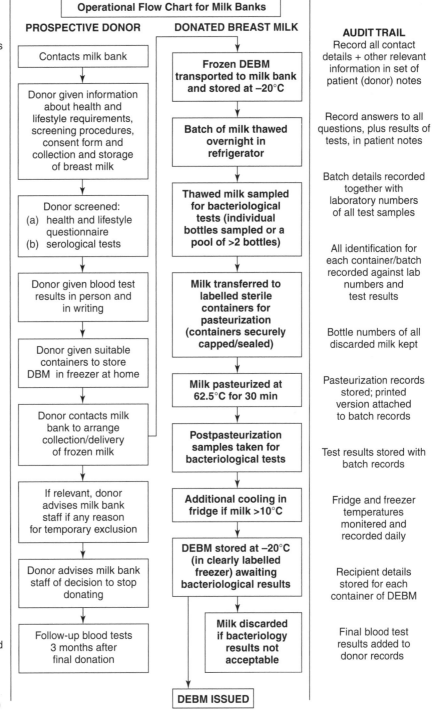

SAFETY MEASURES
NB: Up-to-date guidelines followed at all times

Clear information on donor selection and blood tests given. Opportunity to ask questions

Laminar flow cabinet used for handling and sampling the DBM

Prospective donors able to self-exclude without prejudice

Donor excluded if health, lifestyle or serology tests do not meet standards required

Bacteriological tests ensure milk not heavily contaminated or contaminated with pathogens

DEBM stored in sterile containers provided by milk bank

Heat treatment to give added protection against bacterial and viral infection

Temporary exclusion on grounds of medication, vaccination, illness, etc.

Frozen DEBM transferred to milk bank freezer (freezers labelled and organized to separate milk in different stages of milk-banking process)

Operational Flow Chart for Milk Banks

PROSPECTIVE DONOR

Contacts milk bank

Donor given information about health and lifestyle requirements, screening procedures, consent form and collection and storage of breast milk

Donor screened:
(a) health and lifestyle questionnaire
(b) serological tests

Donor given blood test results in person and in writing

Donor given suitable containers to store DBM in freezer at home

Donor contacts milk bank to arrange collection/delivery of frozen milk

If relevant, donor advises milk bank staff if any reason for temporary exclusion

Donor advises milk bank staff of decision to stop donating

Follow-up blood tests 3 months after final donation

DONATED BREAST MILK

Frozen DEBM transported to milk bank and stored at –20°C

Batch of milk thawed overnight in refrigerator

Thawed milk sampled for bacteriological tests (individual bottles sampled or a pool of >2 bottles)

Milk transferred to labelled sterile containers for pasteurization (containers securely capped/sealed)

Milk pasteurized at 62.5°C for 30 min

Postpasteurization samples taken for bacteriological tests

Additional cooling in fridge if milk >10°C

DEBM stored at –20°C (in clearly labelled freezer) awaiting bacteriological results

Milk discarded if bacteriology results not acceptable

DEBM ISSUED

AUDIT TRAIL
Record all contact details + other relevant information in set of patient (donor) notes

Record answers to all questions, plus results of tests, in patient notes

Batch details recorded together with laboratory numbers of all test samples

All identification for each container/batch recorded against lab numbers and test results

Bottle numbers of all discarded milk kept

Pasteurization records stored; printed version attached to batch records

Test results stored with batch records

Fridge and freezer temperatures monitered and recorded daily

Recipient details stored for each container of DEBM

Final blood test results added to donor records

Figure 6.5 Flowchart showing main procedures for archiving, with suggestions for points of audit. DEBM, donor expressed breast milk

accredited training at the moment; however most established milk banks will welcome new staff and offer the opportunity to visit and spend time in a milk bank. UKAMB (or HMBANA in the USA and Canada) may also be consulted about training opportunities. In Brazil, milk bank staff are trained to a high standard with regular updates.

OBTAINING DONOR BREAST MILK FROM A MILK BANK IN THE UK

If an NNU without access to its own dedicated milk bank requires supplies of DEBM, the first port of call is either a local milk bank known to offer surplus milk to other units or the UKAMB headquarters. The UKAMB will be able to suggest the nearest milk bank with a current surplus. The NNU should first ensure that the milk bank operates within the UKAMB guidelines. Milk banks usually make a charge for donor milk to cover some of the costs incurred in providing tested, screened and processed DEBM. This varies between milk banks.

THE FUTURE FOR HUMAN MILK BANKS

The use of DEBM in the UK is increasing and the future promises to be interesting as moves are made to provide an equitable service to all infants with a clinical requirement for DEBM. Since the early 1990s milk banks have been opening or reopening. The creation of regional banks in the UK would offer a strategically better response to the growing demand for DEBM as well as an overall cost saving.[26] They would require fewer staff and less equipment and resources. The monitoring of milk banks and their inspection, currently under the governance of the individual trust, could be nationally organized, which in turn would provide the transparency that is currently lacking. However, even in the absence of a national system, milk banks should be subject to inspection and accreditation. The tested and processed breast milk provided by milk banks is fed to some of the sickest and most vulnerable infants. Any measures that ensure its safety without compromising its availability are to be welcomed. Closer links, information-sharing and co-operation between national associations are desirable. In Europe it is unlikely that milk banking will continue to escape European Union scrutiny, especially as tissue banking currently awaits the finalized European Union directive on the quality and safety of tissues and cells.

SUMMARY

Human milk banking has seen a global re-surgence of interest in the past decade. This is partly as a result of the proven clinical benefits attributed to its use. Milk banks should operate according to national accredited guidelines that cover donor recruitment and selection, donor screening, including serology, bacteriology testing of the milk and its heat treatment. Where DEBM is obtained from a milk bank, the prescriber should ascertain that the milk bank operates according to these guidelines.

References

1. Human Milk Banking Association of North America. Guidelines for the establishment and operation of a donor human milk bank. Available online at: www.hmbana.com.
2. Williams AS. Women and childbirth in the twentieth century. Sutton; 1997.
3. Department of Health and Social Security. PL/CMO (88)13, PL/CNO (88) 7, dated 27 April 1988.
4. Department of Health and Social Security. PL/CMO (89) 4, PL/CNO (89) 3, dated 4 July 1989.
5. Lucas A, Cole TJ. Breast milk and neonatal necrotising enterocolitis. Lancet 1990; 336:1519–1523.
6. United Kingdom Association for Milk Banking (UKAMB). Available online at: www.ukamb.org.
7. Department of Health and Social Services Breast-feeding Strategy Group for Northern Ireland. Breast-feeding strategy for Northern Ireland. Belfast: Department of Health and Social Services; 1999.
8. Lucas A. AIDS and human milk banking. In: Proceedings of the 19th RCOG Study Group. Royal

College of Obstetricians and Gynaecologists 1988:271–281.

9. Naryanan I, Prakash K, Murthy NS et al. Randomised controlled trial of effect of raw and Holder pasteurised human milk and of formula supplements on the incidence of neonatal infection. Lancet 1984; ii:1111–1112.

10. Lucas A, Cole TJ. Breast milk and neonatal necrotising enterocolitis. Lancet 1990; 336: 1519–1523.

11. Singhal A, Cole TJ, Lucas A. Early nutrition in preterm infants and later blood pressure: two cohorts after randomised trials. Lancet 2001; 357:413–419.

12. Singhal A, Fewtrell M, Cole TJ et al. Low nutrient intake and early growth for later insulin resistance in adolescents born preterm. Lancet 2003; 361:1089–1097.

13. McGuire W, Anthony MY. Donor human milk versus formula for preventing necrotising enterocolitis in preterm infants: a systematic review. Arch Dis Child Fetal Neonatal Ed 2003; 88:F11–F14.

14. Bisquera JA, Cooper TR, Berseth CL. Impact of necrotising enterocolitis on length of stay and hospital charges in very low birth weight infants. Pediatrics 2002; 109:423–428.

15. Guidelines for the establishment and operation of human milk banks in the UK. British Paediatric Association; 1994.

16. Guidelines for the establishment and operation of human milk banks in the UK, 2nd edn. Royal College of Paediatrics and Child Health and United Kingdom Association for Milk Banking; 1999.

17. Guidelines for the establishment and operation of human milk banks in the UK, 3rd edn. United Kingdom Association for Milk Banking; 2003.

18. Department of Health. Transmissible spongiform encephalopathy agents: safe working and the prevention of infection. Infection control of CJD and related disorders in the healthcare setting. Available online at: www.doh.gov.uk/cjd/tseguidance/.

19. The gift relationship by Richard Titmuss, Ed Ann Oakley and John Ashton. LSE Books; 1997.

20. United Kingdom Association for Milk Banking leaflets. Could you be a breast milk donor? Blood tests for breast milk donors. Donating milk, your questions answered.

21. Department of Health. Guidelines for pretest discussion on HIV testing. Department of Health; 1996.

22. Friis H, Andersen HK. Rate of inactivation of cytomegalovirus in raw banked milk during storage at –20°C and pasteurisation. Br Med J Clin Res Edn 1982; 285:1604–1605.

23. Atkinson A, Balmer S. UK milk banking practices. UKAMB Newslett 2003; October:5.

24. Lynch PLM, O'Kane MJ, O'Donohoe J et al. Determination of the total protein and triglyceride content of human breast milk on the Synchron CX7 Delta analyser. Ann Clin Biochem 2004; 41:61–64.

25. Orloff SL, Wallingford JC, McDougall JS. Inactivation of human immunodeficiency virus type 1 in human milk. Effects of intrinsic factors in human milk and pasteurisation. J Human Lactation 1993; 9:13–17.

26. Weaver G. Human milk banking: the case for a national strategy. MIDIRS Midwifery Dig 2001; 11:381–383.

Chapter 7

Enteral feeding

Caroline King

SUMMARY OF RECOMMENDATIONS

Type of milk
- Recommended milks in order of preference:
  - Mother's own freshly expressed
  - Mother's own refrigerated expressed
  - Mother's own frozen expressed
  - Donor expressed breast milk (DEBM)
  - Preterm formula.
- Hydrolysed protein formula:
  - There is little evidence that hydrolysed formula is protective for the preterm gut
  - There is some evidence that hydrolysed formula may lead to more rapid gastric emptying
  - Soya-based formulas are not recommended
- Other enteral liquids:
  - Avoid the use of hypo- and hyperosmolar liquids in the neonatal period

When to start
- As soon as clinical condition allows; aim to start within the first few days
- Delaying enteral feeds is unphysiological and may predispose to bacterial translocation

Minimal enteral feeding
- Give minimal enteral feeds (MEF) to high-risk infants
- Delay increasing feed volume for several days in those considered at the highest risk for gastrointestinal complications, e.g. necrotizing enterocolitis (NEC)

- Aim for a total exceeding 100 ml over the first 6 days

Rate of increase and frequency of feeds
- After a period of MEF:
  - Keep feed increases to < 20 ml/kg per 24 h if the infant is at high risk of NEC
  - Increase > 20 ml/kg per 24 h and < 35 ml/kg per h if the risk of NEC is uncertain
- Increase according to clinical judgement when there is no increased risk of NEC
- Ensure gastric residues are fully collected and recorded
- Do not withhold feeds when there are small to moderate (< 3 ml/h) gastric residues
- Tailor the frequency of feeds to the size of the infant

Continuous versus bolus feeds
- Give bolus feeds initially
- In severe respiratory instability or gastro-oesophageal reflux, try continuous feeds
- If human milk is given by continuous tube feed:
  - do not give < 4 ml/h
  - tilt syringe to allow fat delivery first
  - keep tubing to a minimum length
  - if supplements have been added to milk, ensure that they are well mixed and that the syringe contents are regularly agitated during delivery but do not allow to froth
  - change syringe, tubing and milk every 4 h

Feed intolerance
- Diagnosis can include gastric aspirates > 2 ml in infants < 750 g weight and > 3 ml in infants > 750 g weight; however, the whole clinical picture must be evaluated
- High-risk infants include those who are very preterm, asphyxiated or on morphine
- The risk can be reduced with early enteral feeding of breast milk
- In the absence of breast milk, the use of hydrolysed protein and lactose-free formulas requires more investigation

Necrotizing enterocolitis
- Main risk factors include prematurity, formula feeding, abnormal gut blood flow and high-osmolar enteral liquids

- Risk can be reduced by using breast milk and following a standardized feeding protocol
- There are guidelines to suggest recommencing enteral feeding 2–3 days after mild or suspected NEC and 7–14 days after confirmed NEC

Pre- and probiotics
- Human milk has abundant prebiotics and has a profile that is not equalled by recently developed formulas
- Human milk promotes a beneficial gut flora in the absence of antibiotic therapy and it has not been possible to replicate this with experimental use of probiotics
- Further work is needed to establish the safety of probiotics in preterm neonates

TYPE OF MILK

Mother's own milk

In Chapter 1 the advantages of using human milk are discussed: the milk of choice is mother's own, freshly expressed. As it is not always practical to use fresh milk, any excess should be refrigerated or frozen for later use according to recognized guidelines.[1]

Donor expressed breast milk

When a mother is too ill or unable to express her own milk, DEBM from a milk bank is the next best alternative. DEBM can reduce time to full enteral feeds, thus potentially leading to a decrease in the amount of parenteral nutrition needed.[2] This would make it economically worthwhile to give DEBM to all infants receiving intensive care, if supplies allow.

Even when DEBM is available, it is vitally important that mothers are encouraged to produce their own milk. Fresh milk loses some important components on pasteurization (see Chapter 3).

In practice donor milk only should be used until the baby is tolerating full feeds, then the baby should be graded on to an appropriate formula. However, when it is medically indicated and supplies are adequate, a baby may continue on a proportion (e.g. one-quarter DEBM to three-quarters formula) of donor milk as anecdotally this has been seen to maintain feed tolerance and possibly continue to protect against sepsis and NEC.

Hydrolysed protein formula

Partially hydrolysed feeds (also known as semi-elemental) are indicated when there is strongly suspected malabsorption and/or lactose intolerance, as well as in the rare event of suspected cow's milk protein intolerance.[3] When human milk is unavailable it is currently uncertain which is the best milk to use for feed initiation, particularly in infants who are at high risk of gastrointestinal problems. There is some evidence that a feed based on hydrolysed rather than whole cow's milk protein may lead to significantly shorter gastrointestinal transit time in premature infants.[4,5]

However there may be drawbacks with respect to absorption and assimilation of the nitrogen[6,7] and calcium and phosphorus[6] in these formulas. This may explain the lack of improvement in nutrient balance that has been reported.[8] To overcome this problem a higher-nitrogen version has been evaluated.

With a hydrolysed preterm formula which provided 10–12% more nitrogen than a whole-protein control, serum amino acids[9,10] and nitrogen accretion[10] were similar to controls. In addition equivalent bone mineral density has been shown when hydrolysed formulas contain approximately 15% more calcium than controls.[11]

Other concerns are the observation that in animal experiments intestinal immunoglobulin G levels were significantly lower with hydrolysed protein feeding[12] and that the presence of peptides rather than whole protein in the gut may lead to accelerated destruction of epidermal growth factor (EGF).[13] This is of concern as EGF may be important for gut integrity (see Chapter 1). These feeds should not be used for long-term feeding unless designed for the nutritional needs of the preterm infant.

Soya formulas

These are not recommended for preterm infants, as they have not been designed to satisfy the nutritional needs of this population. In addition soya protein is potentially allergenic. Recently concerns have been raised about the phyto-oestrogen content, leading to UK government recommendations that soya formulas should not be given as the main drink to infants < 1 year unless medically indicated.[14]

Other enteral liquids

Both hypo- and hyperosmolar solutions such as water and glucose solutions should be used with caution during the neonatal period when the gut is at its most vulnerable. Hypo-osmolar solutions may draw solute into the gut lumen due to its low tonicity, while hyperosmolar solutions may increase the risk of NEC (see below).

WHEN TO START

Introduction

Enteral feeding should start as soon as the baby's clinical condition is considered sufficiently stable. However, for the reasons outlined below, some enteral feed should be given within the first few days, even if it is only 1–2 ml.

Physiology

Withholding enteral nutrition from birth is unphysiological as the fetus swallows amniotic fluid for a large part of gestation. A significant reduction in size and weight of gastrointestinal-related organs has been demonstrated following oesophageal ligation in fetal animals.[15]

Maturation of gut motor function

Concerns about the immaturity of the preterm gut has led to cautious feeding regimens in the past; however it has now been shown that maturation of the gastrointestinal tract can be accelerated by early feeding. Enteral feeds have been shown to result in a recognized postprandial motor response in the small intestine, independent of postconceptional age.[16] This is important as the intestine of a 25-week gestation infant is structurally mature with respect to digestion and absorption compared to motor responses and it is the motor responses that are likely to be a key factor, resulting in poor tolerance of enteral nutrition.[17] Some have found that intakes as low as 20 ml/kg triggered accelerated maturation of motor function.[18]

Maturation of gut digestive function

Initiation of enteral feeds on day 4 was associated with later decrease in intestinal permeability[19] and increased lactase activity:[20] this was true in bolus and continuous-fed infants, with breast milk giving significant advantages over formula.

Feed tolerance

A systematic review of the area was limited in its recommendations due to the small number of studies available for scrutiny. However the trend was for earlier feeding to help earlier tolerance of feeds.[21]

Bacterial translocation and sepsis

It is well recognized that lack of luminal nutrients leads to gut atrophy.[22] There is evidence that a further sequela in certain circumstances is increased gut permeability leading to bacterial translocation – the crossing of viable bacteria across the gut mucosa to enter the systemic circulation.[23] This in turn has been associated with systemic infection.[24]

Parenteral nutrition is associated with an increased risk of sepsis and has been shown to impair cytokine production (by infant blood) in vitro.[25] However, even small volumes of enteral feed in postsurgical term infants were shown to normalize an abnormal immune function as compared with controls.[26] Reviews of early enteral feeding are available.[27,28]

MINIMAL ENTERAL FEEDING

Definition

MEF, or trophic feeding, as it is also known, is proposed as a method of priming the gut of the smallest and sickest infants while most of their nutrition is derived from parenteral nutrition. In the following papers feed volumes ranged from 2 to 24 ml/kg per day for a period ranging approximately from 4 to 14 days.[29–35]

Benefits

MEF has been reported to lead to less dependence on parenteral nutrition and earlier discharge.[32,36] Positive effects well beyond the period of MEF have been recorded, i.e. reduced whole-gut transit time.[35] Other work has shown the following benefits of early MEF: lower peak bilirubin levels, lower alkaline phosphatase levels and more rapid tolerance of full enteral feeds,[30] enhanced gut motility,[35] less feed intolerance,[31] increased lactase activity,[37] less hyperglycaemia,[38] alleviation of cholestasis[39] and improved weight gain,[40,41] with no increase in risk of NEC. The association of MEF with reduced rates of sepsis[36] may be due to reduced rates of bacterial translocation (see above).

One recent study found an increased risk of NEC in a group randomized to feed advancement of 20 ml/kg per day compared to a group who remained on trophic volumes of 20 ml/kg per day for 10 days from the day of starting feeds.[42] However, another group found no increase in NEC with early introduction of small volumes and progressive increase reaching full feeds by around day 15.[43] Unfortunately the two groups of infants were not comparable; however the experience of Berseth et al.[42] may suggest that trophic feeds should be started early but not increased for the first few days in those infants who are considered to be at the highest risk of NEC.

A systematic review of the area looking at papers published before 1997 concluded that MEF was associated with a decrease in days to full enteral feeding and in the length of hospitalization.[44] More recent reviews have concluded that MEF leads to multiple benefits with no adverse effects reported so far.[45,46]

Endocrine effects

It has been found that a mean total of 24 ml over the first few days after birth led to significant increase in plasma levels of enteroglucagon, gastrin and gastric-inhibitory polypeptide compared to no enteral feeds. After a mean volume of 96 ml, over the first few days, maximal postnatal levels of these hormones had been achieved.[47] Greater volumes were needed to increase neurotensin and motilin. Enteroglucagon is a trophic hormone for the small intestine, gastrin stimulates the growth of gastric mucosa and exocrine pancrease, while gastric-inhibitory peptide may have a role in initiation of the enteroinsular axis and hence glucose tolerance. Slightly larger volumes (30–40% of total volume) have been needed to increase mucosal mass in animal studies,[48,49] whereas only 10% of total volume was needed to accelerate maturation of motor function.[48]

RATE OF INCREASE AND FREQUENCY OF FEEDS

Rate of increase and risk of NEC

A study showing an association between early enteral feeding and NEC despite the use of human milk employed a relatively rapid increase in enteral feeding.[50] This has been associated with increased rates of NEC, regardless of the type of milk used.[51–55] Some suggest that there may be a volume threshold before NEC occurs;[56] infants developed NEC in this study after exceeding 100 ml/kg. However the type of milk fed was not specified, and thus the protective effect of breast milk could not be evaluated.

A possible mechanism is the introduction of quantities of lactose that exceed the baby's ability to digest due to low lactase activity: this could then be a substrate of pathogenic bacterial overgrowth. However, one study comparing a lactose-free with a standard preterm formula did not show any reduction in NEC.[57]

Recommended rates of increase

Once the period of MEF is completed it may be an advantage to keep the increase in feeding increments < 20 ml/kg per day in babies who are at highest risk of NEC. An association with increased risk of NEC has been shown on feed regimens where volumes increase > 20 ml/kg per day.[52–54,58] However in a recent study of relatively well neonates (500–1500 g birth weight) advancing enteral feeds from around day 4–5 by 15 ml/kg per day gave no advantage over 35 ml/kg per day.[59] All infants were fed a lower-energy density formula until full feeds then switched to a preterm formula.

In a similar study daily increments of 30 ml/kg per day compared to 20 ml resulted in earlier full enteral nutrition and discharge.[60] However, infant characteristics were not given.

Feed frequency

There are no experimental data to guide the choice of feed frequency; however it is common practice to start the smallest babies on hourly feeds and increase to 3- or 4-hourly intervals as the infant grows.[61] This may be acceptable for formula-fed infants, but those on breast milk and with certain conditions may do better on more frequent feeds. At around term date the fully breast-fed infant will take feeds at a frequency dictated to some degree by the mother's breast capacity (see Chapter 4). In practice this is often 2–3-hourly and could be hourly for brief periods, depending on the infant's size and growth rate. For the preterm infant it will be essential to go to the mother's breast this frequently to keep her milk supply adequate to match the baby's needs. If tube feeds have been reduced to 4-hourly, there will need to be a substantial change in feeding pattern once the baby goes to the breast exclusively for nutrition. For this reason it may be an easier transition if tube feeds are kept at 2–3-hourly rather than moving to 4-hourly.

Infants with respiratory problems and those with gastro-oesophageal reflux disease may show some improvement if feed frequency is increased, as this will reduce the degree of stomach distension at each feed due to the smaller volume administered.

Box 7.1 shows a suggested framework for feed frequency.

CONTINUOUS VERSUS BOLUS FEEDS

Evidence for advantage of bolus feeds

A meta-analysis with strict entry criteria was unable to reach a conclusion about the optimal method of feeding;[62] however, discussion of the other studies discussed below points towards the benefits of bolus feeding.

Animal studies have demonstrated greater small intestinal weight after bolus feeding.[63] Although gut hormone levels are similar during bolus versus continuous feeding in animals[64] and preprandial in human neonates,[65] it may be that the cyclic surges with bolus feeding confer the advantage.[65]

Continuous feeds have been shown to reduce energy expenditure slightly ($\downarrow$ 4%)[66] and improve weight gain in some very-low-birth-weight infants ($\uparrow$ 3.6 g/kg per day).[67] However, these improvements are marginal and may be of little clinical significance. More recent work has not found any difference in weight gain.[34,68–70]

Indications for continuous feeding

Continuous feeds may be useful in infants with gut resections[71] and those with severe respiratory problems.[72,73] Continuous feeding is necessary when a tube has been placed nasojejunally; however, this method of feeding is not recommended due to adverse side-effects.[74,75]

When human milk is administered continuously or via slow infusion the syringe must be positioned to allow delivery of the fat portion first[76] as there is a risk of large fat loss.[77] Administration of volumes < 4 ml/h human milk will also lead to unacceptably high losses of fat.[77] If the milk is fortified it should be shaken regularly to prevent poor delivery of sedimented minerals. Avoid prolonged vigorous shaking as this may denature some proteins.

Box 7.1   Early enteral feeding framework

The following is a framework for guidance only: each baby will need an individual feeding plan depending on the individual clinical condition.

Birth weight < 1000 g
- Enteral feeding will usually be as an adjunct to total parenteral nutrition for the first 1–3 weeks in this group of babies
- From day 2, give approximately 1 ml/kg 4-hourly for the first 24 h
- Increase by going to 3-hourly then 2-hourly
- Keep increases < 20 ml/kg per 24 h
- *An increase of 1 ml/feed per 24 h on 2-hourly feeds is equivalent to an increase of 12 ml/kg per day in a 1000-g baby*
- *An increase of 1 ml/feed per 24 h on 2-hourly feeds is equivalent to an increase of 24 ml/kg*

per day in a 500-g baby, and would be excessive
- Wait until the infant is around 1500 g before going to 3-hourly feeds
- Keep infants on breast milk where their mothers wish to breast-feed at a feed interval of 3-hourly maximum

Birth weight 1000–1500 g
- If there is an increased risk of necrotizing enterocolitis (NEC), increase < 20 ml/kg per 24 h
- If the risk of NEC is low or uncertain, increase >20 and < 35 ml/kg per 24 h
- If there is no increased risk of NEC, increase according to clinical condition

A significant increase in colony count after 6 h has been shown in simulated continuous feeding of fresh human milk[78] and after 4 h stored at room temperature.[79] However the rise was non-significant in fresh and frozen human milk at 8 h in another clinical study.[80] Despite its bacterial content, some authors found no morbidity in preterm infants associated with their consumption of 'contaminated' human milk.[81,82] However, infrequent changing of feeding equipment may mean that residual contaminated milk in the tubing will pose a risk to the vulnerable neonate.[83,84] To reduce the risk of breast milk contamination, expressing and storage guidelines should be closely followed (see Chapter 6).[1]

FEED INTOLERANCE/GUT MOTILITY

Definition and diagnosis

Large gastric residues are often a sign of feed intolerance. Identification of this sign depends both on what gastric volumes residues might be expected in a healthy infant of the same gestation and what has been 'normal' for the individual infant previously. A fasting basal gastric residue of around 3 ml every 4 h has been found in infants between 28 and 36 weeks' gestation at birth,[85] with residues of over 2 ml in infants < 750 g and 3 ml in infants > 750 g having been found to be a useful clinical indicator of feed tolerance.[86] Bile-stained aspirate alone may not be a sufficient reason to withhold feeds[86] as it may be due to immature gut motility leading to periodic antiperistalsis.[17] It is possible that the stimulation of bile flow may in theory help reduce the risk of cholestasis. No relationship was found between a fixed gastric residual volume of 2–3 ml or the incidence of bile-stained aspirate and the volume of feed achieved by day 14.[86] Diagnosis of feed intolerance depends on the baby's whole clinical picture as well as more direct measures such as vomiting, abdominal discoloration, blood passed per rectum, stool frequency and increasing abdominal girth.

Risk factors for enteral feed intolerance

Prematurity puts infants at risk of large gastric residue.[87] Also, the lower the birth weight, the longer the time to first stool[88,89] and the longer the time to full enteral feeds.[90]

A significantly higher proportion of preterm infants have immature duodenal motor responses to their first feed than term infants.[29] This has been associated with delay in achieving full enteral feeds.[91] Earlier passage of meconium appears to be related to earlier feed tolerance; however it is unclear whether it is the passage of meconium that enhances feed tolerance or vice versa.[92] There is some evidence that the latter is true, as maturation of gut motor activity is accelerated with enteral feeding.[32]

Other high-risk infants include those suffering from birth asphyxia (at risk of slower gastric emptying[93] and greater feeding intolerance),[94] and those receiving morphine, as it is associated with delayed gastrointestinal transit.[95] Infants with cystic periventricular leukomalacia may have poorer enteral feed tolerance.[96]

Approaches to enhancing feed tolerance

Feed tolerance is enhanced with early enteral feeds compared to intravenous nutrition alone (see above). When human milk is given, this will further enhance feed tolerance. The evidence for faster gut transit with a hydrolysed protein feed is discussed above.

Feeding tube contamination is a further possible cause of feed intolerance;[97] formula-fed infants with contaminated tubes had feed intolerance while breast-milk-fed infants did not.

Feed temperature has not been shown to affect tolerance.[98,99]

In one study a lactose-free formula was associated with improved enteral tolerance;[57] however this has not been shown by others.[100] In addition, if human milk is given, lactase activity is induced at an earlier stage.[20]

When an infant is slow to pass first stool, it is sometimes clinical practice to use suppositories, but this has not been formally evaluated for its effect on feed tolerance.

NECROTIZING ENTEROCOLITIS

Prematurity

Many observers have been unable to identify the risk factors associated with the development of NEC.[101] A score for identifying high-risk infants was evaluated and found to be of limited value.[102] Prematurity (independent of birth weight, feeding volumes and type of milk) does seem to be an important risk factor.[103,104]

Enteral feeding

The observation that the vast majority of infants developing NEC have received some enteral feeds triggered a trend to delay enteral feeds in high-risk infants. However most papers relating early enteral feeding to NEC are retrospective studies.[50,52–54] None of the prospective randomized trials showed any significant increase in NEC with early enteral feeding.[30,33,105,106] In fact, one showed a significant decrease.[105]

Breast versus formula milk

See Chapter 1 for the evidence that those infants fed formula milk have a significantly higher risk of NEC independent of other factors. In addition, some studies have shown a dose-dependent protection from human milk. The feeding of a mother's own fresh breast milk to her baby has been recommended as top priority in a recent review.[107] Another possible risk factor for NEC comes from contaminated feeding tubes:[97] in this study, infants on formula had an increased risk of developing NEC whereas those on breast milk did not, despite similar levels of contamination.

Abnormal gut blood flow

In severely growth-retarded infants and those with very poor umbilical blood flows in utero (absent or reversed end-diastolic flows: A/REDF), a more cautious introduction of enteral feeds may be appropriate.[108] This is due to the risk of insult to the gut when there is preferential blood flow to the brain at the expense of the gut (known as brain-sparing). Infants shown to have experienced this are at higher risk of NEC.[109,110]

No prospective randomized studies could be found looking specifically at early versus late enteral feeding in infants with A/REDF. One observational matched case-controlled study found more NEC in the A/REDF group;[111] however these infants received their first enteral feed at an older median age than controls, suggesting no benefit from the delay. Another prospective study tested the tolerance of a standardized early-feeding protocol in very-low-birth-weight infants and found no difference in tolerance between those with normal and those with prenatally determined high risk of poor gut blood flow.[43]

Infants receiving bolus doses of indometacin may have compromised gut blood flow in the following 2-h period[112] and a higher risk of gastroenterologic lesions,[113] NEC and perforation.[114] However a recent paper has shown good tolerance of early low-volume feeds of human milk despite indometacin administration.[115]

Gut blood flow may also be reduced by caffeine.[116,117]

Osmolality

One strategy recommended for the reduction of risk of NEC has been to keep the osmolarity of enteral solutions < 400 mOsm/L (osmolality < 460 mOsm/kg) for neonates.[118,119]

Care should be taken when altering a feed by adding nutritional supplements (e.g. carbohydrate polymers) or increasing its concentration, as the osmolality may increase.[120] In addition many other enteral drugs, including vitamins and iron, have extremely high osmolalities.

See Table 7.1 for various solutions and the minimum amount of human milk that needs to be added to keep the osmolarity < 400 mOsm/L (osmolality < 460 mOsm/kg). See Table 7.2 for the osmolality of some undiluted solutions.

Standardized feeding protocols

As the onset of NEC is often highly unpredictable, it is very difficult to give a inclusive

Table 7.1 Enteral drugs in breast milk and osmolality

Enteral drug	Dose volume (ml)	Minimum amount of expressed breast milk (ml) needed to keep osmolality < 460 mOsm/kg
Sodium iron edetate (5.5 mg Fe/ml)	1	12
Dalivit (multivitamin)	0.6	6
Sodium acid phosphate (0.9 mmol P + 1.5 mmol Na/ml)	0.5	8
6% Sodium chloride (1 mmol Na/ml)	1	7
Folic acid (500 µg/ml)	1	11.5
Chloral hydrate (40 mg/ml)	0.75	9
Caffeine (10 mg/ml)	Reduces osmolality	No minimum amount of milk needed
Ranitidine*	Isotonic	No minimum amount of milk needed
Infant Gaviscon*	1 sachet in 100 ml	338 mOsm/kg
	1 sachet in 50 ml	360 mOsm/lg

Adapted from Srinivasan et al.[121]
NB Osmolality measured immediately on mixing
*Unpublished data

Table 7.2 Osmolality of some solutions

Solution	Osmolality (mOsm/kg)
Sodium iron edetate	3200
Dalivit	2333
Sodium acid phosphate	1540
6% Sodium chloride	1870
Folic acid	3410
Chloral hydrate	3780
Glucose 5%	278
Glucose 10%	535
Glucose 50%	2775

checklist that will identify infants who go on to develop the disease. A large number of the risk factors apply to many of the infants on a neonatal unit. However there appears to be some benefit to following a standardized feeding protocol in the reduction of incidence.[122] The study by Kamitsuka et al.[122] was a cohort study that retrospectively assessed rates of NEC; it was found that the reduction in risk of developing NEC was independent of birth weight, prenatal steroids, breast milk, timing of first feed and number of days to reach full feeds.

Enteral feeding after NEC

This area remains contentious and to a large degree will depend upon individual assessment. Guidelines suggest recommencing enteral nutrition 2–3 days after mild or suspected NEC, and 7–14 days after confirmed NEC.[123] Restarting enteral feeds 3 days after diagnosis of NEC been tried and compared with historical controls and appeared to lead to shorter time to full enteral feeds, less need for central venous lines and a shorter hospital stay.[124] However, as the authors remark, the safety of this very early restarting of feeds needs to be evaluated in a large controlled trial.

PRE- AND PROBIOTICS

Prebiotics

Oligosaccharides (known as prebiotics) are complex carbohydrates that appear both to encourage the development of a desirable gastrointestinal flora and to reduce the risk of enteric infection by preventing the adherence of bacteria to the gut wall.[125]

They are abundant in breast milk:[126] higher amounts are found in early milk;[127] although preterm milk has not been found to be a richer source than term milk.[128]

Preterm infants fed formula supplemented with oligosaccharides had significantly increased levels of bifidobacteria[129] but no difference was noted in growth or gastrointestinal tolerance, or levels of other bacteria. These supplemented formulas contain a small fraction of the different types of oligosaccharides present in human milk.[126] Supplementation of formula-fed infants with prebiotics holds less risk than with probiotics (see below); nevertheless, more studies are needed to demonstrate benefits.

Probiotics

There has been an increase in the use of viable organisms (known as probiotics) in those who are at risk of abnormal gut flora.[130]

Preterm infants form such a group, as they are at risk of having lower numbers of different strains in their stool compared to healthy term infants in the first few weeks.[131] In an observational study by Gewolb et al.[131] it was also noted that feeding breast milk and reduced antibiotic administration had separate but interactive positive effects on the gut flora.

Several groups have investigated the effects of adding probiotics to formula-fed babies:[132,133] only one has shown any benefit so far.[134]

There remains the risk of septicaemia from the probiotic itself; this may be particularly the case with those that are not normally found in the gut,[135,136] but it is unlikely with commensal organisms.[137] Further work is needed to establish the safety of the administration of live microorganisms to immunocompromised patients such as preterm and sick neonates.[138] At present, breast milk remains the preferred feed to encourage the development of a normal gut flora.[131]

References

1. United Kingdom Association for Milk Banking. Guidelines for the collection, storage and handling of breast milk for a mother's own baby in hospital, 2nd edn. London: Queen Charlotte's and Chelsea Hospital; 2001.

2. Lucas A. AIDS and human milk banking. Procedings of the 19th Royal College of Obstetricians and Gynaecologists study group 1988; 271–281.

3. D'Netto MA, Herson VC, Hussain N et al. Allergic gastroenteropathy in preterm infants. J Pediatr 2000; 137:480–486.

4. Mihatsch WA, Hogel J, Pohlandt F. Hydrolysed protein accelerates the gastrointestinal transport of formula in preterm infants. Acta Paediatr 2001; 90:196–198.

5. Mihatsch WA, Franz AR, Hogel J et al. Hydrolyzed protein accelerates feeding advancement in very low birth weight infants. Pediatrics 2002; 110:1199–1203.

6. Rigo J, Salle BL, Picaud JC et al. Nutritional evaluation of protein hydrolysate formulas. Eur J Clin Nutr 1995; 49 (suppl. 1):S26–S38.

7. Decsi T, Veitl V, Burus I. Plasma amino acid concentrations, indexes of protein metabolism and growth in healthy, full-term infants fed partially hydrolyzed infant formula. J Pediatr Gastroenterol Nutr 1998; 27:12–16.

8. Cooke RJ, Rasgilly L, Wareham P. Nutrient balance in preterm infants fed a partially hydrolysed whey (PHW) infant formula. Pediatr Res 1994; 36:11A.

9. Mihatsch WA, Pohlandt F. Protein hydrolysate formula maintains homeostasis of plasma amino acids in preterm infants. J Pediatr Gastroenterol Nutr 1999; 29:406–410.

10. Picaud JC, Rigo J, Normand S et al. Nutritional efficacy of preterm formula with a partially hydrolyzed protein source: a randomized pilot study. J Pediatr Gastroenterol Nutr 2001; 32:555–561.

11. Picaud JC, Lapillonne A, Rigo J et al. Nitrogen utilization and bone mineralization in very low birth weight infants fed partially hydrolyzed preterm formula. Semin Perinatol 2002; 26:439–446.

12. Kinouchi T, Koizumi K, Kuwata T et al. Evaluation of the development of intestinal function in rats reared on hydrolyzed or native protein-based milk formula. J Pediatr Gastroenterol Nutr 1999; 29:155–162.

13. Playford RJ, Woodman AC, Clark P et al. Effect of luminal growth factor preservation on intestinal growth. Lancet 1993; 341:843–848.

14. Chief Medical Officer Update 37 Jan 2004 (Dept of Health).

15. Sangild PT, Schmidt M, Elnif J et al. Prenatal development of gastrointestinal function in the pig and the effects of fetal esophageal obstruction. Pediatr Res 2002; 52:416–424.

16. Bissett WM, Watt J, Rivers RPA et al. Post-prandial motor response of the small intestine to enteral feeds in preterm infants. Arch Dis Child 1989; 64:1356–1361.

17. Newell S. Gastrointestinal function and its ontogeny: how should we feed the preterm infant? Semin Neonatol 1996; 1:59–66.

18. Bisquera JA, Berseth CL. Large feeding volumes do not induce greater maturation of small intestine motor patterns in preterm infants than small volumes do. Pediatr Res 2001; 49:260A. .

19. Shulman RJ, Schanler RJ, Lau C et al. Early feeding, antenatal glucocorticoids, and human milk decrease intestinal permeability in preterm infants. Pediatr Res 1998; 44:519–523.

20. Shulman RJ, Schanler RJ, Lau C et al. Early feeding, feeding tolerance, and lactase activity in preterm infants. J Pediatr 1998; 133:645–649.

21. Kennedy KA, Tyson JE, Chamnanvanikij S. Early versus delayed initiation of progressive enteral feedings for parenterally fed low birth weight or preterm infants. Cochrane Database Syst Rev 2000; 2:CD001970.

22. Heird WC. Effects of total parenteral alimentation on intestinal function. In: Sunshine P, ed. Gastrointestinal function and neonatal nutrition. Columbus, OH: Ross Labs; 16:1977.

23. Alverdy JC, Aoys E, Moss GS. Total parenteral nutrition promotes bacterial translocation from the gut. Surgery 1988; 104:185–190.

24. Deitch EA. The role of intestinal barrier failure and bacterial translocation in the development of systemic infection and multiple organ failure. Arch Surg 1990; 125:403–404.

25. Okada Y, Papp E, Klein NJ et al. Total parenteral nutrition directly impairs cytokine production after bacterial challenge. J Pediatr Surg 1999; 34:277–280.

26. Okada Y, Klein N, van Saene HK et al. Small volumes of enteral feedings normalise immune function in infants receiving parenteral nutrition. J Pediatr Surg 1998; 33:16–19.

27. Williams AF. Early enteral feeding of the preterm infant. Arch Dis Child Fetal Neonatal Ed 2000; 83(3):F219-F220.

28. Cooke RJ, Embleton ND. Feeding issues in preterm infants. Arch Dis Child Fetal Neonatal Ed 2000; 83:F215–F218.

29. Al Tawil Y, Berseth CL. Gestational and postnatal maturation of duodenal motor responses to intragastric feeding. J Pediatr 1996; 129:374–381.

30. Dunn L, Hulman S, Weiner J et al. Beneficial effects of early hypocaloric enteral feeding on neonatal gastrointestinal function: preliminary report of a randomized trial. J Pediatr 1988; 112:622–629.

31. Meetze WH, Valentine C, McGuigan JE. Gastrointestinal priming prior to full enteral nutrition in very low birth weight infants. J Pediatr Gastroenterol Nutr 1992; 15:163–170.

32. Berseth CL. Effect of early feeding on maturation of the preterm infant's small intestine. J Pediatr 1992; 120:947–953.

33. Slagle TA, Gross SJ. Effect of early low-volume enteral substrate on subsequent feeding tolerance in very low birth weight infants. J Pediatr 1988; 113:526–531.

34. Schanler RJ, Shulman RJ, Lau C et al. Feeding strategies for premature infants: randomized trial of gastrointestinal priming and tube-feeding method [see comments]. Pediatrics 1999; 103:434–439.

35. McClure RJ, Newell SJ. Randomised controlled trial of trophic feeding and gut motility. Arch Dis Child Fetal Neonatal Ed 1999; 80:F54–F58.

36. McClure RJ, Newell SJ. Randomised controlled study of clinical outcome following trophic feeding. Arch Dis Child Fetal Neonatal Ed 2000; 82:F29–F33.

37. McClure RJ, Newell SJ. Randomized controlled study of digestive enzyme activity following trophic feeding. Acta Paediatr 2002; 91:292–296.

38. Beccerra M, Ambiados S, Kuntsman G. Feeding VLBW infants: effect of early enteral stimulation. Pediatr Res 1996; 39:304A.

39. Merrit RJ. Cholestasis associated with total parenteral nutrition. J Pediatr Gastroenterol Nutr 1980; 5:9–22.

40. Ehrenkranz R, Younes N, Fanaroff AA et al. Effect of nutritional practices on daily weight gain in VLBW infants. Pediatr Res 1996; 39:308A.

41. Troche B, Harvey WK, Engle WD et al. Early minimal feedings promote growth in critically ill premature infants. Biol Neonate 1995; 67:172–181.

42. Berseth CL, Bisquera JA, Paje VU. Prolonging small feeding volumes early in life decreases the incidence of necrotizing enterocolitis in very low birth weight infants. Pediatrics 2003; 111:529–534.

43. Mihatsch WA, Pohlandt F, Franz AR et al. Early feeding advancement in very low-birth-weight infants with intrauterine growth retardation and increased umbilical artery resistance. J Pediatr Gastroenterol Nutr 2002; 35:144–148.

44. Tyson JE, Kennedy KA. Minimal enteral nutrition for promoting feeding tolerance and preventing morbidity in parenterally fed infants. Cochrane Database Syst Rev 2000; 2:CD000504.

45. McClure RJ. Trophic feeding of the preterm infant. Acta Paediatr 2001 (suppl.); 90436:19–21.

46. Ziegler EE. Trophic feeds. In: Zeigler EE, Lucas A, Moro G, eds. Nutrition of the very low birthweight infant, vol. 43. Nestle Nutrition Workshop Series. Philadelphia, PA: Nestec, Vevey/Lippincott Williams & Wilkins; 1999:233–244.

47. Lucas A, Bloom SR, Aynsley Green A. Gut hormones and 'minimal enteral feeding'. Acta Paediatr Scand 1986; 75:719–723.

48. Owens L, Burrin DG, Berseth CL. Minimal enteral feeding induces maturation of intestinal motor function but not mucosal growth in neonatal dogs. J Nutr 2002; 132:2717–2722.

49. Burrin DG, Stoll B, Jiang R et al. Minimal enteral nutrient requirements for intestinal growth in neonatal piglets: how much is enough? Am J Clin Nutr 2000; 71:1603–1610.

50. Eyal F, Sagi E, Arad I et al. Necrotizing enterocolitis in the very low birth weight infant: expressed breast milk feeding compared with parenteral feeding. Arch Dis Child 1982; 57:274–276.

51. Covert RF, Neu J, Elliott MJ et al. Factors associated with age of onset of necrotizing enterocolitis. Am J Perinatol 1989; 6:455–460.

52. Anderson DM, Kliegman RM. The relationship of neonatal alimentation practices to the occurrence of endemic necrotizing enterocolitis. Am J Perinatol 1991; 8:62–67.

53. Goldman HI. Feeding and necrotizing enterocolitis. Am J Dis Child 1980; 134:553–555.

54. Uauy RD, Fanaroff AA, Korones SB. Necrotizing enterocolitis in very low birth weight infants. Biodemographic and clinical correlates. J Pediatr 1991; 119:630–638.

55. McKeown RE, Marsh D, Amarnath U. Role of delayed feeding and of feeding increments in necrotizing enterocolitis. J Pediatr 1992; 121:764–770.

56. Owens L, Berseth CL. Is there a volume threshold for enteral feeding and necrotizing enterocolitis? Pediatr Res 1995; 37:315A.

57. Griffin M, Hansen J. Can the elimination of lactose from formula improve feeding tolerance in premature infants? J Pediatr 1999; 135:587–592.

58. Book LS, Herbst JJ, Jung AL. Comparison of fast and slow feeding rate schedules to the development of necrotizing enterocolitis. J Pediatr 1976; 89:463–466.

59. Rayyis SF, Ambalavanan N, Wright L, Carlo WA. Randomized trial of "slow" versus "fast" feed advancements on the incidence of necrotizing enterocolitis in very low birth weight infants. J Pediatr 1999; 134:293–297.

60. Caple J, Amentrout D, Huseby V et al. The effect of feeding volume on the clinical outcome in premature infants. Pediatr Res 1997; 41:229A.

61. Yu VY. Enteral feeding in the preterm infant. Early Hum Dev 1999; 56:89–115.

62. Premji S, Chessell L. Continuous nasogastric milk feeding versus intermittent bolus milk feeding for premature infants less than 1500 grams. Cochrane Database Syst Rev 2003; 1:CD001819.

63. Shulman RJ, Redel CA, Stathos TH. Bolus vs continuous feedings stimulate small intestinal growth and development in the newborn pig. Pediatr Gastroenterol Nutr 1994; 18:350–354.

64. van Goudoever JB, Stoll B, Hartmann B et al. Secretion of trophic gut peptides is not different in bolus- and continuously fed piglets. J Nutr 2001; 131:729–732.

65. Aynsley-Green A, Adrian TE, Bloom SR. Feeding and the development of enteroinsular hormone release in the preterm infants: effects of continuous intragastric infusion of human milk compared with intermittent boluses. Acta Paediatr Scand 1982; 71:379–383.

66. Grant J, Denne SC. Effect of intermittent vs continuous enteral feeding on energy expenditure in premature infants. J Pediatr 1991; 118:928–932.

67. Toce SS, Keenan WJ, Homan SM. Enteral feeding in very-low-birth-weight infants. A comparison of two nasogastric methods. Am J Dis Child 1987; 141:439–444.

68. Silvestre MA, Morbach CA, Brans YW et al. A prospective randomized trial comparing continuous versus intermittent feeding methods in very low birth weight neonates [see comments]. J Pediatr 1996; 128:748–752.

69. Akintorin SM, Kamat M, Pildes RS et al. A prospective randomized trial of feeding methods in very low birth weight infants. Pediatrics 1997; 100:E4.

70. Dollberg S, Kuint J, Mazkereth R et al. Feeding tolerance in preterm infants: randomized trial of bolus and continuous feeding. J Am Coll Nutr 2000; 19:797–800.

71. King C. Neonatal unit short bowel policy. London: Nutrition and Dietetic Department Hammersmith Hospital; 2001.

72. Blondheim O, Abbasi S, Fox WW et al. Effect of enteral gavage feeding rate on pulmonary functions of very low birth weight infants. J Pediatr 1993; 122:751–755.

73. Macagno F, Demarini S. Techniques of enteral feeding in the newborn. Acta Paediatr Suppl 1994; 402:11–13.

74. Macdonald PD, Skeoch CH, Carse H et al. Randomised trial of continuous nasogastric, bolus nasogastric, and transpyloric feeding in infants of birth weight under 1400 g. Arch Dis Child 1992; 67:429–431.

75. McGuire W, McEwan P. Transpyloric versus gastric tube feeding for preterm infants. Cochrane Database Syst Rev 2002; 3:CD003487.

76. Narayanan I, Singh B, Harvey D. Fat loss during feeding of human milk. Arch Dis Child 1984; 59:475–477.

77. Greer FR, McCormick A, Loker J. Changes in fat concentration of human milk during delivery by intermittent bolus and continuous mechanical pump infusion. J Pediatr 1984; 105:745–749.

78. Lemons PM, Miller K, Eitzen H et al. Bacterial growth in human milk during continuous feeding. Am J Perinatol 1983; 1:76–80.

79. Nwankwo MU, Offor E, Okolo AA et al. Bacterial growth in expressed breast-milk. Ann Trop Paediatr 1988; 8:92–95.

80. Hernandez J, Lemons P, Lemons J et al. Effect of storage processes on the bacterial growth-inhibiting activity of human breast milk. Pediatrics 1979; 63:597–601.

81. Narayanan I, Prakash K, Pratharkar, Gujral. A planned prospective evaluation of the anti-infective property of varying quantities of expressed human milk. Acta Paediatr Scand 1982; 71:441–445.

82. Law BJ, Urias BA, Lertzman J et al. Is ingestion of milk-associated bacteria by premature infants fed raw human milk controlled by routine bacteriologic screening? J Clin Microbiol 1989; 27:1560–1566.

83. Graham JC, Morgan S, Ford M et al. Sepsis and ECMO: beware the breast milk. J Hosp Infect 1999; 43:75–76.

84. Botsford KB, Weinstein RA, Boyer KM et al. Gram-negative bacilli in human milk feedings: quantitation and clinical consequences for premature infants. J Pediatr 1986; 109:707–710.

85. Malhotra AK, Deorari AK, Paul VK et al. Gastric residuals in preterm babies. J Trop Pediatr 1992; 38:262–264.

86. Mihatsch WA, von Schoenaich P, Fahnenstich H et al. The significance of gastric residuals in the early enteral feeding advancement of extremely low birth weight infants. Pediatrics 2002; 109:457–459.

87. Gupta M, Brans YW. Gastric retention in neonates. Pediatrics 1978; 62:26–29.

88. Siddiqui K, Fiumara A. Effect of birthweight and perinatal events on the passage of the first meconium. Pediatr Res 1997; 41:178A.

89. Mittal M, Dhanireddy R. Gut transit time (GT) in very low birth weight infants. Pediatr Res 1997; 41:86A.

90. Euler AR, Stanto RS. What factors affect time to full enteral feeds in preterm infants? Pediatr Res 1999; 45:281A.

91. Paie V, Berseth CL. The presence of an immature duodenal motor response to feeding in preterm infants predicts a delay in achieving full enteral feeds. Pediatr Res 2000; 47:167A.

92. Mihatsch WA, Franz AR, Lindner W et al. Meconium passage in extremely low birthweight infants and its relation to very early enteral nutrition. Acta Paediatr 2001; 90:409–411.

93. Boccia G, Salvia G, Minella R et al. Birth asphyxia alters gastric emptying times and gastric electrical activity in term and preterm neonates. J Pediatr Gastroenterol Nutr 1999; 28:548A.

94. Berseth CL, McCoy HH. Birth asphyxia alters neonatal intestinal motility in term neonates. Pediatrics 1992; 90:669–673.

95. Berseth CL. Chronic therapeutic morphine administration alters small intestine motor patterns and gastroanal transit in preterm infants. Pediatr Res 1996; 39:305A.

96. Murase M, Ishida A, Momota T. Early gastrointestinal function and nutritional status in preterm infants with cystic periventricular leukomalacia. Biol Neonate 2002; 82:78–83.

97. Mehall JR, Kite CA, Saltzman DA et al. Prospective study of the incidence and complications of bacterial contamination of enteral feeding in neonates. J Pediatr Surg 2002; 37:1177–1182.

98. Blumenthal I, Lealman GT, Shoesmith DR. Effect of feed temperature and phototherapy on gastric emptying in the neonate. Arch Dis Child 1980; 55:562–564.

99. Costalos C, Ross I, Campbell AG et al. Is it necessary to warm infants' feeds? Arch Dis Child 1979; 54:899–901.

100. Hall RT, Callenbach JC, Sheehan MB et al. Comparison of calcium- and phosphorus-supplemented soy isolate formula with whey-predominant premature formula in very low birth weight infants. J Pediatr Gastroenterol Nutr 1984; 3:571–576.

101. Kliegman RM, Hack M, Jones P et al. Epidemiologic study of necrotizing enterocolitis among low-birth-weight infants. Absence of identifiable risk factors. J Pediatr 1982; 100:440–444.

102. McKeown RE, Marsh TD, Garrison CZ et al. The prognostic value of a risk score for necrotizing enterocolitis. Paediatr Perinat Epidemiol 1994; 8:156–165.

103. Anderson CL, Collin MF, O'Keefe JP et al. A widespread epidemic of mild necrotizing enterocolitis of unknown cause. Am J Dis Child 1984; 138:979–983.

104. De Curtis M, Paone C, Vetrano G et al. A case control study of necrotizing enterocolitis occurring over 8 years in a neonatal intensive care unit. Eur J Pediatr 1987; 146:398–400.

105. La-Gamma EF, Ostertag SG, Birenbaum MNS. Failure of delayed oral feedings to prevent necrotizing enterocolitis. Results of a study in very low birth weight neonates. Am J Dis Child 1985; 139:385–389.

106. Ostertag SG, La-Gamma EF, Reisen CE et al. Early enteral feeding does not affect the incidence of necrotizing enterocolitis. Paediatrics 1986; 77:275–280.

107. Lonnerdal B. Nutritional and physiologic significance of human milk proteins. Am J Clin Nutr 2003; 77:1537S–1543S.

108. Crissinger KD. Regulation of hemodynamics and oxygenation in developing intestine: insight into the pathogenesis of necrotizing enterocolitis. Acta Paediatr 1994; 396 (suppl.):8–10.

109. Hackett GA, Campbell S, Gamsu H et al. Doppler studies in the growth retarded fetus and prediction of neonatal necrotizing enterocolitis, haemorrhage, and neonatal morbidity. Br Med J Clin Res Ed 1987; 294:13–16.

110. Malcolm G, Ellwood D, Devonald K et al. Absent or reversed end diastolic flow velocity in the umbilical artery and necrotizing enterocolitis [see comments]. Arch Dis Child 1991; 66:805–807.

111. McDonnell M, Serra Serra V, Gaffney G et al. Neonatal outcome after pregnancy complicated by abnormal velocity waveforms in the umbilical artery. Arch Dis Child 1994; 70:F84–F89.

112. Christmann V, Liem KD, Semmekrot BA et al. Changes in cerebral, renal and mesenteric blood flow velocity during continuous and bolus infusion of indomethacin. Acta Paediatr 2002; 91:440–446.

113. Ojala R, Ruuska T, Karikoski R et al. Gastroesophageal endoscopic findings and gastrointestinal symptoms in preterm neonates with and without perinatal indomethacin exposure. J Pediatr Gastroenterol Nutr 2001; 32:182–188.

114. Fujii AM, Brown E, Mirochnick M et al. Neonatal necrotizing enterocolitis with intestinal perforation in extremely premature infants receiving early indomethacin treatment for patent ductus arteriosus. J Perinatol 2002; 22:535–540.

115. Bellander M, Ley D, Polberger S et al. Tolerance to early human milk feeding is not compromised by indomethacin in preterm infants with persistent ductus arteriosus. Acta Paediatr 2003; 92:1074–1078.

116. Hoecker C, Nelle M, Poeschl J et al. Caffeine impairs cerebral and intestinal blood flow velocity in preterm infants. Pediatrics 2002; 109:784–787.

117. Lane AJ, Coombs RC, Evans DH et al. Effect of caffeine on neonatal splanchnic blood flow. Arch Dis Child Fetal Neonatal Ed 1999; 80:F128–F129.

118. Barness LA, Mauer AM, Holliday MA et al. Commentary on breast feeding and infant formulas,including proposed standards for formulas. Pediatrics 1976; 57:278–285.

119. Willis DM, Chabot J, Radde IC et al. Unsuspected hyperosmolality of oral solutions contributing to necrotizing enterocolitis in very-low-birth-weight infants. Pediatrics 1977; 60:535–538.

120. Koo WW, Poh D, Leong M et al. Osmotic load from glucose polymers. J Parenter Enteral Nutr 1991; 15:144–147.

121. Srinivasan L, Bokiniec R, King C et al. Increased osmolality of breast milk with therapeutic additives. Arch Dis Child 2004; 89:F514–F517.

122. Kamitsuka MD, Horton MK, Williams MA. The incidence of necrotizing enterocolitis after introducing standardized feeding schedules for infants between 1250 and 2500 grams and less than 35 weeks of gestation. Pediatrics 2000; 105:379–384.

123. Tsang RC, Lucas A., Uauy R et al. Nutritional needs of the preterm infant: scientific basis and practical guidelines. Williams & Wilkins; 1993.

124. Bohnhurst B, Muller S, Dordelmann M et al. Early feeding after necrotizing enterocolitis in preterm infants. J Paediatr 2003; Oct:143(4):484–487.

125. Delzenne NM. Oligosaccharides: state of the art. Proc Nutr Soc 2003; 62:177–182.

126. Brand Miller JB, McVeagh P. Human milk oligosaccharides: 130 reasons to breast-feed. Br J Nutr 1999; 82:333–335.

127. Coppa GV, Pierani P, Zampini L et al. Oligosaccharides in human milk during different phases of lactation. Acta Paediatr 1999; 88 (suppl.):89–94.

128. Nakhla T, Fu D, Zopf D et al. Neutral oligosaccharide content of preterm human milk. Br J Nutr 1999; 82:361–367.

129. Boehm G, Lidestri M, Casetta P et al. Supplementation of a bovine milk formula with an oligosaccharide mixture increases counts of faecal bifidobacteria in preterm infants. Arch Dis Child Fetal Neonatal Ed 2002; 86:F178–F181.

130. Mountzouris KC, McCartney AL, Gibson GR. Intestinal microflora of human infants and current trends for its nutritional modulation. Br J Nutr 2002; 87:405–420.

131. Gewolb IH, Schwalbe RS, Taciak VL et al. Stool microflora in extremely low birthweight infants. Arch Dis Child Fetal Neonatal Ed 1999; 80:F167–F173.

132. Dani C, Biadaioli R, Bertini G et al. Probiotics feeding in prevention of urinary tract infection, bacterial sepsis and necrotizing enterocolitis in preterm infants. A prospective double-blind study. Biol Neonate 2002; 82:103–108.

133. Costalos C, Skouteri V, Gounaris A et al. Enteral feeding of premature infants with *Saccharomyces boulardii*. Early Hum Dev 2003; 74:89–96.

134. Kitajima H, Sumida Y, Tanaka R et al. Early administration of *Bifidobacterium breve* to preterm infants: randomised controlled trial. Arch Dis Child Fetal Neonatal Ed 1997; 76:F101–F107.

135. Pletincx M, Legein J, Vandenplas Y. Fungemia with *Saccharomyces boulardii* in a 1-year-old girl with protracted diarrhea. J Pediatr Gastroenterol Nutr 1995; 21:113–115.

136. Perapoch J, Planes AM, Querol A et al. Fungemia with *Saccharomyces cerevisiae* in two newborns, only one of whom had been treated with ultra-levura. Eur J Clin Microbiol Infect Dis 2000; 19:468–470.

137. Borriello SP, Hammes WP, Holzapfel W et al. Safety of probiotics that contain lactobacilli or bifidobacteria. Clin Infect Dis 2003; 36:775–780.

138. Millar M, Wilks M, Costeloe K. Probiotics for preterm infants? Arch Dis Child Fetal Neonatal Ed 2003; 88:F354–F358.

Background reading

Rennie J, Roberton NRC. Textbook of neonatology. Churchill Livingstone; 1999.

Tsang RC, Uauy R, Koletzko B et al., eds. Nutritional needs of the preterm infant. Scientific basis and practical guidelines, 2nd edn. Cincinnati, OH: Digital Educational; 2004.

Chapter 8

Growth and outcome

Caroline King

SUMMARY OF RECOMMENDATIONS

Monitoring growth
- Plot weight, head circumference and length on a centile chart weekly
- Weigh as necessary for an estimation of fluid balance but plot weekly for growth assessment
- When possible, the same observer should measure head circumference
- It is essential for at least one, if not both, observers to remain consistent for length measurements
- Use the most appropriate chart for plotting preterm growth

Poor growth
Diagnosis
- progressive weight loss over several days, other than the early postnatal period, when diuresis is expected
  or
- when weight, length and/or head circumference velocity decrease over 1 week
  or
- when weight velocity alone decreases over 2 weeks

Factors associated with poor growth
- inadequate nutritional input
- poor fat absorption
- chronic lung and cardiac disease
- corticosteroid treatment
- fluid restriction
- increased metabolic rate

- sodium depletion
- low-fat breast milk
- inactivity

Postdischarge nutrition

- Exclusive breast-feeding should be encouraged postdischarge with supplements of a multivitamin containing vitamin D and an iron supplement
- A phosphorus supplement may be needed until approximately 1 month postterm in breast-fed infants with serum levels < 1.5 mmol/l at discharge
- Formula-fed infants who are growth-restricted at discharge should have a nutrient-enriched postdischarge formula (NEPF) until 3 months corrected age
- Formula-fed infants who are not growth-restricted at discharge would benefit from a NEPF until approximately 1 month corrected age
- After discontinuing the NEPF, an iron-supplemented term formula is recommended until 12–18 months corrected age, depending on the adequacy of the weaning diet
- At 12–18 months, corrected cow's milk can be given as the main drink with a vitamin D supplement until school age
- On discharge all mothers should be given written information on the appropriate weaning of their preterm infant on to solid foods

INTRODUCTION

Growth is at its most rapid in the youngest individuals of all species. However when infants are born with life-threatening illness, attention is drawn away from promoting growth to life-saving therapy. Nevertheless, during this time long-term problems may be avoided if growth can be monitored. This may help to focus on optimizing nutrition and avoiding growth failure and nutritional deficiencies. Growth can most easily be monitored by measuring weight; however it is important to put this into context by looking at both length and head growth at

the same time. Whereas weight can fluctuate rapidly according to fluid balance, length and head circumference give better indications of true growth. The regular plotting of each of these anthropometric measurements on to appropriate growth charts is invaluable for growth assessment.

Poor growth has been associated with adverse outcomes in preterm infants and may be particularly detrimental in the most immature individuals. However, the vast majority of studies in this area are observational and therefore do not prove a causal link. There is evidence that in more mature infants fed breast milk, poor early growth does not predict later disadvantage. Similar randomized controlled studies have not been carried out in less mature infants.

Undernutrition could theoretically have an adverse effect on the respiratory and immune function of the preterm human infant. However when an infant demonstrates good gains in length, this will be mirrored by growth of internal organs, including the lungs; this is likely to enhance recovery and function.

In this chapter there will be a discussion of the best approach to infants who show poor growth on the neonatal unit and have not recovered by discharge.

EFFECTS OF EARLY POOR GROWTH

Short-term

The direct evidence is limited; however there may be an increased risk of sepsis.[1] Also there is a theoretical risk that undernutrition could have adverse effects on the respiratory and immune function, as demonstrated in animal models[2] and older human subjects,[3] although this has not been formally tested in preterm infants.

Some researchers have advocated an aggressive nutritional approach to prevent poor growth and any consequences arising from it.[4] A randomized controlled trial that involved the optimization of parenteral and enteral feeding from birth onwards reduced the risk of having a growth parameter < 10th centile at discharge and of infection while hospitalized. However enhanced nutrition has not been shown to reduce the risk of chronic lung disease or length of time in hospital.[1]

Finally poor growth may delay discharge; this would deny an infant the advantage of earlier close contact with its family.

Long-term

Many studies report that poor growth is associated with poorer neurodevelopmental outcome.[5-7] Those with intrauterine growth retardation (IUGR) have been shown to do worse developmentally than those who are appropriately grown.[8] Growth restrictions that are symmetrical compared to asymmetrical may result in an added penalty.[9] However, more recent data highlight the role for adverse events in the neonatal period on later outcome, independently of growth.[10]

Not all groups have seen the association between poor neonatal growth and poor neurodevelopment at 1 year.[11] Furthermore, in one of the studies that did, it was documented that their undernourished group had significantly smaller head circumferences at birth and were ventilated for significantly longer[12] – factors that could have had a detrimental effect on outcome independently of growth. There is evidence from a randomized controlled trial that breast milk can ameliorate the detrimental effects of poor early growth in moderately preterm infants (born at around 30 weeks' gestation and 1300 g at birth). In this trial[13] the developmental outcome at 18 months was compared, involving infants fed unfortified donor breast milk or preterm formula as sole diets or as supplements to maternal expressed breast milk in the neonatal period. Equivalent developmental outcome was found.[13] This occurred despite the comparatively low nutritional content of some of the breast milk used, which led to very poor growth in the neonatal period. Donor milk at that time and at this particular centre comprised drip milk, which is known to be very low in fat (see Chapter 3). Other publications from the same series of trials suggest that early malnutrition is indeed detrimental

to later neurodevelopmental outcome but only in formula-fed infants.[14,15] At 18 months both sexes did significantly worse after being randomized to a term compared to preterm formula in the neonatal period; boys, and those born small for gestational age, fared the worst.[14] By 7–8 years no differences remained for girls, while they did for boys.[15] The study period in which formula was fed lasted for an average of only 4 weeks, and although infants fed term formula grew very poorly in the neonatal period, they had caught up with the preterm formula group by 9 months.

These studies were carried out over 20 years ago, making comparison with babies managed under today's nutritional protocols difficult. There is an urgent need for randomized controlled trials to assess the long-term effects of early aggressive nutrition in smaller, more preterm infants than those in the Lucas cohort, and to confirm whether breast milk also ameliorates the adverse effects of poor growth in these infants. Currently there is more widespread use of parenteral nutrition, earlier enteral feeding and recognition that unfortified human milk and term formulas are not adequate for very preterm infants. Thus, infants are less likely to grow poorly purely through lack of nutrition; although this does still occur. The remit of this publication does not cover parenteral nutrition, which is the mainstay of early nutritional support, often for many weeks, in infants < 1000 g at birth. Nowadays those infants whose growth is poor at discharge have usually been very sick during their hospitalization; with evidence pointing to independent roles for neonatal morbidity and nutrition on later cognitive outcome.[12] Although there has been a widespread recognition that poor growth in the neonatal period needs to be addressed, the debate remains as to long-term outcomes. Recent data from the cohort studied by Alan Lucas and his team indicate that early rapid growth may increase the risk factors for cardiovascular disease later in life.[16-19] However a specific role for the type of enteral feed will be restricted to moderately preterm infants as they will be less dependent on parenteral nutrition than those who are born very preterm. For these larger,

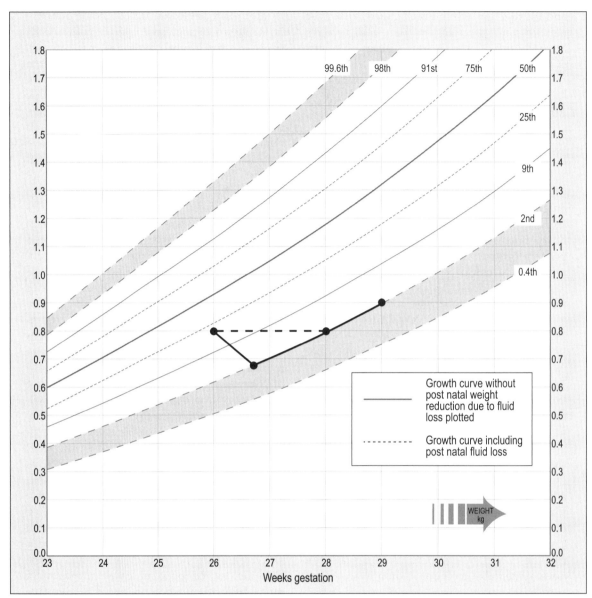

Figure 8.1 Difference if weight is plotted at the nadir compared with weekly from birth. EDD, estimated date of delivery.

moderately preterm infants, early rapid growth is more likely in those fed preterm formula compared to those on human milk.

MONITORING GROWTH

Weight

The need to monitor weight to estimate fluid balance should be distinguished from growth-monitoring. During the first 1–3 weeks most preterm infants experience a weight decline which appears to be due to a contraction of the extracellular fluid space via isotonic diuresis,[20] with the smallest infants undergoing the largest losses. Thus, during this period it is useful to plot the lowest weight an infant reaches: this then helps to establish the pattern of growth once weight gain recommences, and helps in the interpretation of later weights (Fig. 8.1). As can be seen from Figure 8.1, if the early weight loss is not plotted, growth appears poor over the first few weeks. After this early weight loss it is best to plot subsequent weights no more frequently than weekly on a centile chart. The weight of any attached equipment should be documented.

A weight gain of 15 g/kg per day has often been quoted as desirable but to grow along each different centile line requires a different amount of weight gain per kg. Many set their aim at continuing growth at intrauterine rates; however the more immature the infant, the more difficult this is to achieve. A more realistic

aim is to keep infants on the centile to which they drop after the early diuresis, assuming that this early weight loss is not excessive, i.e. limited to around 6% of birth weight. The definition of poor growth can be problematic and will remain a major discussion point.

As the baby stabilizes and approaches discharge, weighing needs to be once weekly. Weight gain appears to have a periodic pattern that is unique to each individual irrespective of short-term changes in energy input.[21] This means that more frequent plotting will include times of slower growth, adding unnecessarily to parental and neonatal unit staff anxiety (Fig. 8.2). As infants are making the transition from tube to exclusive breastfeeding, weight velocity may slow down temporarily; preparing parents and staff for this should avoid unnecessary concern.

Head circumference

Head circumference should be measured and plotted weekly, preferably by the same observer using a new paper tape or a non-stretch plasticized tape (Fig. 8.3). This tape is available from the UK Child Growth Foundation (see Resources). The measurement of head circumference gives valuable information on cerebral growth with respect to cerebral insult, as well as nutritional adequacy.[22] Head growth continues while weight falters in moderate undernutrition.[23] However even head growth may be held back when undernutrition is severe.[24]

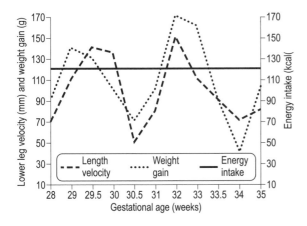

Figure 8.2 Energy intake and growth. (Courtesy of Alan Gibson, Sheffield, UK.)

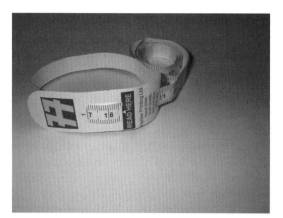

Figure 8.3   Lasso head circumference tape.

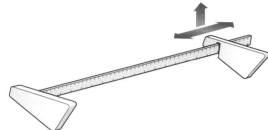

Figure 8.4(a)   Pedobaby ruler.

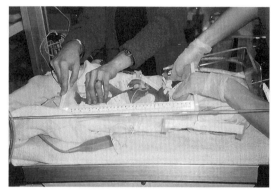

Figure 8.4(b)   Pedobaby ruler in use on a ventilated baby.

Length

Length measurement is essential for accurate growth assessment, as it reflects both skeletal and organ growth. It should be measured and plotted weekly until 40 weeks postconceptual age, then every 2 weeks until discharge. Accuracy is only ensured if the same two observers can do the measurement as there is great variability between individuals performing this measurement. If this is not possible, having the same observer at the baby's feet reduces error. A simple rigid plastic measure such as the Pedobaby 2 is very useful in unstable and ventilated babies as well as stable babies nursed in incubators (Fig. 8.4). It measures up to 50 cm and is available from Harlow Printing (see Resources). A tape measure lined up along the length of the baby is highly inaccurate and should never be used for clinical measurements.

Growth charts

It is advisable to use growth charts based on large recent data sets, as they will reflect the current growth trajectory of preterm infants. In the UK the Child Growth Foundation has developed a growth chart for preterm infants based on data collected predominantly in the 1980s (see Resources); however, centiles for length below 35 weeks' gestation are not included. Until more up-to-date length data are available, the length centiles on an earlier chart published in 1988[25] (available from Castlemead

Publications: see Resources) or those from the chart described below[26] are suitable.

The most commonly used charts in the USA appear to be those of Babson and Benda, and Lubchenco. However, they are both based on infants born before 1975. Recently recommendations have been made to use more up-to-date charts;[27] the charts of choice are those published in late 2003.[26] These include cross-sectional data from several large contemporary data sets of fetal growth (from Canada, Sweden and Australia) and data from the charts produced by the US Centers for Disease Control. These charts span from 22 to 50 weeks postconceptual age and can be freely printed from the internet. Figure 8.5 shows the growth chart with (Fig. 8.5b) and without (Fig. 8.5a) data from the longitudinal growth of preterm infants (both ill and well)[28] superimposed. The early deviation downwards of weight, length and head circumference of the infants studied by Ehrenkranz et al.[28] can quite clearly be seen, highlighting the differences in longitudinal versus cross-sectional growth curves.

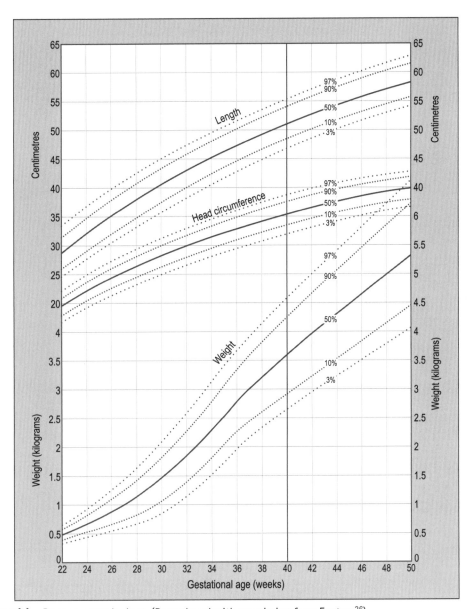

Figure 8.5(a)   Preterm growth chart. (Reproduced with permission from Fenton.[26])

There is some debate about how long to continue correcting for prematurity: up to 3 years has been suggested;[29] however 2 years appears to be sufficient.

Diagnosis of poor growth

The following guidelines provide a framework for defining when significant poor growth is occurring:

- when weight *loss* occurs progressively over several days (other than in the early postnatal period when a diuresis is expected)
- when weight, length and/or head circumference *velocity* decreases over 1 week
- when weight *velocity* alone decreases over 2 weeks

N.B.: Decreased growth velocity occurs when growth continues but at a lower rate than is needed to follow centile lines.

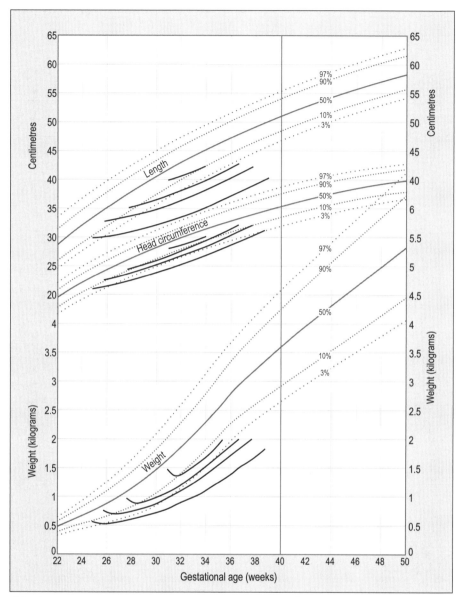

Figure 8.5(b) Data from the longitudinal growth of preterm infants (both ill and well) superimposed on the charts of Fenton.[26,28]

POOR GROWTH: CAUSES AND REMEDIES (CASE STUDY)

It has been shown that, as a population, those born preterm are significantly less likely to have followed their growth trajectory, as predicted by ultrasound measurements made at < 20 weeks' gestation, than infants born at term.[30] This suggests a high rate of IUGR in the preterm population; in addition there is a well-recognized risk of postnatal growth failure, particularly in critically ill preterm infants.[28,31] This adds considerably to the amount of catch-up growth an infant may need to make, although many will achieve this without the aid of specialized nutritional advice.[32,33]

Case study

A female infant was born at 27 weeks and 5 days gestation, weighing 1200 g. It was a spontaneous delivery with no identifiable precipitating factors. The infant's mother received two doses of antenatal steroids prior to delivery and the infant received a dose of surfactant within 1 h of delivery. She was extubated to nasal continuous positive airway pressure (CPAP) after receiving the surfactant and had an uneventful respiratory course, being weaned into room air before discharge home.

The baby's mother was able to express breast milk to supply all her infant's needs. She was encouraged to hold her baby skin to skin as soon as the infant was stable on CPAP. Every effort was made to feed freshly expressed milk. Parenteral nutrition (PN) was given from day 1. After 2 days at 5–10 ml/kg, breast milk was increased by 20 ml/kg per day and PN was decreased until a volume of 120 ml/kg breast milk and 30 ml PN was achieved, when the PN was then stopped. Breast milk intake was then increased to a total of 180 ml/kg over the next 3 days. A multivitamin containing 400 IU vitamin D and 5000 IU vitamin A was given once PN was stopped (while the infant was on unfortified breast milk). A sodium supplement was given for borderline hyponatraemia for the first 4 days after stopping PN and a phosphate supplement from the end of the first week to a week after starting breast-milk fortifier.

The growth chart (Fig. 8.6) shows the infant's weight progress, with values for serum urea superimposed and indications of when fortifier was given.

Urea started within the normal range but fell to below normal by 3 weeks old, when PN was no longer being given and the infant was solely on her mother's milk. Although weight gain began following a centile line, it remained 2 below the birth centile. Milk intake was increased to 200 ml/kg and after a further week, urea rose slightly but was still below normal with no increase in weight velocity. A decision was made to start breast-milk fortifier: it was started at half-strength for 24 h, then increased to full-strength and the multivitamin stopped as the fortifier used contained adequate vitamins. The serum urea began to rise and weight velocity improved, so further changes were not made. Four weeks after starting the fortifier, the infant's weight velocity was increasing and serum urea was rising; her weight gain stabilized along the 50th centile, which was considered acceptable as it was just 1 centile below that at birth. An iron supplement was started at 4 weeks as the unit policy was not to use a fortifier that contained iron.

With this management protocol the infant experienced a smooth transition to full enteral feeds. She avoided any episodes of sepsis and made an uneventful transition from respiratory support to room air.

Some of the reasons for poor growth and possible remedies are now discussed. See also the summary outlined in Table 8.1 and useful texts cited in the section on background reading.

Inadequate nutrient input

This has frequently been noted in the post-partum period,[34,35] with observational studies highlighting the need for both adequate pro-tein[36] and energy.[31] In the early postnatal period metabolic instability may restrict the amount of parenteral nutrition delivered, leading to early growth failure. Later on enteral feeds may be reduced due to many reasons, including feed intolerance, suspected NEC or severe gastro-oesophageal reflux.

- As discussed previously, close attention to optimizing the delivery of parenteral nutrition and enteral feeding can improve the rate of growth.[1]

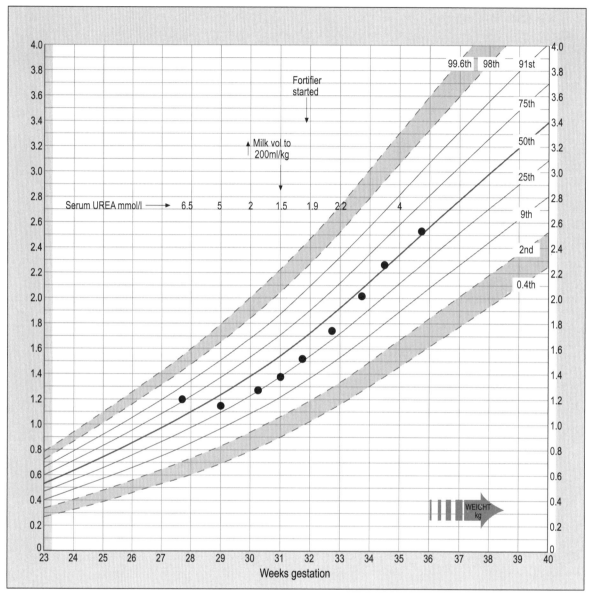

Figure 8.6 Growth chart showing the infant's weight progress with values for serum urea superimposed and indications of when parenteral nutrition was given. EDD, estimated date of delivery.

- A deficit in protein is most likely to occur in breast-milk-fed infants below 1500 g birth weight after the first weeks. (See Chapter 3 for a protocol to assess protein adequacy and on when to begin breast milk fortification.) When poor protein intake is remedied 1 week's delay in growth acceleration is likely.[37]
- Preterm infants who are demand-feeding have been shown to adjust the volume they take of feeds of different energy values to allow a constant energy intake.[38,39] Thus caution is required when adding energy supplements alone to feeds of demand-feeding infants; the volume taken may be reduced and, as a result, less protein, minerals and vitamins would be taken.
- In addition if an infant is on term formula or mature breast milk, the addition of energy

Table 8.1 Poor growth – causes and remedies

Possible causes of poor growth	Remedies

Inadequate nutrient input	• Optimize delivery of parenteral nutrition and enteral feeding
	• Ensure timely breast-milk fortification
	• Caution is required when adding energy supplements alone:
	  to feeds of demand-feeding infants
	  to term formula or mature breast milk

Immature digestion and absorption	• No benefit has been found in the use of medium-chain triglycerides • When maternal expressed breast milk is unavailable and the infant is on donor breast milk, change to preterm formula in infants who are at low risk of necrotizing enterocolitis
Chronic lung disease/cardiac disease	• If a high nutrient density is tried, it should be for a trial period only and it should be discontinued if no improved growth is seen
Fluid restriction	• Ensure that fluid restriction is clinically necessary and, where possible, negotiate a liberalization of fluid input as soon as feasible
Increase in energy expenditure	• Ensure that the infant is kept in a thermoneutral environment • In an infant who is not growing well, and in whom other possible causes have been excluded, ensure that methylxanthine dose is not excessive
Inadequate sodium replacement	• After early postnatal diuresis has occurred, monitor serum sodium levels and supplementation when necessary • Monitor serum sodium levels carefully during diuretic therapy
Low-fat breast milk	• Evaluate milk expression technique • Consider the creamatocrit technique • Consider preferential feeding of hindmilk • Help women who are producing well in excess of their infant's requirements to reduce the volume expressed gradually
Postnatal steroids	• Additional energy supplements are not recommended • Additional protein is not recommended • Ensure liberalization of nutritional input after steroids are finished to allow catch-up growth
Inactivity	• Consideration of very gentle passive exercise may be a worthwhile therapy if further evidence shows benefits and no harm

alone will lower the nutrient value per unit of energy.[40] This has been illustrated in term infants in whom energy-supplemented feeds led to poorer growth and lower albumin levels.[41]

Immature digestion and absorption

In the first weeks postnatally, very-low-birth-weight infants who are receiving substantial amounts of enteral feed may show poor weight gain as a function of immature digestion and poor absorption of dietary fat. This is most likely to occur in infants who are fed formula (see Chapter 1). Infants on DEBM experience lower fat absorption due to destruction of the milk-borne lipase during pasteurization.[42]

● Strategies have been employed to try and overcome fat malabsorption by using medium-chain triglycerides in addition to, or to replace, long-chain triglycerides; however a systematic review found no evidence of benefit in the studies carried out so far.[43]

- Those at high risk of NEC may be better served by the protection conferred by DEBM, despite the risk of temporary slower growth rates compared to formula feeding. The relative risks should be assessed by the clinical team in individual cases.

Chronic lung disease/cardiac disease

Infants developing chronic lung disease often grow poorly.[44] This may be the result of inadequate intake early on during their hospitalization[45] and increased energy expenditure later on.[46,47] However not all infants with chronic lung disease have increased requirements and a blanket prescription for increased nutrition in all of these infants should be avoided. Increased metabolic rate may also be associated with cardiac disease and these infants are often fluid-restricted.[48,49]

- Despite the apparent need for additional nutrition in infants who have developed chronic lung disease, two trials of high nutrient density versus standard formula did not show any difference in growth or respiratory outcome.[50,51] If this approach is tried it should be for a trial period only and discontinued if no improved growth is seen.
- In infants with chronic lung disease or a cardiac condition where it is suspected that energy expenditure is raised above normal, energy supplementation will need to be considered. Supplementation should be for a defined trial period and its efficacy should be evaluated before continuing. When energy alone is considered as a supplement, it is vital that other nutrients continue to be given in adequate amounts (see above with regard to volume adjustment in infants given energy-supplemented feeds). It is the author's experience that, with the declining incidence of severe chronic lung disease and more careful attention to nutrition from earlier postnatally, there is virtually no place for the use of energy supplements in these infants.

Fluid restriction

A systematic review has suggested that fluid restriction may be beneficial for lung function.[52] However the effect of sodium intake independent of fluid intake does not seem to have been taken into consideration. There is good evidence that early excessive sodium intake given before the immediate postnatal diuresis may be more damaging than liberal fluid intake with respect to later lung function.[53] It is practice on the author's unit to wait until there has been an approximately 6% reduction in birth weight until sodium supplementation is begun postnatally. Fluid restriction inevitably also restricts nutritional intake and is probably responsible for a large proportion of early growth-faltering.

- Ensure that fluid restriction is clinically necessary and, where possible, negotiate a liberalization of fluid input as soon as feasible. As an approximate guide, babies on human milk usually require a minimum of 180 ml/kg and can tolerate up to 220 ml/kg, although this should rarely be needed. In contrast, preterm formulas are designed to provide recommended intakes when fed at 150 ml/kg.

Increase in energy expenditure

There are situations where an iatrogenic increase in energy expenditure can occur; for example, both cold stress and the use of methylxanthines may lead to an increased metabolic rate and result in poor weight gain.[54,55] The latter may not often be a clinically significant factor but may occasionally be worth considering. Infants with certain cardiac conditions and some with chronic lung disease can have increased energy expenditure (see above).

- Ensure that the infant is kept in a thermo-neutral environment
- In an infant who is not growing well, and in whom other possible causes have been excluded, ensure that the methylxanthine dose is not excessive

- If energy supplementation is considered, see under *Chronic lung disease/cardiac disease* above

Inadequate sodium replacement

Infants born < 32 weeks' gestation have high sodium requirements because of immature renal function and can need large amounts of sodium supplements to maintain normal serum levels. However it is practice on the author's unit to wait until there has been an approximately 6% reduction in birth weight until sodium supplementation is begun postnatally.[53] In addition some infants with chronic lung disease have courses of diuretics, which could lead to hyponatraemia due to inadequate sodium replacement.

Poor growth can be a consequence of chronic hyponatraemia.[56] In addition, neurodevelopment disadvantage at 10–13 years was shown in a group of infants randomized to diets without sodium supplementation compared to those who were supplemented for only 10 days in the early neonatal period.[57] Although some infants require high intakes of sodium, this has not been shown to have a detrimental effect on blood pressure later in childhood.[58]

- Sodium administration should be avoided before the early postnatal diuresis has occurred; thereafter close monitoring of serum sodium levels is required, with supplementation when necessary
- It is vital to have a record of the infant's serum sodium levels before starting diuretics and to continue monitoring so that timely sodium replacement can be started if needed

Low-fat breast milk

When an otherwise well infant is growing poorly despite a normal or raised serum urea level, the infant may be receiving insufficient non-protein energy. Due to the changing composition of breast milk, if the breast is not emptied during expression mostly foremilk will be collected; this is low-fat (see Chapter 4). In addition a personal observation of the author is that a few women produce copious amounts of low-fat milk, as judged by poor weight gain despite normal urea levels and a good volume of enteral intake.

- Evaluate the milk expression technique (the creamatocrit technique could be used: see Chapter 3)
- Consider a preferential feeding of hindmilk or at least the stored milk with the largest fat layer (see Chapter 3)
- Help women who are producing well in excess of their infant's requirements gradually to reduce the volume expressed. This must be done carefully to ensure that a adequate supply is maintained (see Chapter 5)

Postnatal steroids

The use of postnatal steroids in infants who are at risk of chronic lung disease is associated with poor growth. Dexamethasone treatment and ventilation appear to reduce growth independently; in particular, length is affected.[31,59] Weight gain is also impaired during steroid treatment but not to the same extent as length.[59] This puts these infants at risk of excessive adiposity if an energy supplement is given. This drug can lead to increased catabolism whereby the protein breakdown rate is accelerated,[60] hence an increased protein intake is not likely to be utilized but may add a metabolic stress. This drug treatment is discussed due to its profound effects on growth; however its use has declined drastically due to unacceptable long-term side-effects.[61] If in future different steroid doses from those used in the studies mentioned are used, the effect on growth and metabolism may be different and should be investigated.

- Additional energy supplements are not recommended
- Additional protein is not recommended
- Ensure liberalization of nutritional input after steroids are finished to allow catch-up growth

Inactivity

It is possible that prolonged periods of inactivity in preterm infants are detrimental to both weight gain and bone health. A systematic review found evidence for a very small effect of massage on weight gain but the reviewers felt that overall the evidence was not strong enough to justify the nursing time necessary.[62] However a subsequent paper has found improved weight gain;[63] this has also been seen with passive physical activity.[64,65] There are also benefits with respect to bone mineralization (see Chapter 2).

- It may be worthwhile considering gentle passive exercise if further evidence shows benefits and no harm

POSTDISCHARGE NUTRITION

Introduction

Until relatively recently there were few recommendations concerning the growth and nutrition of preterm babies after they had been discharged from the neonatal unit. This was an area that had a dearth of investigations, making it difficult to establish aims. Now postdischarge nutrition has come under more scrutiny as there are concerns that it may have repercussions for longer-term health.[66] Optimizing nutritional status and growth are the main aims. It is becoming apparent that deviation from optimal growth both through under- and overnutrition may have long-term adverse consequences. In term infants the contribution of poor growth, both in utero and after delivery, to chronic diseases of adulthood is currently a hotly debated topic. In addition, excessive weight gain, with its risk for obesity later in childhood, is now a concern. It is recognized that by the time of discharge many preterm infants demonstrate poor growth. This may be caused by an accumulating nutritional deficiency caused by poor nutritional management while hospitalized;[34,36,67] however the role of severe illness on growth needs further examination. Interestingly, it appears that growth restriction in the neonatal period is not necessarily a predictor of continued poor growth postdischarge, as most infants catch up without the aid of specialized nutrition.[32,33] Infants whose mothers wish to

breastfeed have to make the transition from prescribed amounts of milk by tube to demand-feeding at the breast. During the latter process the difficulty involved in estimating volume taken can lead to anxiety. Many mother-infant pairs do not manage this transition but if they do, it has been reported that infants grow more slowly initially; however later catch-up growth can be expected. For formula-fed infants it used to be accepted practice to transfer babies on discharge from a highly nutrient-dense preterm formula to standard nutrient-density term formula. This has been shown to result in poorer short-term length gain in the immediate post-discharge period.[68]

For both breast- and formula-fed infants there are various implications for postdischarge nutrition. Two significant ones are firstly, the demonstration of an increased demand for nutrients, as shown by very-high-volume consumption;[69] and secondly, an accelerated rate of bone mineralization at approximately 42–43 weeks' postconceptual age.[70]

For the breast-fed infant a crucial factor may be the achievement by the mother of successful lactation before the infant feeds exclusively at the breast. Rather than producing just enough milk for the needs her infant had while in hospital, she may need to produce significantly more. This will then help her to keep up with her baby's demands for catch-up growth. When faltering growth occurs in breast-fed babies, postdischarge supplementation of maternal expressed breast milk with breast-milk fortifier has been advocated.[71] However the rationale for this is debatable and will be discussed later.

Formula-fed infants now have the alternative of NEPF rather than term formula at discharge. These formulas are designed to bridge the gap between term and preterm formulas and allow an infant to ingest comparable amounts of nutrients in a smaller volume than would be necessary for term formula (see Table 8.2 for a comparison of postdischarge formulas).

There have been several recent reviews of postdischarge nutrition, which give useful additional knowledge on this area. Both breast- and formula-fed infants are discussed and the need for further studies to elucidate long-term

Table 8.2 Postdischarge formulas

Nutrients per 100 ml	Nutriprem 2 (Cow & Gate)	Premcare (Farley's)	Neosure Advance (Ross)	Enfacare (Mead Johnson)
Energy (kcal) (×4.18 = kJ)	75	72	74	74
Protein (g)	2	1.8	1.9	2.1
Fat (g)	4.1	4	4	3.9
AA, DHA	✓	✓	✓	✓
Carbohydrate (g)	7.4	7.2	7.6	7.7
Minerals				
Sodium (mg)	26	22	24	26
Potassium (mg)	77	77	105	78
Chloride (mg)	46	46	58	58
Calcium (mg)	94	70	78	89
Phosphorus (mg)	50	35	46	49
Ca : P ratio	2:1	2:1	1.7:1	1.8:1
Magnesium (mg)	7	5.2	6.6	5.9
Iron (mg)	1.2	0.65	1.3	1.3
Zinc (mg)	0.7	0.6	0.9	0.9
Copper (µg)	60	57	89	89
Iodine (µg)	20	7.3	11	15
Manganese (µg)	7	5	7.4	11
Selenium (µg)	1.9	1.3	1.7	2.1
Vitamins				
Vitamin A (µg)[a]	99	100	102	99
Vitamin D (µg)[a]	1.6	1.3	1.3	1.5
Vitamin E (TE) (mg)[a]	1.9	1.5	2.6	3
Vitamin K (µg)	5.9	6.0	8	5.9
Thiamin B_1 (mg)	0.09	0.09	0.16	0.15
Riboflavin B_2 (mg)	0.11	0.1	0.11	0.15
Niacin (NE) (mg)	1.7	1.0	1.44	1.5
Pantothenic acid (mg)	0.62	0.4	0.59	0.63
Pyridoxine B_6 (mg)	0.08	0.08	0.07	0.07
Folic acid (µg)	20	25	18	19
Vitamin B_{12} (µg)	0.28	0.2	0.3	0.22
Biotin (µg)	3	1.1	6.6	4.4
Vitamin C (mg)	16	15	11	12
Other				
Choline (mg)	32	5.1	12	18
Taurine (mg)	4.9	5.1	NS	4.4
Inositol (mg)	29	–	4.4	22
Carnitine (mg)	–	1.1	NS	1.48
Nucleotides (mg)	1.8	–	NS	3.36
Beta-carotene (µg)	6.6	6	NS	–
Osmolality (mOsm/kg)	290	280	250	230
Potential renal solute load (mOsm/L)	124	116	NS	NS

_ Not present.
[a] Conversion factors: vitamin A: µg ÷ 0.3 = IU; vitamin D: µg ÷ 40 = IU. 1 IU vitamin E = 1 mg d, Lα tocopherol acetate.
AA, arachidonic acid; DHA, docosahexaenoic acid; NS, not specified.

This information is correct at the time of publication but may change: please check with the manufacturers

outcomes is highlighted. The lack of consensus concerning the use of postdischarge formulas endorses the recommendation for further work, as recommendations for their use range from only 2 months postdischarge to the whole of the first year.[72–77]

LONG-TERM OUTCOMES OF POOR GROWTH POSTDISCHARGE

Term infants

Severe malnutrition in the fetal and neonatal period is associated with long-term adverse effects, with respect both to neurodevelopmental outcome and long-term morbidity.

The Barker or fetal origins hypothesis suggests that growth in utero can predict the risk of adult disease in term infants.[78–80] However the link with later blood pressure and cholesterol levels may be weak.[81,82]

With respect to growth during the first year, an association has been shown between poor weight gain and later risk of coronary heart disease, independent of birth weight.[83,84]

However it increasingly appears that restricted growth in utero followed by catch-up growth and later obesity may be more important triggers of later morbidity in term infants.[84–87] Recently it has been hypothesized that it is not just catch-up growth but any accelerated growth in infancy that may lead to an increased risk of later chronic disease in adulthood.[18]

Preterm infants

An observational study has shown an association between poor neurodevelopmental outcome and slow growth from term (i.e. at around the time of discharge) to 8 months;[88] this was irrespective of growth from birth to term. Most other studies do not distinguish between poor growth pre- or postterm and report that poor growth is associated with poorer neurodevelopmental outcome (see section above on growth during hospitalization for a dis-

cussion of the implications of poor growth during this period).

There is contradictory evidence concerning the appearance of risk factors for cardio-vascular disease: some researchers have shown that they are increased in those born preterm irrespective of growth,[89,90] while others have shown that they are not increased unless there is IUGR.[91] However one study showed that the more weight gained from 18 months, the higher the risk of raised insulin levels.[92] As for term infants, accelerated growth in the early neonatal period has been proposed as a risk factor for later disease.[19]

Summary

There is evidence that being born preterm, high-risk and/or small for gestational age is associated with developmental delay and cardiovascular risk factors. Poor postnatal growth may be an independent risk factor for a poor developmental outcome, irrespective of intrauterine growth. However increased weight gain during childhood, particularly after infancy, may increase the chances of adverse cardiovascular health.

Most studies are weakened by the fact that they are observational, and despite controlling for as many confounding factors as possible, there is the risk that growth is simply associated with other factors that lead to, rather than cause, poor outcome.

A significant number of small-for-gestational-age infants catch up in the first year and appear to have a good outcome.[88] Of those small-for-gestational-age infants who remain small and those average-for-gestational-age infants who grow poorly after discharge, a vital but as yet unanswered question is: does the enhancement of catch-up growth after discharge give any health advantages?

Further studies are needed to establish the optimum rate of growth for preterm infants postdischarge and to discover if the age at which catch-up growth occurs is important. These studies should address, in particular, growth and the risk of later chronic disease.

BREASTFEEDING POSTDISCHARGE

Growth

Many studies investigating the effects of post-discharge formula have included a breast-fed control group.[93–96] By its very nature it is impossible to randomize babies to breast milk postdischarge, so all these studies will be confounded by factors associated with a mother's choice and ability to sustain breastfeeding after hospitalization. In most of these studies the breast-fed group were a similar size to the formula-fed groups at study entry but grew more slowly subsequently. In general those babies that were breast-fed tended to grow at a similar rate to those on term formula;[96,97] however both groups grew more slowly than babies on an enriched formula. Despite this initial lag in weight gain, the breast-fed infants showed catch-up growth.[93,98,99] It is important to note that poor early head growth reported in some breast-fed infants did not predict later neurodevelopment disadvantage.[99]

When faltering growth occurs in breast-fed babies it has been suggested that there should be continued supplementation of maternal expressed breast milk with breast-milk fortifier to improve nutritional intake.[71] However this requires that the infant take the fortified breast milk by bottle, with the result that, although milk supply is maintained via milk expression, the opportunity for mother and infant to establish breastfeeding is denied. This approach seems unjustified in view of the limited evidence that promoting growth is beneficial. As above, it may interfere with the establishment of breastfeeding. During the time of rapid bone mineralization (from the last trimester to just beyond term date), supplemental phosphate may help growth[100] as well as bone mineralization.

Neurodevelopmental outcome

In all studies carried out so far, the breast-fed control group has usually fared better than their formula-fed counterparts, whatever their growth performance (see Chapter 1).

Bone health

There is some evidence that additional phosphate is needed to help growth and bone mineralization in the immediate postdischarge period.[100] This coincides with a period spanning approximately 1 month of corrected age, when a period of enhanced bone mineral accretion has been demonstrated.[70] However, unsupplemented infants will eventually catch up.[101,102] When mineral-supplemented human milk was given during hospitalization, bone mineral density was positively related to length of breastfeeding postdischarge,[102] although a mechanism for this finding has not yet been established. Furthermore at 12-year follow-up early mineral intake or type of milk had no effect on height[103] or bone mineral density.[104] Infants who are exclusively breastfeeding should have a vitamin D supplement as their needs will exceed the low levels supplied in breast milk.

Despite the evidence showing that bone mineralization in breast-fed preterm infants eventually shows catch-up, it is still vitally important to ensure adequate mineral supplementation in the early neonatal period to reduce the risk of severe osteopenia and fractures (see Chapter 2).

Iron

Preterm and low-birth-weight infants have much depleted iron stores compared to term infants and require iron supplementation at an earlier age than term infants (see Chapter 2). Due to the low levels in breast milk, those who are breast-fed postdischarge will need an iron supplement until their weaning diet contains sufficient iron.

Zinc

A study to evaluate zinc status in preterm babies found satisfactory levels in breast-fed infants to 6 months.[105] This suggests that, for most babies, zinc supplementation is not needed postdischarge. However there have been reports of zinc deficiency in human-milk-fed preterm infants (see Chapter 2); thus it is important to ensure a good dietary source in weaning foods.

Maintenance of lactation

If a mother's milk production is optimized during the early weeks of expression, this will put her in a better position to meet her infant's needs at discharge and beyond. It will also help her to cope with the demand if her baby needs to make catch-up growth. Babies are often discharged apparently fully breastfeeding but soon fail to thrive; this in turn leads to a feeling of failure, with mothers blaming their milk as not 'good enough' for their infant. However it is more likely that it is a problem of quantity rather than quality, with women having difficulty increasing their milk volumes to match their infant's increasing requirements.

Summary

It is unlikely that there is any benefit to be gained from postdischarge supplementation of exclusively breast-fed infants with nutrients other than iron, vitamins and possibly phosphorus. Despite poorer growth in the neonatal period, infants fed human milk while hospitalized and for the first few months postdischarge had no long-term growth or bone mineralization disadvantages, but have shown developmental advantages.

NUTRIENT–ENRICHED POSTDISCHARGE FORMULA

Growth

Many studies evaluating NEPF have shown improved growth, but often this occurred in the first month or two, with no additional advantage thereafter.[39,94,106–108] However, one research group found no differences in growth.[109] Many other observational studies show continued catch-up growth beyond 6 months in those fed

breast milk or standard term formula in the early postdischarge period.[110,111]

In many of the studies using postdischarge formula, the growth advantage was restricted to boys; no mechanism for this discrepancy in response to enhanced nutrition has yet been evaluated. Alan Lucas and his group have made similar findings during their evaluation of early postnatal nutrition (see above).

Neurodevelopmental outcome

Despite the improved growth demonstrated in some studies, there has not been a concomitant improvement in neurodevelopmental outcome.[94,112,113] It will be important to see if growth advantages shown by the studies discussed above are maintained and if they translate into any other tangible benefits.

Protein

A common finding was that growth rates in infants fed NEPF were often greater despite a similar intake of total energy, leading to suggestions that increased protein may have been the growth-promoting factor. This has been tested and no differences in growth attributable to different protein intakes were found at 12-week follow-up.[114] More worryingly, in term small-for-gestational-age girls, poorer neurodevelopmental assessment was found at 9 months when fed NEPF compared to those on term formula, although there was no difference at 18 months.[115]

Nutrient–enriched feeds designed for term infants

The use of nutrient-enriched prescribable ready-to-feed formulas has been advocated for preterm infants postdischarge. However, these formulas have not been evaluated in this population and have several potential drawbacks. They are not designed with the needs of the preterm infant in mind, for whom additional calcium, phosphorus, zinc and iron may be an advantage.

Bone health

Improved bone mineral status has been found in infants randomized to formulas with higher calcium and phosphorus compared to term formula in the postdischarge period.[116,117] However in follow-up studies spanning several years, all babies eventually appear to attain the same bone mineral status as their term-born counterparts. Body size and therefore growth itself have an important effect on bone mineralization independently of mineral intake.[100,103,104] Postdischarge feeds containing vitamin D in the range 40–80 IU/100 ml were found to lead to satisfactory status of this vitamin throughout the first year.[118]

Iron

In one study, formulas containing either 1.3 or 2 mg iron/100 ml up to 1 year both led to satisfactory iron nutritional status and development in infants around 1400 g birth weight and 32 weeks' gestation.[119] It is to be noted that there was a trend towards lower zinc and copper levels in the infants on the higher iron formula at 12 months. In another study, 1 mg/100 ml of iron was sufficient for a group of relatively well preterm infants.[120]

Zinc

It has been suggested that formula-fed infants would benefit from a milk containing 1.2 mg/100 ml through infancy to make up for early losses in gut secretions coupled with high requirements.[121] However, the possible interactions with other divalent metals must be considered (see above); thus, levels as high as 1.2 mg/100 ml may be excessive unless balanced with adequate iron and copper. In practice the zinc levels seen in current NEPF seem reasonable, including the ratios of zinc, iron and copper.

Selenium

There are data indicating that a selenium-supplemented formula would be useful, as status is poor until solids are started in preterm infants fed unsupplemented milks.[122]

Summary

In formula-fed babies it appears that in the first few months postdischarge, catch-up growth can be accelerated with the use of enriched formulas, and that growth-restricted infants may benefit most. Nevertheless, many infants will make catch-up growth without this intervention, and so far significant developmental benefits have not been demonstrated. There is a need for continued observation of the outcome of feeding nutrient-enriched feeds postdischarge.

RECOMMENDATIONS FOR POSTDISCHARGE NUTRITION

Breast-fed

The following recommendations are based on the author's practice; individual infants may require different treatment. Preterm infants who are exclusively breast-fed at discharge will need both iron and vitamin D supplements. A phosphate supplement postdischarge should be considered in infants with serum levels < 1.5. It may be useful to continue this supplement until approximately 1 month of corrected age. A dose of vitamin D 200-400 IU/day should be aimed for. This may be best provided as part of a multivitamin supplement; although there may not be a specific need for the other vitamins, their provision would act as a safety net to ensure adequate intake. Vitamin supplements in addition to this should be discouraged unless a specific need is identified, since there may be a risk of excessive intake.[96,123] Other published recommendations advise that around 2 mg/kg iron is continued postdischarge. For many infants, less iron is probably sufficient and there is an advantage to giving a single dose which provides 2 mg/kg at discharge, but not adjusting it with growth, so that the infant 'grows out' of the dose, with the weaning diet gradually taking over supply. When an infant is shown to be on a nutritionally balanced weaning diet (or, at one year corrected age), the iron supplements can be stopped. An infant who continues to be breast-fed during the first year and who goes directly on to unmodified cow's milk should continue on vitamin D until school age, following government guidelines in the UK[124] and USA.[125] If breast-feeding is replaced by an infant formula, the vitamin D can be stopped but will need to be restarted when unmodified cow's milk is the main drink and continued as above. Infant formula should continue to 12–18 months' corrected age depending on the adequacy of the weaning diet.

Formula-fed

The following recommendations are based on the author's practice; individual infants may require different treatment. Formula-fed infants who have not made catch-up growth by discharge should transfer from preterm formula to an NEPF until approximately 3 months corrected age. Formula-fed infants who are not growth-restricted at discharge would benefit from an NEPF until approximately 1 month corrected age, as it will provide more calcium and phosphorus to aid bone mineralization. It would be an advantage for the feed to contain at least 1 mg/100 ml iron, as this will remove the need for iron supplements in most infants. Additional vitamins should be discouraged unless a specific need is identified since there may be a risk of excessive intake.[96,123]

The NEPF should be replaced with a standard term formula which should be used until 12–18 months' corrected age, depending on the adequacy of the weaning diet. It is important that unmodified cow's milk is not introduced before 12–18 months as there is a risk of iron deficiency.[126] With timely and balanced weaning on to solid foods there should not be any need for supplementary vitamins or iron.[127]

Once unmodified cow's milk is the main milk drink, all infants should receive children's vitamin drops containing vitamin D until school age, according to the government guidelines in the UK[124] and USA.[125]

Weaning on to solids

Despite the lack of randomized controlled trials in this area, parents will need practical advice. Using the available data, a weaning leaflet has been designed for preterm infants; it is available from the UK neonatal charity BLISS (see Resources).

Conclusion

Initially, nutritional input needs to be optimized, taking into consideration the risks and benefits of promoting early rapid growth. The ultimate feeding and nutritional goal is to achieve baby-led demand-feeding to enable catch-up growth to occur if necessary. With demand-feeding most infants who are born small-for-gestational-age do manage to catch up within the first year. There remain questions about the desirability of accelerating growth in those who are already growing satisfactorily, and about the predisposition to later chronic disease.

References

1. Wilson DC, Cairns P, Halliday HL et al. Randomised controlled trial of an aggressive nutritional regimen in sick very low birthweight infants. Arch Dis Child Fetal Neonatal Ed 1997; 77:F4–11.

2. Kalenga M. Lung growth and development during experimental malnutrition. Pediatr Pulmonol 1997; 16 (suppl.):165–166.

3. Ong TJ, Mehta A, Ogston S et al. Prediction of lung function in the inadequately nourished. Arch Dis Child 1998; 79:18–21.

4. Thureen PJ, Hay W-WJ. Early aggressive nutrition in preterm infants. Semin Neonatol 2001; 6:403–415.

5. Powls A, Botting N, Cooke RW et al. Growth impairment in very low birthweight children at 12 years: correlation with perinatal and outcome variables. Arch Dis Child Fetal Neonatal Ed 1996; 75:F152–F157.

6. Brandt I, Sticker EJ, Lentze MJ. Catch-up growth of head circumference of very low birth weight, small

for gestational age preterm infants and mental development to adulthood. J Pediatr 2003; 142:463–468.

7. Cooke RW, Foulder-Hughes L. Growth impairment in the very preterm and cognitive and motor performance at 7 years. Arch Dis Child 2003; 88:482–487.

8. Matilainen R, Heinonen K, Siren-Tiusanen H. Effect of intrauterine growth retardation (IUGR) on the psychological performance of preterm children at preschool age. J Child Psychol Psychiatry 1988; 29:601–609.

9. Martikainen MA. Effects of intrauterine growth retardation and its subtypes on the development of the preterm infant. Early Hum Dev 1992; 28:7–17.

10. Gutbrod T, Wolke D, Soehne B et al. Effects of gestation and birth weight on the growth and development of very low birthweight small for gestational age infants: a matched group comparison. Arch Dis Child Fetal Neonatal Ed 2000; 82:F208–F214.

11. Davidson S, Schrayer A, Wielunsky E et al. Energy intake, growth, and development in ventilated very-low-birth-weight infants with and without bronchopulmonary dysplasia. Am J Dis Child 1990; 144:553–559.

12. Hayakawa M, Okumura A, Hayakawa F et al. Nutritional state and growth and functional maturation of the brain in extremely low birth weight infants. Pediatrics 2003; 111:991–995.

13. Lucas A, Morley R, Cole TJ et al. A randomised multicentred study of human milk vs formula and later development in preterm infants. Arch Dis Child 1994; 70:F141–F146.

14. Lucas A, Morley R, Cole TJ et al. Early diet in preterm babies and developmental status at 18 months. Lancet 1990; 335:1477–1481.

15. Lucas A, Morley R, Cole T. Randomised trial of early diet in preterm babies and later intelligence quotient. Br Med J 1998; 317:1481–1487.

16. Singhal A, Cole TJ, Fewtrell M et al. Breastmilk feeding and lipoprotein profile in adolescents born preterm: follow-up of a prospective randomised study. Lancet 2004; 363:1571–1578.

17. Singhal A, Fewtrell M, Cole TJ et al. Low nutrient intake and early growth for later insulin resistance in adolescents born preterm. Lancet 2003; 361:1089–1097.

18. Singhal A, Cole TJ, Fewtrell M et al. Is slower early growth beneficial for long-term cardiovascular health? Circulation 2004; 109:1108–1113.

19. Singhal A, Lucas A. Early origins of cardiovascular disease: is there a unifying hypothesis? Lancet 2004; 363:1642–1645.

20. Bauer K, Versmold H. Postnatal weight loss in preterm neonates less than 1500 g is due to isotonic dehydration of the extracellular volume. Acta Paediatr Scand 1989; 360 (suppl.):37–42.

21. Gibson AT. Early postnatal growth – what should we measure? Why should we bother? In: Controversies in nutrition: feeding the preterm infant (abstract). London: Hammersmith Hospital; 1994.

22. Lindley AA, Benson JE, Grimes C et al. The relationship in neonates between clinically measured head circumference and brain volume estimated from head CT-scans. Early Hum Dev 1999; 56:17–29.

23. Radmacher P, Gilliatt N, Rafail S et al. Changes in weight and head circumference during the first postnatal weeks in very very low birth weight infants. Pediatr Res 2004; 43:267A.

24. Marks KH, Maisels MJ, Moore E et al. Head growth in sick premature infants: a longitudinal study. J Pediatr 1979; 94:282–285.

25. Keen DV, Pearse RG. Weight, length, and head circumference curves for boys and girls of between 20 and 42 weeks' gestation. Arch Dis Child 1988; 63:1170–1172.

26. Fenton TR. A new growth chart for preterm babies: Babson and Benda's chart updated with recent data and a new format. BMC Pediatr 2003; 3:13.

27. Sherry B, Mei Z, Grummer-Strawn L et al. Evaluation of and recommendations for growth references for very low birth weight (< or =1500 grams) infants in the United States. Pediatrics 2003; 111:750–758.

28. Ehrenkranz RA, Younes N, Lemons JA et al. Longitudinal growth of hospitalized very low birth weight infants. Pediatrics 1999; 104:280–289.

29. Wang Z, Sauve RS. Assessment of postneonatal growth in VLBW infants: selection of growth references and age adjustment for prematurity. Can J Public Health 1998; 89:109–114.

30. Bukowski R, Gahn D, Denning J et al. Impairment of growth in fetuses destined to deliver preterm. Am J Obstet Gynecol 2001; 185:463–467.

31. Berry MA, Abrahamowicz M, Usher RH. Factors associated with growth of extremely premature infants during initial hospitalization. Pediatrics 1997; 100:640–646.

32. Morley R, Lucas A. Randomized diet in the neonatal period and growth performance until 7.5–8 y of age in preterm children. Am J Clin Nutr 2000; 71:822–828.

33. Gargus R, Vohr BR, Tucker R et al. Impact of early growth velocity on post natal growth in ELBW infants born AGA. Pediatr Res 2003; 53:406A.

34. Embleton NE, Pang N, Cooke RJ. Postnatal malnutrition and growth retardation: an inevitable consequence of current recommendations in preterm infants? Pediatrics 2001; 107:270–273.

35. Fenton TR, McMillan DD, Sauve RS. Nutrition and growth analysis of very low birth weight infants. Pediatrics 1990; 86:378–383.

36. Carlson SJ, Ziegler EE. Nutrient intakes and growth of very low birth weight infants. J Perinatol 1998; 18:252–258.

37. Georgieff MK, Sasanow SR, Pereira GR. Serum transthyretin levels and protein intake as predictors of weight gain velocity in premature infants. J Pediatr Gastroenterol Nutr 1987; 6:775–779.

38. Brooke OG, Kinsey JM. High energy feeding in small for gestation infants. Arch Dis Child 1985; 60:42–46.

39. Cooke RJ, Griffin IJ, McCormick K et al. Feeding preterm infants after hospital discharge: effect of dietary manipulation on nutrient intake and growth. Pediatr Res 1998; 43:355–360.

40. Cooke RJ, McCormick K, Griffin IJ et al. Feeding preterm infants after hospital discharge: effect of diet on body composition. Pediatr Res 1999; 46:461–464.

41. Clarke S, MacDonald A, Booth IW. Impaired growth and nitrogen deficiency in infants receiving an energy supplemented standard infant formula. 50th Study day. Paediatric Group BDA (April) 1999;01.

42. Williamson S, Finucane E, Ellis H. Effect of heat treatment of human milk absorption of nitrogen, fat, sodium, calcium and phosphorus by preterm infants. Arch Dis Child 1978; 53:553–563.

43. Klenoff-Brumberg HL, Genen LH. High versus low medium chain triglyceride content of formula for promoting short term growth of preterm infants. Cochrane Database Syst Rev 2003; 1:CD002777.

44. Ryan S. Nutrition in neonatal chronic lung disease. Eur J Pediatr 1998; 157 (suppl. 1):S19–S22.

45. deRegnier RA, Guilbert TW, Mills MM et al. Growth failure and altered body composition are established by one month of age in infants with bronchopulmonary dysplasia. J Nutr 1996; 126:168–175.

46. de Meer K, Westerterp KR, Houwen RH et al. Total energy expenditure in infants with bronchopulmonary dysplasia is associated with respiratory status. Eur J Pediatr 1997; 156:299–304.

47. Leitch CA, Denne SC. Increased energy expenditure in premature infants with chronic lung disease. Pediatr Res 2000; 47:291A.

48. Schwarz SM, Gewitz MH, See CC et al. Enteral nutrition in infants with congenital heart disease and growth failure. Pediatrics 1990; 86:368–373.

49. Yahav J, Avigad S, Frand M et al. Assessment of intestinal and cardiorespiratory function in children with congenital heart disease on high-caloric formulas. J Pediatr Gastroenterol Nutr 1985; 4:778–785.

50. Fewtrell MS, Adams C, Wilson DC et al. Randomized trial of high nutrient density formula versus standard formula in chronic lung disease. Acta Paediatr 1997; 86:577–582.

51. Moyer-Mileur L, Chan GM, Ammon BB et al. Growth and tolerance of calorically dense, high fat feeding in infants with bronchopulmonary dysplasia (BPD). Pediatr Res 1994; 35:317A.

52. Bell EF, Acarregui MJ. Restricted versus liberal water intake for preventing morbidity and mortality in preterm infants. Cochrane Database Syst Rev 2001; 3:CD000503.

53. Modi N. Clinical implications of postnatal alterations in body water distribution. Semin Neonatol 2003; 8:301–306.

54. Sauer PJ, Dane HJ, Visser HK. Longitudinal studies on metabolic rate, heat loss, and energy cost of growth in low birth weight infants. Pediatr Res 1984; 18:254–259.

55. Bauer J, Maier K, Linderkamp O et al. Effect of caffeine on oxygen consumption and metabolic rate in very low birth weight infants with idiopathic apnea. Pediatrics 2001; 107:660–663.

56. Haycock GB. The influence of sodium on growth in infancy. Pediatr Nephrol 1993; 7:871–875.

57. Al Dahhan J, Jannoun L, Haycock GB. Effect of salt supplementation of newborn premature infants on neurodevelopmental outcome at 10-13 years of age. Arch Dis Child Fetal Neonatal Ed 2002; 86:F120–F123.

58. Lucas A, Morley R. Does early nutrition in infants born before term programme later blood pressure? Br Med J 1994; 309:304–308.

59. Gibson AT, Pearse RG, Wales JKH. Growth retardation after dexamethasone administrating assessment by knemometry. Arch Dis Child 1993; 69:505–509.

60. Van-Goudoever J, Wattimena JDL, Carnielli V. The effect of dexamethasone on protein metabolism in infants with bronchopulomary dysplasis. J Pediatr 1994; 124:112–118.

61. Halliday HL. Postnatal steroids and chronic lung disease in the newborn. Paediatr Respir Rev 2004; 5 (suppl. A):S245–S248.

62. Vickers A, Ohlsson A, Lacy JB et al. Massage for promoting growth and development of preterm and/or low birth-weight infants. Cochrane Database Syst Rev 2000; 2:CD000390.

63. Ferber SG, Kuint J, Weller A et al. Massage therapy by mothers and trained professionals enhances weight gain in preterm infants. Early Hum Dev 2002; 67:37–45.

64. Moyer-Mileur LJ, Brunstetter V, McNaught TP et al. Daily physical activity program increases bone mineralization and growth in preterm very low birth weight infants. Pediatrics 2000; 106:1088–1092.

65. Eliakim A, Dolfin T, Weiss E et al. The effects of exercise on body weight and circulating leptin in premature infants. J Perinatol 2002; 22:550–554.

66. Lucas A, Hay W, Atkinson SA et al. Posthospital nutrition in the preterm infant. Ross Products Division; 1996.

67. Ernst KD, Radmacher PG, Rafail ST et al. Postnatal malnutrition of extremely low birth-weight infants with catch-up growth postdischarge. J Perinatol 2003; 23:477–482.

68. Nicholl RM, Gamsu H. Effect on growth of changing to full term milk in VLBW babies at the time of discharge. Presented at the Paediatric Research Society meeting Glasgow Sept 13th 1996.

69. Lucas A, King F, Bishop NB. Postdischarge formula consumption in infants born preterm. Arch Dis Child 1992; 67:691–692.

70. Congdon PJ, Horsman A, Ryan SW. Bone mineral repletion in preterm infants after 40 weeks post-conception. Arch Dis Child 1990; 65:1038–1042.

71. Hall RT. Nutritional follow-up of the breastfeeding premature infant after hospital discharge. Pediatr Clin North Am 2001; 48:453–460.

72. Fewtrell MS. Growth and nutrition after discharge. Semin Neonatol 2003; 8:169–176.

73. Greer FR. Feeding the preterm infant after hospital discharge. Pediatr Ann 2001; 30:658–665.

74. Griffin IJ. Postdischarge nutrition for high risk neonates. Clin Perinatol 2002; 29:327–344.

75. Heird WC. Determination of nutritional requirements in preterm infants, with special reference to 'catch-up' growth. Semin Neonatol 2001; 6:365–375.

76. Picaud JC. Formula-fed preterm neonates. Minerva Pediatr 2003; 55:217–229.

77. De Curtis M, Pieltain C, Rigo J. Nutrition of preterm infants on discharge from hospital. In: Raiha NCR, Ruballelli FF, eds. Infant formula; closer to the reference, vol. 47. Nestle Nutrition Workshop Series. Philadelphia, PA: Lippincott Williams & Wilkins; 2002:149–163.

78. Barker DJ, Gluckman PD, Godfrey KM et al. Fetal nutrition and cardiovascular disease in adult life. Lancet 1993; 341:938–941.

79. Leeson CP, Whincup PH, Cook DG et al. Flow-mediated dilation in 9- to 11-year-old children: the influence of intrauterine and childhood factors. Circulation 1997; 96:2233–2238.

80. Leon DA, Lithell HO, Vagero D et al. Reduced fetal growth rate and increased risk of death from ischaemic heart disease: cohort study of 15 000 Swedish men and women born 1915-29. Br Med J 1998; 317:241–245.

81. Huxley R, Neil A, Collins R. Unravelling the fetal origins hypothesis: is there really an inverse association between birthweight and subsequent blood pressure? Lancet 2002; 360:659–665.

82. Owen CG, Whincup PH, Odoki K et al. Birth weight and blood cholesterol level: a study in adolescents and systematic review. Pediatrics 2003; 111:1081–1089.

83. Fall CH, Vijayakumar M, Barker DJ et al. Weight in infancy and prevalence of coronary heart disease in adult life. Br Med J 1995; 310:17–19.

84. Eriksson JG, Forsen T, Tuomilehto J et al. Early growth and coronary heart disease in later life: longitudinal study. Br Med J 2001; 322:949–953.

85. Cianfarani S, Germani D, Branca F. Low birthweight and adult insulin resistance: the "catch-up growth" hypothesis. Arch Dis Child 1999; 81:F71–F73.

86. Adair LS, Cole TJ. Rapid child growth raises blood pressure in adolescent boys who were thin at birth. Hypertension 2003; 41:451–456.

87. Hales CN, Ozanne SE. The dangerous road of catch-up growth. J Physiol 2003; 547:5–10.

88. Hack M, Merkatz IR, Gordon D et al. The prognostic significance of postnatal growth in very low-birth weight infants. Am J Obstet Gynecol 1982; 143:693–699.

89. Stevenson CJ, West CR, Pharoah PO. Dermatoglyphic patterns, very low birth weight, and blood pressure in adolescence. Arch Dis Child Fetal Neonatal Ed 2001; 84:F18-F22.

90. Irving RJ, Belton NR, Elton RA et al. Adult cardiovascular risk factors in premature babies. Lancet 2000; 355:2135–2136.

91. Singhal A, Kattenhorn M, Cole TJ et al. Preterm birth, vascular function, and risk factors for atherosclerosis. Lancet 2001; 358:1159–1160.

92. Fewtrell MS, Doherty C, Cole TJ et al. Effects of size at birth, gestational age and early growth in preterm infants on glucose and insulin concentrations at 9–12 years. Diabetologia 2000; 43:714–717.

93. Chan GM, Borschel MW, Jacobs JR. Effects of human milk or formula feeding on the growth, behavior, and protein status of preterm infants discharged from the newborn intensive care unit. Am J Clin Nutr 1994; 60:710–716.

94. Lucas A, Fewtrell MS, Morley R et al. Randomized trial of nutrient-enriched formula versus standard formula for postdischarge preterm infants. Pediatrics 2001; 108:703–711.

95. Wauben IP, Atkinson SA, Grad TL et al. Moderate nutrient supplementation of mother's milk for preterm infants supports adequate bone mass and short-term growth: a randomized, controlled trial. Am J Clin Nutr 1998; 67:465–472.

96. Wheeler RE, Hall RT. Feeding of premature infant formula after hospital discharge of infants weighing less than 1800 grams at birth. J Perinatol 1996; 16:111–116.

97. Chan GM. Growth and bone mineral status of discharged very low birth weight infants fed different formulas or human milk. J Pediatr 1993; 123:439–443.

98. Ng S, Randall-Simpson J, Marchment B et al. The influence of breast compared to formula feeding of preterm infants to three months corrected age on growth and body composition to one year. Pediatr Res 1998; 43:266A.

99. Worrell LA, Thorp JW, Tucker R et al. The effects of the introduction of a high-nutrient transitional formula on growth and development of very-low-birth-weight infants. J Perinatol 2002; 22:112–119.

100. Faerk J, Petersen S, Peitersen B et al. Diet and bone mineral content at term in premature infants. Pediatr Res 2000; 47:148–156.

101. Schanler RJ, Burns PA, Abrams SA et al. Bone mineralization outcomes in human milk-fed preterm infants. Pediatr Res 1992; 31:583–586.

102. Backstrom MC, Maki R, Kuusela AL et al. The long-term effect of early mineral, vitamin D, and breast milk intake on bone mineral status in 9- to 11-year-old children born prematurely. J Pediatr Gastroenterol Nutr 1999; 29:575–582.

103. Fewtrell MS, Cole TJ, Bishop NJ et al. Neonatal factors predicting childhood height in preterm infants: evidence for a persisting effect of early metabolic bone disease? J Pediatr 2000; 137:668–673.

104. Fewtrell, Prentice A, Cole TJ et al. Effects of growth during infancy and childhood on bone

mineralization and turnover in preterm children aged 8-12 years. Acta Paediatr 2000; 89:148–153.

105. Wauben I, Gibson R, Atkinson S. Premature infants fed mothers' milk to 6 months corrected age demonstrate adequate growth and zinc status in the first year. Early Hum Dev 1999; 54:181–194.

106. Lucas A, Bishop NJ, King FJ et al. Randomised trial of nutrition for preterm infants after discharge. Arch Dis Child 1992; 67:322–327.

107. Atkinson S, Randall-Simpson J, Chang M et al. Randomised trial of feeding nutrient enriched vs standard formula to premature infants during the first year of life. Pediatr Res 1999; 45:276A.

108. Carver JD, Wu PY, Hall RT et al. Growth of preterm infants fed nutrient-enriched or term formula after hospital discharge. Pediatrics 2001; 107:683–689.

109. De Curtis M, Pieltain C, Rigo J. Body composition in preterm infants fed standard term or enriched formula after hospital discharge. Eur J Nutr 2002; 41:177–182.

110. Qvigstad E, Verloove-Vanhorick SP, Ens-Dokkum MH et al. Prediction of height achievement at five years of age in children born very preterm or with very low birth weight: continuation of catch-up growth after two years of age. Acta Paediatr 1993; 82:444–448.

111. Hirata T, Bosque E. When they grow up: the growth of extremely low birth weight (< or = 1000 gm) infants at adolescence. J Pediatr 1998; 132:1033–1035.

112. Cooke RJ, Embleton ND, Griffin IJ et al. Feeding preterm infants after hospital discharge: growth and development at 18 months of age. Pediatr Res 2001; 49:719–722.

113. Agosti M, Vegni C, Calciolari G et al. Post-discharge nutrition of the very low-birthweight infant: interim results of the multicentric GAMMA study. Acta Paediatr 2003; 91 (suppl.):39–43.

114. Embleton N, Wells J, Cooke R. Randomised trial of protein intake in preterm infants. Pediatr Res 2001; 49:260A.

115. Morley R, Fewtrell MS, Abbott RA et al. Neurodevelopment in children born small for gestational age: a randomized trial of nutrient-enriched versus standard formula and comparison with a reference breastfed group. Pediatrics 2004; 113:515–521.

116. Bishop NJ, King FJ, Lucas A. Increased bone mineral content of preterm infants fed a nutrient enriched formula after discharge from hospital. Arch Dis Child 1993; 68:573–578.

117. Raupp P, Poss G, von Kries R et al. Effect of a calcium and phosphorus-enriched formula on bone mineralization and bone growth in preterm infants after discharge from hospital. Ann Nutr Metab 1997; 41:358–364.

118. Koo W, Hammami M. Vitamin D status of preterm infants fed milks with different vitamin D and mineral content after hospital discharge. Pediatr Res 2003; 53:407A.

119. Friel JK, Andrews WL, Aziz K et al. A randomized trial of two levels of iron supplementation and developmental outcome in low birth weight infants. J Pediatr 2001; 139:254–260.

120. Griffin IJ, Cooke RJ, Reid MM et al. Iron nutritional status in preterm infants fed formulas fortified with iron. Arch Dis Child 1999; 81:F45–F49.

121. Friel JK, Andrews WL. Zinc requirement of premature infants. Nutrition 1994; 10:63–65.

122. Friel JK, Andrews WL, Long DR et al. Selenium status of very low birth weight infants. Pediatr Res 1993; 34:293–296.

123. Nako Y, Fukushima N, Tomomasa T et al. Hypervitaminosis D after prolonged feeding with a premature formula. Pediatrics 1993; 92:862–864.

124. COMA Department of Health. Weaning and the weaning diet. London: HMSO; 1994.

125. Gartner LM, Greer FR. Prevention of rickets and vitamin D deficiency: new guidelines for vitamin D intake. Pediatrics 2003; 111:908–910.

126. Friel JK, Andrews WL, Matthew JD et al. Iron status of very-low-birth-weight infants during the first 15 months of infancy. CMAJ 1990; 143:733–737.

127. King CL. Neonatal unit weaning policy 2005. Dietetics Dept, Hammersmith Hospital, London.

Background reading

Rennie J, Roberton NRC. Textbook of neonatology. Churchill Livingstone; 1999.

Tsang RC, Uauy R, Koletzko B et al., eds. Nutritional needs of the preterm infant. Scientific basis and practical guidelines, 2nd edn. Cincinnati, OH: Digital Educational; 2004.

Chapter 9

Feeding development

Annie Bagnall

INTRODUCTION

At birth the oral cavity of a term infant is anatomically designed primarily for the purpose of feeding. Structures are arranged to ensure that the processes of sucking, swallowing and breathing occur with minimal risk of aspiration. The relative arrangement of structures supports the immature nervous system, which is only able to move in gross motor patterns. During sucking, the tongue, lower lip, mandible and hyoid act as a single motor unit. With increasing maturity, anatomical changes take place to allow more space for the more fine motor, complex actions of chewing and speech.

ANATOMY OF FEEDING

Infant anatomy differs from the adult in the following ways:

- The epiglottis is omega-shaped at birth, providing an umbrella-like covering for the trachea, which directs milk safely away from the airway towards the oesophagus
- The tongue fills the oral cavity, leaving little intraoral space (Fig. 9.1). The tongue has a central groove to facilitate good bolus formation and transport
- The lateral walls are stabilized by sucking or fat pads composed of a discrete mass of fat within the masseter muscle. This provides structural stability for the generation of intraoral suction

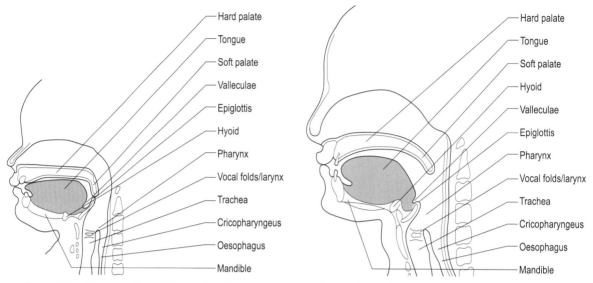

Figure 9.1   Cross-section of the head and neck of a young infant and an adult.

- The soft palate and epiglottis are in approximation, affording anatomical protection of the infant's airway and allowing safe feeding in a reclined position (Fig. 9.1). This anatomical proximity of structures is present until around 6 months of age, when rapid growth moves the soft palate and epiglottis apart. Approximation is observed during the swallow up to 18 months of age.[1]
- The larynx is at an elevated position in the neck, tucked up under the epiglottis, protecting the airway (Fig. 9.1). Minimal laryngeal elevation is required to protect the airway during swallowing.

In medical literature, infants up to 6 months of age are often described as obligate nose-breathers.[2] This theory is based on anatomical structure. The assumption is that the approximation of the soft palate and epiglottis will make oral breathing difficult. However, infants, including preterm infants, have been found to be able to tolerate nasal occlusion and can breathe through their mouths.[3] It may therefore be more accurate to describe them as preferential rather than obligate nose-breathers.[1,2]

The narrowest portion of the nasal airway of an infant is just 20 mm,[2] with mucosal inflammation increasing the risk of nasal occlusion. Infants with nasal congestion or a nasogastric tube, for example, may have difficulty with nasal breathing, which may then impact on their ability to coordinate sucking and swallowing with respiration and consequently on their ability to feed.

ORAL REFLEXES

In the immediate postnatal period oral feeding in the newborn infant is almost entirely reflexive: rooting, attaching, sucking and swallowing do not appear to require suprabulbar activity.[4]

The primitive reflexes involved in feeding begin to develop during the first trimester in utero. As early as the 9th gestational week, the fetus has enough oral development to move its mouth and lower face. Touching the lip region at 11 weeks' gestation leads to swallowing.[5] A more complex reflex response occurs at 14 weeks, in which touching the perioral region leads to head rotation and body stretching (primitive rooting). Development continues to be refined and established during the second and third trimesters. At birth, all reflexes are of brainstem origin, with minimal cortical control.

At term, an infant is equipped with the mature reflexes required for successful feeding.

Although the feeding reflexes are involved in feeding and can inform about the neurological development of an infant, in themselves they cannot predict the readiness of an infant to suck, feed or indicate how efficient an infant will be at feeding. When assessing an infant's non-nutritive suck we must exercise caution. Even if the reflexes are present this may not necessarily indicate that the baby will be able to co-ordinate suck and swallow effectively.[5]

Feeding difficulties may arise when a reflex is poorly developed, hyper- or hyporesponsive, or persists beyond a developmental stage one would expect.

Sucking

Sucking is the first rhythmic behaviour in which the fetus engages and it may contribute to neurological development by facilitating internally regulated rhythms. Rhythmic movement patterns of the jaw and lips that resemble sucking are observed early in the life of the fetus. Jaw-opening movements occur at 10–11 weeks of gestation and rhythmical bursts of opening and closing at 12 weeks.[6] The fetus can be seen to suck on its fingers on ultrasound at 15 weeks' gestation.[7] The phasic bite reflex characterized by rhythmic opening and closing of the jaw in response to stimulation of the gums is present at 28 weeks' gestation.

Preterm infants born between 29 and 30 weeks' gestation are without a rhythmic suck pattern until 33–36 weeks' gestation. At this age a pattern of sucking emerges which is similar to that of full-term infants. However, it is still immature, with an irregular pattern and a slower rate.[8] There is an increase in the number of sucks per burst with increasing postmenstrual age.[9,10] By 28–33 weeks the fetus can generate rhythmic bursts of non-nutritive sucking.[10] Sucking rhythm is essentially complete by 35–36 weeks of postconceptional age, reflecting the infant's increasing organization and regulation of the central nervous system. Disruption in sucking ability may be an indicator of underlying neurological deficits.[11–13]

Sucking maturation as an indicator of underlying neurobehavioural maturation has been studied and is described as an excellent barometer of central nervous system organization.[14] The study of sucking rhythms can be useful clinically as it differs among infants of different gestational ages and in those with additional perinatal complications.

Improved co-ordination of sucking motor patterns observed with increasing postnatal age demonstrates the importance of feedback to the suck central pattern generator and to the orofacial system as a whole.[15] Sensory input in the orofacial area moulds development by way of afferent feedback. Therefore, early sensory experiences are important to later feeding reactions and abilities and may provide some explanation as to the development of oral aversion and poor sucking patterns in some infants.

Human infants suck in two modes: non-nutritive and nutritive sucking. Non-nutritive sucking usually occurs when there is no nutrient flow, i.e. on fingers or a pacifier. Its main function is that of calming the infant. It is organized in a series of short sucking bursts separated by brief pauses. Sucking is rapid and occurs at a rate of two sucks per second.[16] Nutritive sucking, to obtain nourishment, is more continuous and occurs at a slower pace of one suck per second[17] to allow time for co-ordination with swallowing and breathing.

Swallowing

Swallowing of amniotic fluid occurs in utero from 11 to 13 weeks' gestation.[6,18,19]

Fetal swallowing is thought to regulate amniotic fluid volume. Disruption of amniotic fluid volume in utero (for example polyhydramnios) can indicate fetal swallowing problems.

Rooting

The rooting reflex is also known as the mouthing or cardinal points reflex. The maxillary and mandibular divisions of the trigeminal nerve are the first peripheral afferents to develop and achieve functionality in the human fetus. The earliest-appearing reflex consists of flexion of the head and neck in response to mechanical stimulation of the upper lip in the 8-week-old fetus.[18] This is primitive rooting. Touch stimulation in the perioral region elicits rooting, which is a positional response of the lips, face, head and neck to turn towards the nipple to facilitate attachment. A quick and sustained response to touching the cheeks or the corner of the mouth, before a feed is due, is seen by 32 weeks' gestation. Rooting is inhibited by higher cortical pathways and diminishes by 3 months of postnatal age in term infants.[20]

Reflexive tongue movement

Lateral movement of the tongue towards the side of stimulation is present by 28 weeks' gestation. Tongue protrusion in response to anterior touch is present at term but diminishes by 6 months of age in term infants and allows for introduction of solids and a spoon.

Gag, cough and airway protection

The airway is protected by a number of reflexes. Swallowing removes material from around the pharyngeal airway. The cough prevents material entering the airway and can expel aspirated material from below the vocal cords. The gag, which is associated with vocal fold closure, can also prevent aspiration. Gag is discernible at 26–27 weeks' gestation in some infants. However, the protective reflexes of gag and cough are only present in about half of term infants and only 25% of preterm infants.[19] The laryngeal chemoreflex (LCR) is a contraction of the muscles of the larynx, resulting in airway closure. Recent research has emphasized the importance of this reflex in airway protection, particularly in preterm infants. This may be the primary sensory mechanism in infants for defending the airway from aspiration of liquids.[1,21] The LCR is thought to develop initially to prevent the fetus aspirating amniotic fluid. Fetal lung fluid contains chloride, which does not trigger the LCR. It is triggered by the introduction of water or acid into the larynx, stimulating sensory afferents in the superior laryngeal nerves, resulting in vocal cord constriction and pro-

longed apnoea until the stimulus is removed. An apnoeic event is not a problem in the fetus, whose oxygenation is provided by the placenta. However, in the preterm infant this apnoeic reaction can have significant consequences.[21]

Researchers in the adult literature have concluded that the presence of a gag reflex does not protect against aspiration and the absence of a gag reflex does not predict swallowing difficulties.[22,23] A significant proportion of healthy adults have an absent gag reflex.[24] Assessment of the gag reflex therefore may not be the best indicator or predictor of feeding abilities. However, failure of the cough or gag response caused by neurological injury or dampening of the reflexes secondary to recurrent aspiration can result in aspirated material entering the respiratory tract. This may lead to respiratory difficulties or aspiration pneumonia in these infants.[1]

Preterm delivery, the atypical extrauterine environment and invasive interventions in the oral cavity such as intubation and the insertion of gastric tubes may impact on the development of these protective reflexes.

COORDINATION OF SUCKING. SWALLOWING AND BREATHING FOR FEEDING

Three distinct motor acts are coordinated during feeding: (1) sucking; (2) swallowing; and (3) breathing.

Some authors have claimed that swallowing and breathing occur simultaneously. The approximation of epiglottis and larynx may allow separation of the bolus behind the epiglottis in laterally placed food channels while nasal breathing occurs. This theory is still reported in many modern texts but it cannot be substantiated since it has been observed that infants experience a brief cessation of breathing associated with airway closure during the swallow, referred to as swallow apnoea[25] (Fig. 9.2). There is some inefficiency in the timing of airway closure in preterm infants representing immaturity of coordination which may predispose them to aspiration during the swallow.

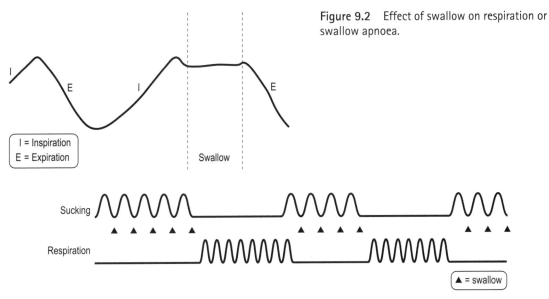

Figure 9.2   Effect of swallow on respiration or swallow apnoea.

Figure 9.3   Immature pattern of sucking.

The duration of each swallow apnoea is significantly greater at 32–37 weeks' gestation compared to preterm infants at term gestational age,[26] also reflecting immature coordination.

In term infants, sucking coordination and oesophageal function continue to mature within the first days after birth.[27] An immature sucking pattern may be a protective function to prevent overloading of the immature oesophagus.

Preterm infants are born before their neurological development is complete. Many are born before they are able to coordinate sucking with swallowing and breathing. Preterm sucking coordination has been studied by a number of authors and increases with gestational age. The majority of experts agree that coordination matures with gestational age and is not fully established before 35–37 weeks' gestation.[16,28,29] However there is ongoing debate as to how much is governed by gestational maturation and how much is determined by experience.

It is important to be able to differentiate between immature sucking patterns and those that are aberrant. Dysfunctional sucking patterns may be an indicator of neurological damage, maternal drug use and obstetric anaesthesia.[30,31]

An immature pattern is characterized by periods of breath-holding/apnoea when short sucking bursts occur. Instead of breathing being coordinated within the sucking burst, it occurs in the pauses (Fig. 9.3). Immature infants have been observed to stop the milk flow from a bottle teat with their tongue tip during pauses in sucking, possibly as a mechanism to protect the airway from the continuous milk flow.[28]

The immature pattern of coordination is not like the mature pattern of the 1:1:1 ratio of suck:swallow:breathe seen in a mature infant.[8,28,32]

The immature suck has short bursts of 4–7 sucks (Fig. 9.3) There is an increase in number of sucks per burst to around 30 by term (Fig. 9.4). With increasing maturation, the frequency of sucking in bursts increases, the number of bursts per minute increases and the interburst variance declines.[8,10,13] Sucking becomes more stable, regular and rhythmic. Sucking is correlated with gender as well as with gestational age. Preterm girls have been found to have a greater amplitude of and frequency of non-nutritive sucking than preterm boys.[33]

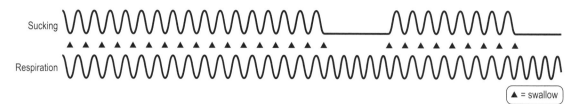

Figure 9.4   Mature pattern of sucking.

There is a pattern to the bursts and pauses over the course of a feed. In the mature pattern, there is an initial continuous sucking burst of at least 30 sucks in which sucking pauses do not exceed 2 seconds.[34] There is then an initial short pause, during which depressed respiration recovers; another burst of sucking begins, shorter than the first continuous burst. The intermittent burst pause pattern then repeats itself throughout the course of the feed, with the bursts gradually becoming shorter. The suck–pause pattern is punctuated by pauses of around 4 seconds (Fig. 9.4).[34]

There is a significant reduction in ventilation during the initial continuous sucking burst of oral feeding in term infants, associated with shorter inspiration and a decrease in breathing frequency (Fig. 9.4). A decrease in ventilation during feeding may be due to swallow apnoea/ breath-holding during the swallow and its resultant slowing of the rate of breathing.

Respiratory recovery occurs during the pauses in the intermittent sucking phase (Fig. 9.4).[35] Poor recovery results in hypoxia, hypercarbia and acidosis and may be manifested clinically by apnoea or bradycardia. Its occurrence depends on the magnitude of the reduction in ventilation and oxygenation and the efficiency of the recovery. Preterm infants have a similar respiratory pattern to term infants; however they have additional decreased tidal volume during the continuous sucking burst which leads to decreased minute ventilation and oxygenation.[34] This may leave them more vulnerable to poor recovery during the later stage of feeding. Consequently they have a greater incidence of desaturation with feeds.[36] Recovery is dependent on postconceptional age.[34] The bulk of apnoea occurs in the initial continuous sucking

phase in term infants[35] but occurs during the intermittent sucking phase in preterm infants.

Apnoea appears to be a factor that influences the length of time it takes premature infants to begin receiving full oral feedings.[37] Infants with immature cardiorespiratory control are more likely to be poor feeders than infants with mature patterns.[38] Monitoring of preterm and term infants has shown that profound cardiorespiratory disturbances can occur during bottle-feeding in preterm infants at a corrected gestational age of 36–42 weeks and in some term infants up to a postconceptional age of 52 weeks.[39,40] Poor co-ordination of sucking and breathing resulting in apnoea and bradycardia has also been detected in infants who had been or were just about to be discharged from hospital.[36] Coordination development may not be complete on discharge from hospital and careful monitoring and assessment of feeding are required before discharge home.

Increasing respiratory drive through artificially elevating the amount of carbon dioxide in inspired air while feeding has been found to decrease sucking and swallowing rates in preterm infants significantly.[41] This suggests that the increased respiratory drive resulting from carbon dioxide chemoreceptor activation has a detrimental effect on feeding. This will further impair feeding in infants with bronchopulmonary dysplasia (BPD), also known as chronic lung disease, who have a higher respiratory drive as a consequence of diminished lung function. In infants with BPD, their lung disease may override the ability to co-ordinate suck, swallow and breathing.[42] Decreasing the rate of milk flow may increase the time available for breathing through a reduction in the number of swallows per unit time. This may be particularly beneficial to the baby with BPD or immature coordination but may increase the time needed to complete a feed.

Recent work has assessed the development of rhythmic sucking patterns in bottle-fed term infants. In the first month of life, sucks and swallows become more rapid and are increasingly organized into runs. Suck rate and length of sucking runs increase in the first month, as does swallow rate and occurrence in runs. The result is that the efficiency of feeding doubles over the first month of life. Infants appear to gain the ability to adjust feeding patterns to improve efficiency by altering the suck-to-swallow ratio. These detailed observations of term sucking rhythms provide a model to compare feeding development in preterm and other high-risk infants.[43] In a group of low-risk preterm infants,[44] increasing gestational age is correlated with a faster and more stable sucking rhythm and with an increasing organization into longer suck and swallow runs. The fact that gestational age is a better predictor than postnatal age lends support to the concept that these patterns are innate and develop in a specific sequence and timeframe rather than being learned behaviours that improve with experience and/or practice.

Future research and literature regarding the nature of the development of suck, swallow, breathe co-ordination in different preterm populations is required to ensure good feeding practices and enable effective intervention for feeding problems. Some experts postulate that neurological maturation is a pre-programmed sequence of events which come together with time to enable efficient oral feeding. The counter view is that, despite the progression of normal development, preterm infants can be encouraged to feed before coordination development is complete and that the combination of practice with maturity may enable them to feed earlier than expected. An infant may not feed in a manner similar to the neurologically mature infant but may feed well enough to facilitate earlier full oral feeding and subsequently earlier discharge home.[45]

There are a substantial number of variables influencing the development of feeding co-ordination. This warrants informed observation and awareness of feeding development to ensure individual infants are provided with the opportunity to feed safely and efficiently. While some infants follow developmental norms and proceed with maturation through the ages and stages of feeding coordination, others, when given earlier opportunities to feed, are home and breastfeeding well before reaching term gestation.

BIOMECHANICS OF SUCKING: COMPRESSION AND SUCTION

An infant relies on two techniques of sucking to receive adequate nutrition efficiently. These are suction and compression.[46–48]

The tongue strips the teat against the hard palate and alveolar ridge to express milk from the teat by positive pressure, known as compression. At the same time a seal is formed anteriorly by the tongue and the alveolar ridge and posteriorly by the base of the tongue and palate. This space forms a sealed vacuum. By moving the tongue down and back, negative pressure is generated to draw milk into the mouth (Fig. 9.5). This is referred to as suction. This resistance can be felt by pulling against it and is described as a baby being attached.[28] Videosonography using an ultrasound probe on the cheek demonstrates tongue movements during suckling. A wave of downward displacement followed by upward displacement is observed, effecting a succession of suction and compression.[17]

There are two phases in development in preterm infants.[49] Initially weak arrhythmic compression predominates and is co-ordinated with swallowing. With increasing maturation the action becomes rhythmic; alternating suction and compression appears that is increasingly co-ordinated with swallowing.

Suction and compression positively correlate with efficiency (ml/min) and proficiency (ml taken in the first 5 min/total volume offered) of feeding but not with gestational age or number of feeds given. Preterm infants can successfully take small volumes when they use only the compression component of sucking. Consideration of suction and compression skills is vital when looking at feeding readiness as oral feeding performance is positively correlated with the maturation of these sucking skills.[50]

The need for early sucking practice, to develop sucking pressures, has been debated by experts in the field. Intraoral sucking pressures increase with advancing gestational age. By utilizing the promotion of non-nutritive sucking they can be advanced,[9] and may make feeding more efficient at an earlier age. Improved suction may also help to correct the high arched palate often seen secondary to oral intubation in the preterm infant by helping to bring the palate back down into place.

Suction and compression are required to obtain an adequate volume of feed per suck. Infants may have absent or reduced suction for a variety of reasons. Preterm infants may not have lateral wall support to generate suction due to absent fat pads. Infants who are reluctant to maintain an anterior seal due to respiratory difficulties, e.g. BPD, may not make a good anterior seal. Some babies who have structural abnormalities preventing an effective seal, e.g. those with cleft palate, cannot generate intraoral suction. For these infants, feeding will be inefficient unless there is compensation for this reduced suction.

SUMMARY

Effective suck-feeding relies on the maturity of feeding reflexes and anatomic structures. The development of co-ordination of sucking, swallowing and respiration occurs late in pregnancy and may be incomplete in preterm infants. For successful feeding the infant needs to root and attach on to the nipple. The tongue and jaw move to compress the nipple against the upper jaw and palate and express milk from the nipple. The sucking reflex then moves the tongue in a peristaltic motion to transport the bolus into the pharynx. The lateral borders of the tongue move up to contact with the palate, creating a central channel for the bolus. Suction is achieved by creating a vacuum in

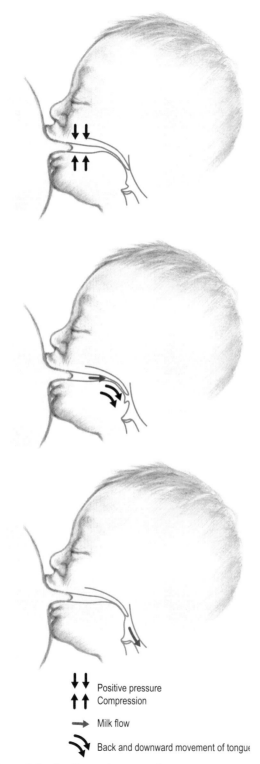

↓↓ Positive pressure
↑↑ Compression

➡ Milk flow

↘ Back and downward movement of tongue

Figure 9.5 Suction and compression.

the mouth. A seal at the front of the mouth (anterior seal) is created by the tongue and the hard palate around the nipple. At the back of the mouth the tongue base and soft palate approximate. Retraction of the tongue base then increases the intraoral space and sucks milk into the mouth. The swallow is triggered at the valleculae, the airway is closed and respiration ceases. The bolus passes safely through the relaxed cricopharyngeal sphincter and into the oesophagus. Oesophageal peristalsis is initiated, the cricopharyngeus returns to its tonic position preventing retrograde flow and respiration resumes. Suck and swallow occur in rhythmic bursts with pauses between bursts allowing recovery of depressed respiration.

In this complex and coordinated action an infant is able to obtain adequate nutrition for growth and development.

Preterm infants are born before their feeding development is complete. Their early delivery, extrauterine environment and associated interventions may impact on the normal progression of development. Therefore, a sound understanding of the development of feeding in utero and in the infant born prematurely underlies good feeding practice on the special care baby unit and facilitates the assessment and management of preterm infants with feeding difficulties.

References

1. Loughlin GM, Lefton-Greif MA. Dysfunctional swallowing and respiratory disease in children. Adv Pediatr 1994; 41:135–162.
2. Bergeson PS, Shaw JC. Are infants really obligatory nasal breathers? Clin Pediatr (Phila) 2001; 40:567–569.
3. deAlmeida VL, Alvaro RA, Haider Z et al. The effect of nasal occlusion on the initiation of oral breathing in preterm infants. Pediatr Pulmonol 1994; 18:374–378.
4. Stevenson RD, Allaire JH. The development of normal feeding and swallowing. Pediatr Clin North Am 1991; 38:1439–1453.
5. Ingram T. Clinical significance of the infantile feeding reflexes. Dev Med Child Neurol 1962; 4:159–169.
6. de Vries JI, Visser GH, Prechtl HF. The emergence of fetal behaviour. I. Qualitative aspects. Early Hum Dev 1982; 7:301–322.
7. Ianniruberto A, Tajani E. Ultrasonographic study of fetal movements. Semin Perinatol 1981; 5:175–181.
8. Wolff PH. The serial organization of sucking in the young infant. Pediatrics 1968; 42:943–956.
9. Bernbaum JC, Pereira GR, Watkins JB et al. Nonnutritive sucking during gavage feeding enhances growth and maturation in premature infants. Pediatrics 1983; 71:41–45.
10. Hack M, Estabrook MM, Robertson SS. Development of sucking rhythm in preterm infants. Early Hum Dev 1985; 11:133–140.
11. Hafstrom M, Kjellmer I. Non-nutritive sucking by infants exposed to pethidine in utero. Acta Paediatr 2000; 89:1196–1200.
12. Hafstrom M, Kjellmer I. Non-nutritive sucking in the healthy pre-term infant. Early Hum Dev 2000; 60:13–24.
13. Hafstrom M, Kjellmer I. Non-nutritive sucking in sick preterm infants. Early Hum Dev 2001; 63(1):37–52.
14. Medoff-Cooper B, Ray W. Neonatal sucking behaviors. Image J Nurs Sch 1995; 27:195–200.
15. Finan DS, Barlow SM. Intrinsic dynamics and mechanosensory modulation of non-nutritive sucking in human infants. Early Hum Dev 1998; 52:181–197.
16. Gryboski JD. Suck and swallow in the premature infant. Pediatrics 1969; 43:96–102.
17. Bosma JF, Hepburn LG, Josell SD et al. Ultrasound demonstration of tongue motions during suckle feeding. Dev Med Child Neurol 1990; 32:223–229.
18. Humphrey T. The development of human fetal activity and its relation to postnatal behavior. Adv Child Dev Behav 1970; 5:1–57.
19. Miller HC, Proud GO, Behrle FC. Variations in the gag, cough and swallow reflexes and tone of the vocal cords as determined by direct laryngoscopy in newborn infants. Yale J Biol Med 1952; 24:284–291.
20. Sheppard JJ, Mysak ED. Ontogeny of infantile oral reflexes and emerging chewing. Child Dev 1984; 55:831–843.
21. Thach BT. Maturation and transformation of reflexes that protect the laryngeal airway from liquid aspiration from fetal to adult life. Am J Med 2001; 111 (suppl. 8A):69S–77S.
22. Bleach NR. The gag reflex and aspiration: a retrospective analysis of 120 patients assessed by videofluoroscopy. Clin Otolaryngol 1993; 18:303–307.
23. Leder SB. Videofluoroscopic evaluation of aspiration with visual examination of the gag reflex and velar movement. Dysphagia 1997; 12:21–23.
24. Davies AE, Kidd D, Stone SP et al. Pharyngeal sensation and gag reflex in healthy subjects. Lancet 1995; 345:487–488.

25. Wilson SL, Thach BT, Brouillette RT et al. Coordination of breathing and swallowing in human infants. J Appl Physiol 1981; 50:851–858.

26. Hanlon MB, Tripp JH, Ellis RE et al. Deglutition apnoea as indicator of maturation of suckle feeding in bottle-fed preterm infants. Dev Med Child Neurol 1997; 39:534–542.

27. Gryboski JD. The swallowing mechanism of the neonate. I. Esophageal and gastric motility. Pediatrics 1965; 35:445–452.

28. Bu'Lock F, Woolridge MW, Baum JD. Development of co-ordination of sucking, swallowing and breathing: ultrasound study of term and preterm infants. Dev Med Child Neurol 1990; 32:669–678.

29. Casaer P, Daniels H, Devlieger H et al. Feeding behaviour in preterm neonates. Early Hum Dev 1982; 7:331–346.

30. Kron RE, Stein M, Goddard KE. Newborn sucking behavior affected by obstetric sedation. Pediatrics 1966; 37:1012–1016.

31. Kron RE, Ipsen J, Goddard KE et al. Consistent individual differences in the nutritive sucking behavior of the human newborn. Newborn sucking behavior affected by obstetric sedation. Psychosom Med 1968; 30:151–161.

32. Weber F, Woolridge MW, Baum JD. An ultrasonographic study of the organisation of sucking and swallowing by newborn infants. Dev Med Child Neurol 1986; 28:19–24.

33. Dubignon J, Campbell D, Curtis M et al. The relation between laboratory measures of sucking, food intake, and perinatal factors during the newborn period. Child Dev 1969; 40:1107–1120.

34. Shivpuri CR, Martin RJ, Carlo WA et al. Decreased ventilation in preterm infants during oral feeding. J Pediatr 1983; 103:285–289.

35. Mathew OP, Clark ML, Pronske ML et al. Breathing pattern and ventilation during oral feeding in term newborn infants. J Pediatr 1985; 106:810–813.

36. Guilleminault C, Coons S. Apnoea and bradycardia during feeding in infants weighing greater than 2000 gm. J Pediatr 1984; 104:932–935.

37. Mandich MB, Ritchie SK, Mullett M. Transition times to oral feeding in premature infants with and

without apnoea. J Obstet Gynecol Neonatal Nurs 1996; 25:771–776.

38. Daniels H, Devlieger H, Casaer P et al. Feeding, behavioural state and cardiorespiratory control. Acta Paediatr Scand 1988; 77:369–373.

39. Rosen CL, Glaze DG, Frost JD Jr. Hypoxemia associated with feeding in the preterm infant and full-term neonate. Am J Dis Child 1984; 138:623–628.

40. Thoyre SM, Carlson J. Occurrence of oxygen desaturation events during preterm infant bottle feeding near discharge. Early Hum Dev 2003; 72:25–36.

41. Timms BJ, DiFiore JM, Martin RJ et al. Increased respiratory drive as an inhibitor of oral feeding of preterm infants. J Pediatr 1993; 123:127–131.

42. Gewolb IH, Bosma JF, Reynolds EW et al. Integration of suck and swallow rhythms during feeding in preterm infants with and without bronchopulmonary dysplasia. Dev Med Child Neurol 2003; 45:344–348.

43. Qureshi MA, Vice FL, Taciak VL et al. Changes in rhythmic suckle feeding patterns in term infants in the first month of life. Dev Med Child Neurol 2002; 44:34–39.

44. Gewolb IH, Vice FL, Schwietzer-Kenney EL et al. Developmental patterns of rhythmic suck and swallow in preterm infants. Dev Med Child Neurol 2001; 43:22–27.

45. Simpson C, Schanler RJ, Lau C. Early introduction of oral feeding in preterm infants. Pediatrics 2002; 110:517–522.

46. Dubignon J, Campbell D. Sucking in the newborn during a feed. J Exp Child Psychol 1969; 7:282–298.

47. Sameroff AJ. The components of sucking in the human newborn. J Exp Child Psychol 1968; 6:607–623.

48. Dubignon JM, Campbell D, Partington MW. The development of non-nutritive sucking in premature infants. Biol Neonat 1969; 14:270–278.

49. Lau C, Sheena HR, Shulman RJ et al. Oral feeding in low birth weight infants. J Pediatr 1997; 130:561–569.

50. Lau C, Alagugurusamy R, Schanler RJ et al. Characterization of the developmental stages of sucking in preterm infants during bottle feeding. Acta Paediatr 2000; 89:846–852.

Chapter 10

Transition from tube to breast

Elizabeth Jones

SUMMARY OF RECOMMENDATIONS

- The transition from nasogastric feeds to established breastfeeding is discussed
- Since it can be a challenge to achieve correct attachment and positioning for preterm infants, management issues will be probed
- Key issues in preterm breastfeeding management, such as milk ejection and milk transfer, will be debated
- Methods to supplement breast feeds, i.e. cup-feeding and the use of the supplementary nursing system, will also be discussed

WHEN TO START AND TRANSITION

Sucking, swallowing and breathing are the cornerstones of infant feeding[1] (see Chapter 9). An infant may experience significant feeding problems if sucking, swallowing and breathing are not smoothly coordinated. Currently, there are few published criteria to indicate when a preterm infant should first be put to the breast. In a survey of 420 neonatal intensive care units (NICUs) in the USA, fewer than 50% identified a specific feeding policy for the initiation of oral feeding. Seventy-five per cent used either gestational age or weight criteria in determining when to initiate oral feeds. Eighty-six per cent also considered infant behaviour when deciding when to start oral feeds.[2] However, 93% of the nurses surveyed reported that the standard practice was to start bottle-feeding before breast-feeding, even if the mother indicated her desire to breastfeed. In many NICUs in the UK and in Sweden, the criterion used to initiate breast-feeding is based exclusively on physiologic stability.[3,4] Feeding bottles are not offered routinely during the transition from tube-feeding to breastfeeding.

In term newborn infants swallowing interrupts breathing, tidal volume, minute ventilation, oxygen saturation and heart rate.[5] The faster the rate of milk flow, the faster the rate of sucking and swallowing.[6] Although milk flows at a relatively constant rate during a bottle feed, the rate of flow during breastfeeding is highly variable. In the past, it was commonly believed that breastfeeding was more tiring than bottle-feeding. In the USA, Meier & Anderson[7] found that preterm infants who served as their own controls for bottle- and breastfeeding sessions demonstrated more stable oxygenation patterns during breast-feeding than bottle-feeding (Fig. 10.1). This study was subsequently replicated by Blaymore-Bier et al.,[8] who found that very-low-birth-weight infants (VLBW) were less likely to have less clinically significant oxygen desaturation during breast- than bottle-feeding. Mathew & Bhatia[9] noted similar findings: infants demonstrated more significant respiratory interruption and episodes of oxygen desaturation during bottle-feeding. Although the term 'nipple/teat' confusion remains a hypothesis, it has been suggested that if bottles are offered routinely, some infants may find it difficult to progress to breastfeeding (see Chapter 11). The results of the above studies appear to indicate that preterm infants are able to progress directly from tube-feeding to breastfeeding without bottles being offered.

Pioneering work in Sweden has been undertaken based on a developmental care approach in which mothers are taught to identify infant behavioural cues in relation to breastfeeding management.[10] Establishing breastfeeding can present a considerable challenge to mothers since preterm infants exhibit high reactivity to stimuli from the neonatal environment, resulting in limited periods of awake, alert behaviour.[11] Als[12] suggests that high-risk infants display their physiological and neurological immaturity in several ways. Cues of stress can be subtle or dramatic, and are not always understood by the caregiver. Motor disorganization can be dramatic, from loss of tone in the face, or finger splay, to strong hyperflexion or hyperextension of limbs and trunk, with diffuse movement. Active gaze or auditory averting can also be a reaction to overstimulation. Staying asleep or inconsolable crying are alternative strategies. All these behaviours are signs of state disorganization. Nyqvist et al.[13] argue that breastfeeding constitutes a complex source of simultaneous stimuli: changes in position, touch, visual contact, listening to the mother's voice, smell and the taste of milk. They suggest that programmes that focus on guiding parents to recognize and respond effectively to their infant's cues in order to prevent under- and overstimulation are important for supporting infant development.

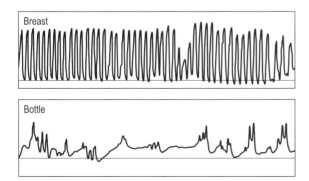

Figure 10.1   Polygraph recording demonstrating the organization of sucking during breastfeeding for a preterm infant. The breastfeeding recording is characterized by a long sucking burst with rhythmic, symmetrical sucks. The bottle-feeding recording is characterized by isolated, arrhythmic sucks. (Reproduced with permission from Meier.[10])

Some of the interventions Nyqvist and colleagues[13] recommend include:

- Encourage kangaroo mother care (KMC) as early as possible
- Plan the day so that the breastfeeding session does not occur after a stressful experience (such as following venepuncture)
- Provide a supportive physical environment (where the infant is protected from distracting sounds, bright lights and activity within the infant's visual field)
- Ensure maternal comfort (e.g. privacy and a comfortable chair)
- Show the mother how to hold her infant in a correct position. Secure support should be provided with 'nesting' (providing an infant with secure physical boundaries such as pillows and fabric rolls) and containment holding
- Continue physiologic monitoring as required
- Stay near the mother to describe her infant's behavioural cues
- Have realistic expectations of the infant's performance, considering the baby's level of maturity and medical status. Explain that the infant may not show the same behaviour every feed or every day

In another study performed by Nyqvist & Ewald,[14] the aim was to explore the influence of infant and maternal factors on the development of preterm infants' breastfeeding and breastfeeding outcome. The sample consisted of 71 preterm infants born between 26 and 35 weeks' gestation. A descriptive, prospective design was used, with direct behavioural observation as the data collection method, based on mothers' assessments according to the Preterm Infant Breastfeeding Behaviour Scale (PIBBS), in which higher scores indicate higher feeding competence. The PIBBS scale includes key items about breastfeeding behaviour such as rooting, areolar grasp, sucking, sucking burst, swallowing, milk ejection reflex (MER) and behavioural state. Multiple regression analyses revealed that variables associated with efficient infant performance included higher birth weight, less need of ventilator and oxygen treatment, higher haemoglobin level, absence of bottle-feeding, no need for apnoea treatment and no suspicion of infection. An earlier gestational age was associated with high PIBBS scores during weeks 32–37; possibly indicating that feeding competence is more influenced by early breastfeeding exposure than by gestational age. Maternal characteristics associated with higher infant competence include previous breastfeeding experience. Fifty-seven infants in the study were discharged fully breastfeeding. The results of this study help to identify barriers that may be associated with a longer transition from tube-feeding to established breastfeeding.

A developmentally based breastfeeding programme was also utilized in an inner-city neonatal unit with a diverse population in the UK.[15] A cohort of 60 infants born before 35 weeks' gestation was studied. The breastfeeding uptake almost doubled, with 95% of infants receiving expressed breast milk and 83% fully or partially breast-fed at discharge. Although it is difficult to assess the effects of developmental intervention programmes, promising results have been obtained, particularly in creating a nurturing environment for both infants and their mothers, and helping parents to let the infant's physiological and behavioural responses guide their interactions.[13] This is a welcome move away from a more traditional and rigid model of medical and nursing care. Although the studies discussed are based on clinical experience, they suggest that positive suggestions related to infant behavioural cues might make a big difference in terms of maternal motivation by allowing a mother to recognize the subtle progression that often occurs from tube- to breastfeeding, especially in VLBW infants. This is particularly helpful in neonatal units where breastfeeding babies are in the minority. Mothers often perceive that bottle-feeding babies are making swifter progress and change the feeding method in order to expedite an earlier infant discharge from hospital.[3]

SUMMARY OF RECOMMENDATIONS

When to start
- when an infant is able to tolerate enteral feeds
- when an infant is able to co-ordinate sucking and swallowing with minimal changes in cardiovascular response

Transition
- Teach the infant to associate the mother with breastfeeding
- Practice KMC
- Maximize maternal milk production
- If the breast is full of milk or the mother's MER is forceful, encourage the mother to express first (2-3 min) to reduce the rate of flow
- Establish realistic expectations
- Provide reassurance and an optimal environment
- Help the mother to acquire a comfortable position
- Use optimal infant positioning ('nesting') and support to the head and neck to avoid airway closure
- Stimulate rooting and latching by teasing the infant's mouth and lips
- Express milk on to the baby's lips
- Trigger the MER
- Offer a few drops of milk orally to stimulate suck and swallow
- Monitor the infant, where appropriate
- Audible swallowing is a sign that milk transfer is occurring
- Do not limit feeds unless clinically indicated

ATTACHMENT AND POSITIONING

Achieving correct attachment positioning while assisting a mother to breastfeed a preterm baby can be a significant challenge, particularly if there is a considerable disparity between the size of an infant's mouth and the mother's breast. In order to achieve effective milk transfer an infant must obtain an adequate seal, sufficient negative pressure and an adequate suckling mechanism.[16,17] Mothers must be supported and guided by neonatal staff during early breast feeds. Infants should be coaxed into a position of flexion with pillows or rolled fabric. Flexion is a key factor to promote a co-ordinated oral response. Hyperextension of the neck during feeding should also be corrected since it reduces jaw stability, increases cheek retraction and reduces the seal between the baby's lips and the mother's breast. Hyperextension will also inhibit the muscle movements needed for swallowing.[18] It is extremely important to remember that the preterm head is heavy in relation to the weak musculature of the neck. Unless a neonate's head and neck is supported with gentle pressure to provide neck stability, undirected head movements can easily collapse the airway, causing apnoea and bradycardia.[19]

The underarm position (sometimes called the 'football hold') is a position that often works very well for premature babies. This position is particularly effective since preterm infants are commonly hypotonic and the muscles that extend the neck are often more developed than those that sustain flexion. (However, a slight degree of flexion is essential to enable effective swallowing and to achieve optimal attachment.) The underarm position gives a mother more control of an infant's head and allows a clear view of the infant's face[17] (Fig. 10.2).

A cross-cradle hold is equally helpful if pillows are used to support the infant so that the baby is level to the breast (Figs 10.3 and 10.4).

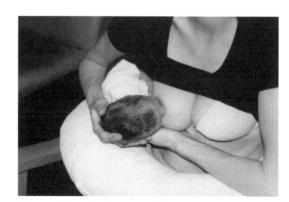

Figure 10.2   Underarm position.

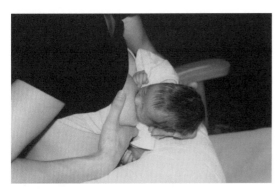

Figure 10.3   Cradle hold.

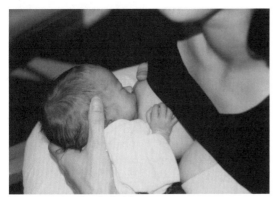

Figure 10.4   Cradle hold.

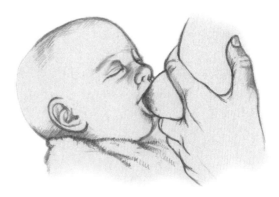

Figure 10.5   V-hold.

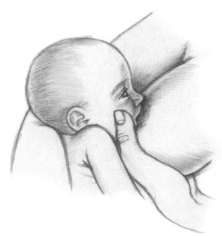

Figure 10.6   Dancer's hand position.

Although positioning is part of the story, attachment is also of critical importance to feeding outcome. Preterm infants are commonly unable sustain enough negative pressure to hold the nipple or areola in place. A 'V-hold' (Figure 10.5) can sometimes be useful to shape and compress the breast, helping to compensate for a small mouth and a weak suckling mechanism. The 'dancer position' (Figure 10.6) is also recommended by the US nurse/midwife Sarah Coulter Danner to provide help to obtain an adequate seal. This position provides both jaw and chin support, and helps to compensate for the lack of buccal pads in the cheeks that provide jaw and cheek stability (see Chapter 11).

It can also be helpful to advise mothers to express before the breast feed to soften the breast, to trigger the MER and to elongate the nipple. Guidance on practical ways to assist a mother to achieve correct attachment and positioning can be found in Figure 10.7 and Boxes 10.1–10.3.

SUMMARY OF RECOMMENDATIONS

Attachment and positioning
- Achieving correct preterm attachment and positioning is a challenge
- To obtain milk transfer an infant must obtain an adequate seal, sufficient negative pressure and an adequate sucking mechanism
- Hyperextension must be corrected and flexion facilitated
- An infant's head and neck must be supported to prevent airway closure
- The underarm position gives a mother more control of the infant's head and a clear view of the infant's face

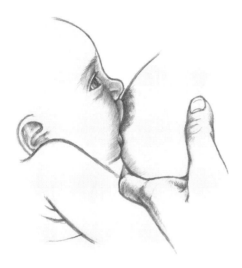

Figure 10.7 Correct attachment. (Adapted from Royal College of Midwives.[19])

Box 10.1 Correct attachment and positioning: the mother's recognition

- She should feel a painless drawing sensation
- If there is any areola visible, she will see more above the top lip than below the bottom lip
- The infant's head is slightly extended
- The infant's chin is in contact with the breast
- As behaviour matures, the suckling pattern changes to a long deep suck with pauses

---

Box 10.2 An observer's recognition of correct positioning

- The infant's mouth is wide open and the baby has a big mouthful of breast tissue
- The infant's chin is touching the breast
- The infant's bottom lip is curled out (this is sometimes difficult to see)

Box 10.3 Recognition of incorrect attachment (for an infant capable of nutritive suckling)

- The infant is continuing to make little suckling movements
- There is no change in rhythm of suckling
- The lips are pursed
- The cheeks draw in during suckling
- There is maternal discomfort
- The infant shows frustration (becoming sleepy, coming off the breast, crying)

- The 'V-hold' can help to shape breast tissue, if necessary
- The 'dancer position' offers jaw and chin support
- Milk expression before feeding will help to elongate the nipple, if appropriate
- Assist the mother to understand the principles of correct attachment and positioning
- Assist a mother to recognize the signs of correct attachment

MILK EJECTION AND MILK TRANSFER

The MER is regulated by the hormone oxytocin. When the nipple is stimulated, the myoepithelial cells (muscle cells) that surround the alveoli contract and milk is propelled towards the nipple. As mentioned in Chapter 5, this reflex can be inhibited by many factors, including emotion, stress and ineffectual infant suckling. Some mothers can distinguish when milk ejection occurs, but many women are unaware of the phenomenon. Up to eight milk ejections can occur during a breast feed, but on average there are 2.5 milk ejections during a term breast feed of approximately 7 min from one breast, resulting in an average milk yield per ejection of 35 g.[20] A healthy term infant typically stimulates milk ejection by sucking rapidly, between 72 and 120 sucks/min, before slowing to 60 sucks/min once milk starts to

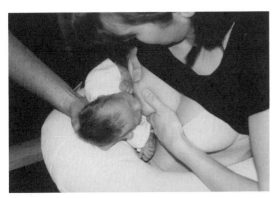

Figure 10.8   Breast compression.

flow. Preterm infants have relatively low suction pressures and a weak, ineffectual sucking mechanism. They are often unable to trigger milk ejection, which will mean that they may have to suck repeatedly until enough milk accumulates in their mouth to trigger a swallowing mechanism. For a baby to obtain enough milk to satisfy infant nutritional requirements, mothers must be taught methods to trigger the MER in conjunction with feeding. Gentle breast compression will also help to facilitate a faster milk flow, which will help an infant to remain interested in feeding (Fig. 10.8).

Some mothers become conditioned to manual expression;[21] even when a preterm infant's suckling pattern matures and becomes functional, mothers experience a delay in milk ejection when an infant is put to the breast. It is not uncommon for a tiny baby to become frustrated after a period of ineffectual suckling and simply to go to sleep before milk flow begins. Using either a breast pump or hand expression to elicit flow is helpful, but will not always remedy the situation. Sometimes it is necessary to place an infant on one breast and the breast pump at the other to provide more intense stimulation. Since suck, swallow, breathe is a chained response, infants often respond with longer bursts of suckling, which helps to promote a co-ordinated suck, swallow, breathe response. Gradually, as the effectiveness of suckling increases, extra mammary stimulation becomes unnecessary as milk ejection becomes conditioned to infant demand.

SUMMARY OF RECOMMENDATIONS

Milk ejection and milk transfer
- The MER facilitates milk transfer
- MER can be inhibited by emotion, stress and ineffectual suckling
- Not all women are aware of MER occurring
- MER results in an average milk yield per ejection of 35 g
- Some mothers need to trigger MER artificially in conjunction with breastfeeds
- MER is a conditioned reflex
- MER may be conditioned to milk expression, not infant suckling

MODIFIED DEMAND-FEEDING

As an infant matures, his ability to breastfeed improves, but there is still often inconsistency in suckling performance both between individual babies and between individual feeds. During the transition from tube-feeding this can be overcome by ensuring that the infant receives the full nutritional requirement either by tube or by cup when the mother is not available to put her baby to the breast. However, during the immediate period before infant discharge and in the postdischarge period this can become more problematic as the infant spends more time at the breast. Although infant consumption during feeds can be estimated by suckling patterns, audible swallowing and breast softening, researchers from the USA report that mothers are often concerned that infants are not receiving an adequate volume of milk by breastfeeding alone.[22,23] Meier et al. suggest that clinicians are commonly unable to recognize the difference between 'getting enough' and insufficient milk supply.[21] In a study focusing on the infant suckling component of milk transfer, Meier and colleagues performed a study[21] to determine whether mothers and investigators could accurately estimate intake during breastfeeding, by utilizing clinical cues that are recommended for this purpose. Test weights were performed before and after feeds by researchers and by mothers. Results indicate that clinical cues alone did not provide an accurate estimate of the milk consumed. Test-weighing using the 'Baby Weigh Scale' provided an accurate estimate of intake and allowed mothers to make individual decisions about supplementing breastfeeding sessions. The baby weigh scale is not marketed in the UK or continental Europe.

Schanler et al.[24] from the USA suggest that milk intake can be estimated in several ways: by observing the infant's suck and swallow, from maternal perceptions of the MER, by the degree of breast fullness and by test-weighing. The researchers argue that test-weighing provides reassurance to mothers who want to know how much milk their baby is receiving during breastfeeding sessions. They also warn that counselling mothers merely to feed on demand in the postdischarge period is extremely unhelpful and may result in infant underconsumption. They advise that the following factors should be considered in the development of a discharge breastfeeding plan: (1) the minimum number of feeds in the 24-h period; (2) the need for supplementary feeds; (3) the need for postfeed breast pumping; and (4) the monitoring of the infant's urination and stooling patterns. They also recommend the practice of test-weighing at home in the immediate postdischarge period to ensure adequacy of milk intake.

This inevitably leads to the question about the psychological effects test-weighing has on mothers. A recent paper published by researchers from Canada[25] sought to determine whether weighing preterm infants before and after breastfeeding affects maternal confidence and competence. Sixty mothers of preterm infants were randomly assigned to a test-weight or non-test-weight group. Maternal confidence and competence were measured four times: (1) 3 days after the initiation of breast-feeding; (2) on discharge; (3) 1 week after discharge; and (4) 4 weeks after discharge. No significant differences in maternal confidence and competence at any of the measurement times were found. When change in maternal perception was examined over time, the results indicate that the levels of competence and confidence in both groups increased significantly. The researchers recommend that the findings of this study call into question claims that such interventions are necessary to develop competence or confidence in mothers of preterm infants.

In the immediate discharge period, support must be available from health care professionals who are skilled in preterm breastfeeding. There is no longer a weight criterion for discharge from many units and often neonates are sent home with a nasogastric tube in situ to establish breastfeeding in the community. Indices used to evaluate breastfeeding for term babies, such as wet and dirty nappies and the pattern of feeds, are not always appropriate for an infant born preterm. Members of voluntary support groups do not always have this knowledge, although it is important to keep them involved and informed regarding local preterm breastfeeding guidelines and protocols. The concerns mothers have about the adequacy of breast feeds are realistic and not just the result of their experience in hospital. The risk of underconsumption is a very real concern, necessitating skilled advice and support. A discharge plan should be made in conjunction with parents to ensure continuity of care and to provide anticipatory advice. Open access to hospital breast-feeding coordinators can also make an enormous difference in emergency situations such as the baby refusing to feed or significant weight loss. Planning well in advance will help to alleviate parental anxiety by providing a raft of practical breastfeeding support.[3]

SUMMARY OF RECOMMENDATIONS

Modified demand–feeding
The following factors should be considered to determine infant intake:
- Assessment of attachment and positioning
- Suck/swallow patterning and audible swallowing
- Maternal perceptions regarding MER
- Degree of breast fullness before and after feeds

- Minimum feeds in 24 h
- Need for supplementation following breast feeds
- Need for milk expression after breast-feed
- Infant excretion patterns
- Discharge planning should include a plan for exclusive demand-feeding
- Provide a postdischarge breastfeeding support network

CUP-FEEDING

Although cup-feeding has been used to supplement breastfeeding infants in the developing world,[26,27] this method of feeding was not reintroduced to the UK until the late 1980s.[28,29] Lang et al.[28] observed mothers cup-feeding low-birth-weight infants in Nepal, and recognized that cup-feeding was a skill that could easily be acquired by preterm infants, at a point in development where it was otherwise thought that feeding tubes were a necessity (Box 10.4). On her return to the UK, she introduced the use of cup-feeding for infants from 30 weeks' postconceptional age in a British NICU.[28] Lang et al.[28] studied 500 babies who received cup feeds on one or more occasions and came to the conclusion that cup-feeding was appropriate for several groups of infants. These were:

- preterm infants who were breast-fed but did not settle after tube feeds
- breastfeeding infants nearing discharge whose mothers were not resident on the neonatal unit
- larger infants born by caesarean section who could not be put to the breast in the immediate period following delivery

A recent study measured sipping, breathing, oxygen saturation and volume of intake during 15 cup-feeding sessions for 8 infants.[31] The results of the study showed that breathing and oxygen saturation remained stable during bursts of laps and sips. The researchers came to the conclusion that cup-feeding as performed in the study is a safe method for feeding preterm infants. However, the authors caution that differentiating between actual intake versus

> ### Box 10.4 Method for cup-feeding[30]
>
> 1. Wrap the baby securely to prevent the baby's hands knocking the cup. Use a terry napkin (diaper) placed under the infant's chin. (This can be weighed both before and after the feed, if necessary)
> 2. Support the baby in a semi-upright sitting position
> 3. If possible, have the cup at least half-full for the beginning of the feed
> 4. The cup should be tipped so that the milk is just touching the baby's lips. Do not pour milk into the baby's mouth
> 5. Direct the rim of the cup towards the corners of the upper lips and gums, with it gently touching or resting on the baby's lower lip. Do not apply pressure to the lower lip
> 6. Leave the cup in the correct position during the feed. Do not keep removing it when the baby stops lapping. It is important to let babies pace their own intake in their own time

spillage of milk merits attention. In a detailed discussion of their findings the authors suggest that 'sipping' was observed more frequently than 'lapping'. They question whether or not 'sipping' is conducive to establishment of breastfeeding, since sipping requires a different mouth action than breast- or bottle-feeding. Further research is needed to clarify this point.

In a prospective randomized cross-over study in the USA, 56 infants ≤ 34 weeks' gestation at birth, whose mothers indicated a desire to breastfeed, were studied.[32] When infants were ≤ 34 weeks' corrected gestational age, the order of the first two non-breast oral feedings was randomized to one cup-feeding and one bottle-feeding. Heart rate, respiratory rate and oxygen saturation were recorded at 1-min intervals for 10 min before and during the feeding. Volume taken, time required to complete a feed, and any apnoea, bradycardia, choking or spitting episodes were recorded. The researchers concluded that during cup feeds infants were physiologically stable with lower heart rates, higher oxygen saturation and less desaturations than during bottle feeds. However, during cup feeds infants took less volume and required a longer feeding time than when bottle-feeding.

In another study from the USA, the researchers compared the amounts ingested, administration time and infant physiologic stability during cup-, bottle- and breastfeeding.[33] A total of 98 term, healthy newborns were randomized to either cup-feeding or bottle-feeding. Twenty-five breast-fed infants were also monitored for heart rate, respiratory rate and oxygen saturation during one feed. Administration times, amounts ingested and infant physiological stability did not differ between the cup and bottle groups. Breastfeeding took longer than cup- or bottle-feeding, but infants experienced less physiologic variability. These data support cup-feeding as an alternative to bottle-feeding for supplying supplements for breast-fed infants.

In conclusion, although cup-feeding appears to be a safe short-term method to supplement preterm breast-fed infants, appropriate training must be in place, since there is a risk of aspiration if a poor technique is used. Milk spillage can also be a significant problem, exposing infants to the risk of underconsumption. The opportunity to establish breastfeeding must be in place since an infant may become addicted to sipping and become unwilling to make the wider jaw excursions needed for correct attachment. Exclusive long-term cup-feeding will also deprive a baby of the sucking experience.[34] In addition, some infants 'fight' the cup, refusing to lap the milk offered. Therefore, the feeding method must be determined individually depending on infant response and circumstances.

SUMMARY OF RECOMMENDATIONS

Cup–feeding
- A series of studies have shown that cup-feeding is a safe method to supplement preterm infants, if appropriate training is in place

Disadvantages include:
- milk loss from spillage

- aspiration is a danger if a poor feeding technique is used
- some infants become addicted to cup-feeding
- some infants 'fight' the cup and want to suck
- long-term exclusive cup-feeding will deprive a baby of the sucking experience

NIPPLE SHIELDS

In a study performed in the USA by Meier et al.,[35] the researchers reported on the breastfeeding outcome for 34 preterm infants whose mothers used ultrathin silicone nipple shields to increase milk transfer. Mean milk transfer was compared for two consecutive breast feeds with and without the nipple shield. Mean milk transfer was significantly greater for feeding with the nipple shield. Mean duration of nipple shield use was 32 days and mean duration of breastfeeding was 169 days. The authors conclude that this study is the first one performed to indicate that nipple shield use increases milk intake without decreasing the total duration of breastfeeding for preterm infants.

The authors also state that, once the shield is placed properly over the nipple and the infant begins to suck, negative pressure appears to be generated and maintained in the small chamber between the tip of the nipple and the interior of the shield. These pressures may compensate for weak infant suction and facilitate the accumulation of milk in the shield during pauses in sucking, making it immediately available to the infant when sucking resumes (Fig. 10.9).

Unfortunately, this was a non-experimental study with no random selection in a clinically selected group of babies, where test feeds were not randomly assigned. However, despite the poor study design, this study indicates that in cases where there is a marked disparity between the size of an infant's mouth and the mother's breast, nipple shields are an effective tool for an infant to obtain an adequate seal, sufficient negative pressure and an adequate suckling mechanism. Mothers must be advised to empty the breast following a feed, since the use of a shield may decrease the amount of milk removed from the breast.[36]

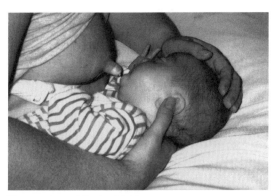

Figure 10.9   Nipple shield.

SUMMARY OF RECOMMENDATIONS

Nipple shields
- Nipple shields should not be offered on a routine basis, but rather weighing up risk versus benefit
- Nipple shields may decrease the amount of milk removed from the breast

BREASTFEEDING SUPPLEMENTER

Breastfeeding supplementers are designed to provide the infant with a steady flow of a supplementary feed while suckling and to provide nipple and breast stimulation. They are particularly useful in a mother with an insufficient milk supply. They help to entice the infant to suck at the breast with a good suckling pattern.

Figure 10.10 shows the supplemental nursing system produced by Medela. It consists of a container to hold milk and thin tubing that is attached to the mother's nipple, paper tape and an adjustable shoulder halter. The rate of milk flow can be determined by the size of tubing. The system was first developed to help adoptive mothers to induce lactation by stimulating a hormonal response to suckling. When the baby suckles at the breast, milk supplements are also delivered (Fig. 10.11; Box 10.5) A system like this can be improvised using a nasogastric tube and a cup.

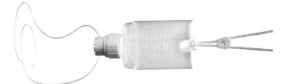

Figure 10.10   Breast-feeding supplementer equipment.

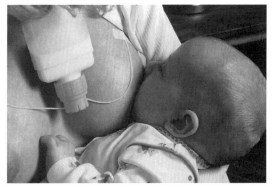

Figure 10.11   Breast-feeding supplementer.

Box 10.5   How to help a mother to use a breast-feeding supplementer

Show the mother how to:
- use a fine nasogastric tube (or other fine plastic tubing) and a cup to hold milk
- cut a small hole in the side of the tube, near the end that goes into the infant's mouth. This helps milk flow
- prepare a cup of milk (expressed or formula) containing the amount an infant will require for one feed
- tape one end of the tube near the nipple, so that the infant suckles at the breast and the tube simultaneously
- put the other end of the tube in a container of milk
- clamp the tube to control the flow of milk
- control the flow of milk so an infant suckles for approximately 30 min to ensure nipple and breast stimulation. (Raising the milk container makes the milk flow faster, while lowering the container will reduce the flow)
- encourage an infant to suckle often
- clean and sterilize both the tube and the milk container before each feed

Feeding-tube systems are extremely useful for infants with weak or disorganized sucking patterns. They avoid the potential threat of nipple/teat confusion by allowing an infant to be coaxed to feed at the breast. Correct breast attachment and suckling will cause milk to flow and will reward an infant for the effort.

Since the tubing is small and very soft, flow is easily controlled. When a nutritive suckling pattern is achieved, further flow is obstructed by suction, allowing milk to be suckled from the breast and not from the storage container. Feeding tubes are not easy to use, and many women find them intrusive and psychologically difficult to accept.

Some babies may become addicted to the device, or may quickly discover that the easiest way to obtain a feed is to grasp the tubing by hand and to place it in the mouth. However, this system has been used very successfully on the NICU at North Staffordshire Maternity Hospital, UK. It was particularly useful in a situation in which a mother wished to relactate.

SUMMARY OF RECOMMENDATIONS

Breastfeeding supplementer
- Breastfeeding supplementers are designed to provide the infant with a steady flow of a supplementary feed during suckling, whilst suckling provides nipple and breast stimulation

References

1. Glass RP, Wolf LS. Coordination of sucking, swallowing and breathing as an etiology for breathing difficulty. J Hum Lact 1994; 10:185–189.
2. Siddell E, Froman RA. A national survey of neonatal intensive-care units: criteria used to determine readiness for oral feeding. JOGNN 1994; 23:783–789.
3. Jones E, Spencer SA. Successful preterm breastfeeding. In: Wickham S, ed. Midwifery best practice. London: Churchill Livingstone; 2003:176–179.
4. Nyqvist KH, Ewald U. Successful breast-feeding in spite of early mother-baby separation for neonatal care. Midwifery 1997; 13:24–31.
5. Mathew OP, Clark ML, Pronske ML et al. Breathing pattern and ventilation during oral feeding in term newborn infants. J Pediatr 1985; 106:810–813.
6. Weber F, Woolridge MW, Baum JD. An ultrasonographic study of the organization of sucking and swallowing by newborn infants. Dev Med Child Neurol 1986; 28:19–24.
7. Meier PP, Anderson GC. Responses of preterm infants to bottle and breast-feeding. Am J Mat Child Nurs 1987; 12:420–423.
8. Blaymore-Bier J, Ferguson A, Anderson L et al. Breastfeeding of very low birth weight infants. Pediatrics 1993; 123:773–778.
9. Mathew OP, Bhatia J. Sucking and breathing patterns during breast- and bottle-feeding in term neonates. Am J Dis Child 1989; 143:588–592.
10. Nyqvist KH, Sjoden PO, Ewald U. The development of preterm infants' breast-feeding behavior. Early Hum Dev 1999; 55:247–264.
11. Cole JG. Using the NBAS with high-risk infants. In: Brazelton TB, Nugent JK, eds. Neonatal behavioral assessment scale, 3rd edn. Cambridge: Cambridge University Press; 1995:126–132.
12. Als H. Toward a synactive theory of development: promise for the assessment and support of infant individuality. Infant Mental Health J 1982; 3:229–243.
13. Nyqvist KH, Ewald U, Sjoden P. Supporting a preterm infant's behaviour during breastfeeding: a case report. J Hum Lact 1996; 12:221–228.
14. Nyqvist KH, Ewald U. Infant and maternal factors in the development of breast-feeding behaviour and breastfeeding outcome in preterm infants. Acta Paediatr 1999; 88:1194–1203.
15. Warren I, Tan GC, Dixon P. Breast-feeding success and early discharge for preterm infants: the result of a dedicated breast-feeding programme. J Neonatal Nurs 2000; 6:43–48.
16. Biancuzzo M. Techniques of delivering human and artificial milk. In: Biancuzzo M, ed. Breastfeeding the newborn. Clinical strategies for nurses, 2nd edn. St Louis, MO: Mosby; 2003:445–464.
17. Biancuzzo M. Strategies for breastfeeding the preterm newborn. In: Biancuzzo M, ed. Breast-feeding the newborn. Clinical strategies for nurses, 2nd edn. St Louis, MO: Mosby; 2003:261–286.
18. Jones E, Spencer SA. Promoting successful preterm breastfeeding (part 2). Pract Midwife 2002; 5:22–24.
19. Neifert M, Seacat J. Practical aspects of breastfeeding the preterm infant. Perin Neonatol 1988; 12:24–28.
20. Ramsay DT, Kent JC, Owens RA et al. Ultrasound imaging of milk ejection in the breast of lactating women. Pediatrics 2004; 113:361–367.
21. Meier PP, Brown LP, Hurst NM. Breastfeeding the preterm infant. In: Riodan J, Auerbach KG, eds. Breastfeeding and human lactation, 2nd edn. Boston MA Sudbury: Jones and Bartlett; 1998:449–481.
22. Kavanaugh K, Mead L, Meier P et al. Getting enough: mothers' concerns about breastfeeding a

preterm infant after discharge. J Obstet Gynecol Neonatal Nurs 1995; 24:23–32.

23. Hill PD, Hanson KS, Mefford AL. Mothers of low birthweight infants: breastfeeding patterns and problems. J Hum Lact 1994; 10:169–176.

24. Schanler RJ, Hurst NM, Lau C. The use of human milk and breastfeeding in premature infants. Clin Perinatol 1999; 26:379–398.

25. Hall WA, Shearer K, Mogan J et al. Weighing preterm infants before and after breastfeeding: does it increase maternal confidence and competence? MCN 2002; 27:318–326.

26. Armstrong HC. Breast-feeding low birthweight babies: advances in Kenya. J Hum Lact 1987; 3:34–37.

27. Muhudhia SO, Musoke RN. Postnatal weight gain of exclusively breast feed preterm African infants. J Trop Pediatr 1989; 35:241–244.

28. Lang S, Lawrence CJ, Orme R'E. Cup-feeding: an alternative method of infant feeding. Arch Dis Chil 1994; 71:365–369.

29. Jones E. Breastfeeding in the preterm infant. Mod Midwife 1994; 4:22–26.

30. Lang S. Alternative methods of feeding and breast-feeding. In: Lang S, ed. Breast-feeding special care babies, 2nd edn. Edinburgh: Baillière Tindall; 2002:202.

31. Dowling DA, Meier PP, DiFiore J et al. Cup-feeding for preterm infants: mechanics and safety. J Hum Lact 2002; 18:13–20.

32. Marinelli KA, Burke GS, Dodd VL. A comparison of the safety of cupfeedings and bottle-feedings in premature infants whose mothers intend to breastfeed. J Perinatol 2001; 21:350–355.

33. Howard CR, de Blieck EA, ten Hoopen CB. Physiologic stability of newborns during cup- and bottle-feeding. Pediatrics 1999; 104:1204–1207.

34. Fisher C, Inch S. Nipple confusion - who is confused? J Pediatr 1996; 129:174–175.

35. Meier PP, Brown LP, Hurst NM. Nipple shields for preterm infants. effect on milk transfer and duration of breastfeeding. J Hum Lact 2000; 16:106–114.

36. Woolridge MW, Baum JD, Drewett RF. Effect of a traditional and of a new nipple shield on sucking patterns and milk flow. Early Hum Dev 1980; 4:357–364.

Chapter 11

Feeding problems

Annie Bagnall

PREMATURITY AND FEEDING PROBLEMS

As described in detail in Chapter 9, feeding reflexes and the ability to co-ordinate sucking with swallowing and respiration reach maturity during the last trimester of pregnancy. Premature infants are at risk of feeding difficulties by nature of their neurological immaturity and they often start oral feeding before they reach term gestational age. Without a mature feeding pattern the baby may demonstrate suboptimal feeding behaviours and will require supplemental tube-feeding. An understanding of the normal development of feeding enables the caregiver to assess a preterm infant's readiness to feed. Gradual introduction of oral feeding is necessary to avoid complications such as aspiration caused by poor co-ordination and/or fatigue.

Coupled with prematurity, feeding problems seen on the special care baby unit (SCBU) often have additional underlying causes, such as neurological impairment, gastro-oesophageal reflux (GOR), respiratory disease and behavioural issues.

If feeding problems do not resolve with maturity or are not treated effectively, they can become behavioural. In clinical data collected from a group of children under 7 years of age attending a behavioural feeding disorders clinic, 50% had required special care after birth and 22% were born prematurely. Other factors such as low birth weight, distress during feeding in the first 6 months of life, prolonged tube-feeding and frequent vomiting were common findings in their case histories.[1] Similar findings were reported in a group of children (age range 4 months to 17 years) referred to a feeding team. Thirty-eight per cent of the children evaluated had a history of prematurity.[2] Many infants who experience feeding difficulties in the neonatal period are at risk of developing protracted feeding problems.

PREVENTING FEEDING PROBLEMS

Infants in utero are in a flexed position and can be seen sucking on their fingers on ultrasound scan and swallowing amniotic fluid. This intrauterine environment gives the baby the opportunity to develop and integrate immature feeding skills. When a baby is delivered prematurely this opportunity is disrupted. Many infants require procedures such as intubation and ventilation, which prevent them from maintaining a flexed position and they are unable to bring their hands to their mouth. Secretions are often suctioned to prevent aspiration during sedation and intubation. Such infants do not get the opportunity to swallow. Some infants suck on their endotracheal tube but this form of sucking practice is atypical of normal oral motor development.

Part of the role of managing feeding difficulties in preterm infants begins at this early stage. The gut may still be too immature to tolerate all their nutritional requirements enterally. In addition, their suck patterns are too immature to feed safely and efficiently, their state too fragile and unstable and the medical interventions too invasive, particularly orally, to consider suck-feeding. However, there are caregiving activities that can normalize their oral experiences and enable them to practise some of the skills they will need for later successful oral feeding.

The oral cavity is one of the most sensitive areas for the infant[3] and yet it is often where many invasive procedures occur. Infants who receive only painful or irritating stimuli in the oral cavity may be at risk of developing later

feeding aversion and oral hyper- or hypo-sensitivity which can interfere with later suck-feeding. Interventions to diminish negative stimulation may reduce the frequency of sensory-based feeding difficulties which commonly occur in preterm infants.

Sick and premature infants may have dampened oral motor reflexes. They do not develop rooting in the marked way that is seen in the term infant. The gag and cough reflex may be suppressed to enable endotracheal and orogastric (OG) or nasogastric (NG) tubes to remain in situ. Positive-pressure ventilation will alter the sensation of the oral pharyngeal cavity and may lead to desensitization of the area where reflexes critical to safe feeding are found, e.g. the site of swallow trigger and gag. The process and extent of how these reflexes recover are unknown. Consideration of this during or after invasive procedures and routine cares may reduce potential complications. The best treatment for feeding difficulties is prevention.[4]

INTUBATION

Oral intubation can cause palatal grooves/high arched palate, gum or lip clefting, laryngeal trauma, subglottic stenosis and subsequent dental complications, all of which can have an impact on the development of successful feeding.[5] The length of time of orotracheal intubation also has an impact on sucking behaviour at 3 months.[5] This may be due to a lack of sucking experience, severity of neonatal illness, intubation injury/palatal groove or neurological status.[6] Palatal grooves make it hard to achieve a good seal between the palate and the tongue.[7]

NASO- AND OROGASTRIC TUBES

Very preterm infants will initially need tube- (gavage) feeding. The longer the periods of no suck-feeding, the poorer the feeding performance later.[8]

Tube-feeding in small compromised infants can have an adverse effect on respiration, affecting compliance of the lung and chest wall and causing a consequent increase in diaphragmatic work; this is thought to be due to the effect of filling the stomach.[9]

One study reported that NG tubes caused nasal obstruction and were found to interfere with respiration, resulting in decreased minute ventilation and increased pulmonary resistance, causing secondary hypoventilation in infants under 2 kg.[10] However, NG tubes are easy to secure and allow the infant to suck-feed. OG tubes have less effect on the respiratory system but may interfere with tongue movement for sucking during oral feeding. Infants over 2 kg tolerate both NG and OG tube placement without difficulty. However, OG tube placement is favoured in infants under 2 kg.[10] There is a lack of consensus on using either NG or OG tubes in feeding very-low-birth-weight (VLBW) infants and each infant must be assessed individually.[11]

There is no research into the effect of NG tubes on swallowing in infants. A study by Huggins et al.[12] looked at the effect in young patients (20–27 years old) using videofluoroscopy. The effect on swallowing depended on the size of the tube and was most impaired with a wide-bore tube (16 French). However, the researchers noted that disruption also occurred with a fine-bore tube (8 French). Pharyngeal swallow was disrupted in terms of earlier swallow initiation, delayed pharyngeal transit times and prolonged opening of the cricopharyngeus. Therefore the presence of an NG tube must be considered as a potential contributing factor to observed feeding difficulties.

Shiao et al.[13] observed feeding performance in infants with or without an NG tube present. The average VLBW infant without an NG tube in situ fed better 71% of the time than with an NG tube in place. In a further study by Shiao et al.,[13] infants who were bottle-fed with an NG tube in situ had more prolonged feed-associated desaturations.

Long-term intubation or use of NG tubes can lead to ulceration, laryngeal injury and pharyngeal discomfort.[14] Trauma to the oral pharyngeal mucosa can lead to the development of sensory-based feeding difficulties, where sensory awareness in the pharynx has become depressed in order to withstand the initial trauma.[15] This is referred to as conditioned dysphagia.[16] Stimulation of the oral area may result in avoidance behaviours such as gagging, vomiting or physically expelling food. Unpleasant experiences or lack of positive experiences associated with eating can result in an infant who exhibits food refusal.[17,18]

PREVENTIVE INTERVENTIONS

Non-nutritive sucking

A substantial amount of work has been published on the topic of non-nutritive sucking (NNS) in the past 30 years. Preterm infants are born before they are able to co-ordinate nutritive sucking safely and efficiently. The benefits of NNS (on a dummy or pacifier) for this population are different than for term babies. Pacifier use has been shown to reduce behavioural distress to painful procedures and to help organize state/physiological stability, particularly during tube feeds.[19–26] The use of NNS is also recommended by some experts as a developmentally supportive response to behavioural cues.[27–29]

NNS may promote easier or more rapid transition from tube- to full-suck feeds as it may accelerate the organization and efficiency of sucking.[20,27,30–34] It can also build an association between sucking and satiation.[27,31]

NNS may stimulate the gastric motor function and therefore facilitate the digestion of enteral feeds. This occurs via activity of vagal mechanisms with stimulation of nerve fibres in the oral cavity. Activation of the vagal nerve influences the levels of gastrointestinal hormones such as gastrin and somatostatin. Secretion of gastrin is necessary for acid secretion, gastric motility and intestinal mucosa growth. A decrease in somatostatin hormone promotes gastric emptying.[34] There is evidence that maturation of gastrointestinal motility can be enhanced by the introduction of enteral feeds (see Chapter 7). However, many preterm infants, particularly the most immature and growth-restricted, develop feed intolerance, which can present as abdominal distension and vomiting. NNS has been hypothesized to improve gastric motility.[31] However two studies[35,36] found no difference in intestinal transit times or energy intakes. In addition, three randomized controlled trials report no effect of NNS on gastric emptying.[34,37,38]

A recent Cochrane review[39] of 20 papers (14 of which were randomized controlled trials) looked at the influence of NNS on weight gain, energy intake, heart rate, oxygen saturation, length of hospital stay, intestinal transit time, age at full oral feeds and any other clinically relevant outcomes. The review found that NNS significantly decreases the length of hospital stay in preterm infants. There was no consistent benefit of NNS with respect to any other major clinical variables. Other positive clinical outcomes were transition from tube to bottle feeds, better bottle-feeding performance and behaviour. The researchers concluded that NNS in preterm infants would appear to have some clinical benefit and does not have any short-term negative outcomes, although longer-term data would be helpful.

A number of feeding experts have expressed concerns regarding pacifier use in term breast-fed infants. They suggest that pacifier use leads to 'nipple teat confusion', which teaches an infant improper breastfeeding suckling techniques. The United Nations Children's Emergency Fund (UNICEF)/World Health Organization recommends avoiding both supplemental feedings as well as artificial teats as part of their 10 steps to successful breastfeeding.[116]

Several retrospective and cohort studies have shown a negative impact of pacifier use on duration and exclusivity of breast-feeding in term babies.[40–44] Two randomized trials demonstrated no effect; however, they were limited to either the first week of life or randomized not to pacifier use but to counselling regarding use.[42,45] Although it can be argued that pacifier use may be a marker for differing attitudes and commitment regarding breastfeeding or differences in the baby's temperament, undoubtedly insufficient breast stimulation and milk removal has a detrimental effect on maternal lactation and breastfeeding duration.[46] There does not appear to be evidence for a biological basis for 'nipple/teat confusion' and this theory remains anecdotal.

In a recently published randomized controlled trial of the effect of bottles, cups and dummies on breastfeeding in preterm infants, the use of dummies was not found to affect breast-feeding habits.[47] Many neonatal feeding experts argue that preterm infants should be given the chance to practise sucking skills as they would in utero.[31] If an infant is stable, a pacifier can be substituted by encouraging an infant to suck the fingers or alternatively NNS can be offered during skin-to-skin/kangaroo activity by offering the emptied breast during tube feeds. During this early period before oral feeding is established, maternal lactation must be sustained by milk expression. It is possible that prolonged pacifier sucking may interfere with the baby's ability to display feeding cues. Therefore, NNS use on the neonatal unit should be a very specific part of the feeding regime and not used indiscriminately or for long periods of time.

As an infant begins to take more oral feeds at around 33 weeks' gestation, the use of NNS is no longer appropriate, unless the baby's clinical condition indicates otherwise. To conclude, in sick and premature infants the careful use of NNS may have advantages for babies that outweigh any possible disadvantages.

Which dummy to use?

There are a variety of shapes, sizes and textures of dummies available commercially and some specialized dummies are produced for medical use.

There are no specific recommendations, although there is some discussion in the literature that can inform individual decision-making. Drosten[48] recommends an orthodontic rather than big ball shape to avoid restricting tongue movement. Webster[29] produced some useful guidelines after nursing consultation in 1999. Tiny dummies such as the 'wee thumbie' continuous positive airway pressure dummy or the preterm NUK™ dummy are only useful for

VLBW babies (see Resources for stockists). It is better for an infant to maintain a wide mouth posture for later establishment of breastfeeding rather than develop a tiny pursed attachment around a small teat.

Babies should not develop a preference for one dummy. Varying dummy use should be considered if illness is prolonged and NNS continues to be indicated. A recent study using an odour-emitting pacifier demonstrated an increase in NNS activity during tube-feeding when breast milk odour was present.[49] Such pacifiers are available commercially and may have a use with preterm infants.

It is vital that a properly manufactured dummy is used. Makeshift pacifiers stuffed with cotton or gauze taped to the plastic collar have been reported as resulting in fatal aspiration and their use should stop.[50]

ADDITIONAL CAUSES OF FEEDING DIFFICULTY IN PRETERM INFANTS

As well as being immature, preterm infants may be predisposed to coexisting factors that may have an impact on feeding.

Neurological impairment

Extreme prematurity (< 25 weeks' gestation) is a risk factor in the development of neurological impairment and developmental disability.[51,52] Neonatal feeding problems may be an early indicator of neurological impairment. Wolff,[53] in a study of infant sucking behaviour, concluded that neurological disease alters the pattern of sucking, resulting in abnormal sucking rhythms.

The sucking reflex, along with normal tongue, lip, jaw and pharyngeal movements needed for sucking and swallowing, is regulated in the central nervous system. Co-ordination of sucking and swallowing depends on intact brainstem pathways and the transmission of nerve impulses through cranial nerves to healthy musculature. Damage to these regulatory centres or pathways may result in feeding difficulties. This could result in failure to thrive and/or recurrent aspiration pneumonia.

A decreased sucking reflex can occur in infants with perinatal hypoxia. They present with slower rates of NNS and tongue and jaw tremors. Abnormalities of the motor cranial nerve nuclei X, XI and XII (bulbar palsy) may lead to weak or poorly sustained sucking. The tone of the tongue may be hypotonic, making it remain flat without a central groove to cup the nipple. A weak suck can reduce the ability to generate suction and result in poor attachment. Infants with neurological impairment may also present with incoordination of sucking, swallowing and respiration. If the brainstem is damaged there may be mistiming of the sucking sequence. If swallowing is incoordinated, coughing, choking and aspiration may occur. Infants with neurological damage are frequently hypersensitive to oral stimulation as it triggers their hyperactive reflex activity, e.g. tongue-thrusting, excessive jaw-opening, jaw-clenching (tonic bite reflex), gagging or neck and body extensor tone/spasm. Infants may have increased muscle tone. A hypertonic tongue is bunched and retracted, which can also interfere with attachment and stripping of the nipple. When there is bilateral damage to the corticospinal tract (psuedobulbar palsy), infants present with spastic weakness of the muscles innervated by the cranial nerves. Due to the extent of the damage, the feeding prognosis for these infants is poor and they often experience recurrent episodes of aspiration. Oral motor features are tongue-thrusting and hyperactive gag. Poor co-ordination is often seen as sucking returns after severe birth asphyxia. Infants who sustain unilateral cerebral insults in the perinatal period (e.g. infarcts or parenchymal haemorrhages) may have suppression of sucking at first but do not usually develop incoordinated sucking and swallowing.[54]

The prognosis with feeding depends on the underlying neurological impairment. Improvement can occur due to further maturation of the central nervous system. However some children will require long-term supplemental feeding for safe and efficient feeding, e.g. gastrostomy.

There is little information regarding the success of breastfeeding in infants with neurological impairment: This may be due to prolonged neonatal illness, poor sucking or unsafe swallow co-ordination. Due to the potential risk of aspiration and the limitations of assessment techniques, an infant with neurological problems may be bottle-fed. However, a neurologically impaired child and mother will still benefit from kangaroo/skin-to-skin contact and breastfeeding should not be ruled out. An infant may in fact be better able to pause and co-ordinate swallowing from the breast, i.e. from a milk source that is not rapid and free-flowing, like some bottles. However, cup-feeding may be contraindicated as the infant has reduced ability to protect the airway from aspiration and may not co-ordinate lapping with swallowing and breathing.

Respiratory difficulties

Preterm infants, particularly those who require long-term mechanical ventilation secondary to respiratory distress syndrome are at risk of developing bronchopulmonary dysplasia (BPD), also known as chronic lung disease. Other respiratory difficulties, such as tracheobronchomalacia, can occur after intubation.

Infants who develop BPD weigh less at birth than age-matched controls and typically have lower energy intakes due to later establishment of enteral feeds.[55] Some infants with BPD may have higher calorie requirements due to chronic hypoxaemia and increased energy expenditure with the work of respiration. Studies in oxygen-dependent infants with BPD have shown that some of them have increased energy expenditure.[56,57] It is therefore essential that they receive adequate nutrition (see Chapter 8).

Infants who develop BPD are at high risk of adverse oral experiences and GOR.[59] They often have longer transition times from tube on to oral feeding.[60,61] These can result in sensory-aversive feeding difficulties such as food refusal and gagging and these infants are at risk of long-term feeding problems.

Infants with BPD have a high prevalence of suck–swallow–breathe coordination difficulties.[62–65] In an infant with respiratory compromise, the respiratory suppression that occurs during the continuous sucking burst may not be well tolerated or sustainable for an entire feed. The infant may not recover respiration adequately in the pauses and may fatigue before a feed is completed. Furthermore, when the respiratory drive is increased by artificially elevating the amount of carbon dioxide in inspired air, sucking and swallowing rates have been found to decrease.[66] This suggests that the increased respiratory drive resulting from carbon dioxide chemoreceptor activation has a detrimental effect on feeding. This has added consequences for infants with BPD who have a higher respiratory drive due to diminished lung function. Infants with BPD have been found to have more desaturation events during feedings.[67] Feeding for these infants may be further inhibited, leading to poor growth and development.

In a study by Gewolb et al.,[68] anticipated maturational patterns of suckle and swallow rhythms did not occur in preterm infants with BPD. There was not only a lag in development of suck/swallow stability but it appeared to get worse as the babies got older. The researchers hypothesized that this may reflect the impact of tachypnoea and respiratory factors but concluded that it may also predict neurological impairment risk factors for these infants.

Desaturation events during feeding can persist once infants are weaned from oxygen and discharged home.[69] They correlate with larger volumes consumed and faster intake, implying that some infants with BPD may feed slowly to avoid desaturations. Desaturations can be prevented by the feeder with interventions such as pacing or slowing the rate of flow of the teat. Prolonging the use of supplemental oxygen when feeding may also reduce the risk of desaturations with feeds as supplemental oxygen during feeding may be helpful in minimizing hypoxaemia-induced respiratory depression.[70–72] Infants with BPD who were breast-fed have been found to have higher oxygen saturations during feeding than bottle-fed infants.[6]

In studies looking at parent–child feeding interaction, mothers of VLBW infants spent more time prompting their infants to feed when their infants engaged in non-feeding behaviour. Despite this encouragement, the VLBW infants with BPD took in less formula and spent less time sucking.[69]

These infants can be particularly difficult to feed and it is essential that families receive adequate support in their feeding practice.[63]

Gastrointestinal problems

GOR is common in young infants and most outgrow it. It can range from mild and benign through to life-threatening and is termed GOR disease (GORD) at this end of the spectrum. Oesophageal peristalsis, lower oesophageal sphincter competence and the anatomy of the oesophagus mature with postnatal age, reducing the incidence of GOR.[73] In preterm infants, the tone may be lower and progression through this development may be slower. The incidence of GOR in VLBW preterm infants has been reported to be as high as 85% of subjects studied and was unrelated to postconceptual age.[74]

Reflux of gastric contents can elicit the laryngeal chemoreflex, resulting in apnoea and bradycardia.[75] Severe GOR can result in vomiting but symptoms can also be more discrete and are not always clinically apparent.[74] In persistent GOR, crying, arching and food refusal are common. A learned association of feeding with the pain of oesophagitis can lead to feeding aversion.[73]

GOR is known to be a contributing factor in respiratory disease due in part to aspiration[76,77] and can exacerbate chronic lung disease. Infants with coexisting neurological impairment have an increased chance of having GOR.[78] In the infant requiring NG tube-feeding, GOR may be worse due to an increased number of transient relaxations of the lower oesophageal sphincter, the physiological mechanism responsible for most reflux episodes.[79]

Feeding difficulties are common in the infant with GORD. A controlled study of 6-month-old term infants with GORD found that a significant proportion of subjects had moderate to severe oral motor dysfunction. They presented with oral hypersensitivity and immature lip,

tongue and jaw control. This resulted in food refusal and more food loss during mealtimes. The infants had significantly more panic reactions and choking episodes. Videofluoroscopy showed marked oral phase problems, with a substantial number of infants being aversive to the procedure. Some infants had compensatory abnormal head extension that increased the risk of aspiration. Infants with GORD had lower energy intakes than controls and consumed less than their recommended daily intake. Infants were more demanding, had fewer vocalizations and were more difficult to feed. Mothers reported more negative feelings and found feeding less enjoyable and rewarding. The authors concluded that significant morbidity was associated with GORD in relation to the infant-feeding experience for mother and child.[80] Once infants have a disrupted development of feeding they may acquire maladaptive behavioural patterns.[2]

Optimal diagnosis and treatment of GOR are essential to avoid long-lasting behavioural feeding difficulties. Recent research has questioned the validity and reliability of using pH monitoring to detect GOR in preterm infants.[81] Current clinical management, particularly the use of cisapride, remains controversial. An increased incidence of coughing has been recorded when infants are given thickened feeds.[82] This may be due to its effect on gastric emptying and precipitation of later GOR. Currently there are significant variations in practice.[83] Further studies regarding optimal assessment and treatment of GOR are vital for the effective management and to prevent feeding problems developing.[73,77,78]

Other gastrointestinal problems common to preterm infants can also contribute to feeding difficulties. Necrotizing enterocolitis may lead to prolonged periods of nil by mouth, resulting in delayed sucking and sensory-aversive feeding difficulties.

Other coexisting factors that can cause feeding difficulties are cardiac anomalies or jaundice leading to fatigue with feeding. Coexisting developmental syndromes or structural abnormalities such as tongue-tie, macroglossia, choanal atresia, micrognathia or cleft palate may also have an impact on feeding but are beyond the scope of this chapter. However, it is important to ascertain, where possible, the cause of the feeding difficulty to enable effective treatment.

Feeding problems are frequently multifactorial and therefore detailed multidisciplinary assessment is essential.

ASSESSMENT OF FEEDING PROBLEMS

Case history

Assessment begins by taking a case history from the medical notes and reports from carers. This includes factors that may influence feeding performance, such as perinatal events and chronological and gestational age. Other factors known to influence feeding performance, e.g. respiratory, neurological, gastroenterological and cardiac status, should also be noted. The course of medical intervention, including ventilation and feeding history, will give an indication of other factors that may predispose the infant to feeding problems.

Pre-feeding assessment/oral examination

Before feeding, the resting respiratory rate should be assessed. Tachypnoea with a respiratory rate above 60 breaths/min can have a profound effect on the ability to feed orally[84] and may preclude oral feeding. If the infant commences oral feeding with rapid breathing, the baby will be unable to increase the respiratory rate to compensate for swallow apnoea. This can lead to difficulties with co-ordination, resulting in fatigue and aspiration during feeds. An oral examination assesses oral structures, shape, symmetry and muscular ability. A note should be made of any structural abnormalities of the lips, tongue, palate and buccal musculature. An assessor must wear gloves when doing an oral evaluation and a pen torch is useful in visualizing structures. Tongue depressors can be used but are often too large

and are an invasive start to an oral feed. Such rigorous oral examination may only be required where structural problems are strongly suspected.

Typical observations in a preterm oral assessment are that the tongue tip is held in an elevated, retracted position[18] and fat/sucking pads are absent.

It is important to assess perioral sensitivity and rooting. Rooting is unlikely to be elicited more than 30 min before a feed is due. Term infants born by elective caesarean section have been found to have a weaker rooting response,[85] as have preterm infants who have received numerous oral-based interventions. This may have an impact on an infant's ability to attach to a nipple or teat.

Assessing the gag may be an invasive first approach with a preterm infant with feeding difficulties. Asking caregivers about their observations of an infant's gag function during suction or tube changes can avoid the need for invasive assessment. However, for the infant with neurological impairment, who may not yet be having suck feeds, it is a vital first step to inform on the safety of swallow trials.

The frequency of suctioning of saliva required and the presence of drooling give an indication of spontaneous swallow functioning.

Non-nutritive sucking

Before a feed it is important to elicit NNS to assess initiation, strength and rhythm. This is best done with a gloved finger in order to feel tongue compression or stripping and the suction efficiency.

Objective and quantitative techniques to assess compression and suction during NNS have been used in the research literature but are either too invasive and cumbersome or not yet available for routine use in clinical evaluation.[86,87]

Atypical oral motor patterns and abnormalities of tone or movement can be felt, for example tongue retraction or tremor, wide jaw excursion or jaw clenching and arrhythmic tongue or jaw movement. These are often associated with neurological impairment and have a negative impact on feeding.

Feeding observation

Where possible, a feeding evaluation should be performed by an observer experienced in preterm feeding development. In the UK in the SCBU this is often a specialist speech and language therapist or a trained nurse or specialist midwife.

Feeding assessment must include a feeding observation by an experienced practitioner as reports on an infant's feeding behaviour from an inexperienced observer may not be accurate. Observations can be made during breast- or bottle-feeding. It may be useful to observe the feeding process rather than being the feeder, as this enables more careful observation. An infant should be assessed while being fed in the usual circumstances, i.e. the same position and type of teat. Some feeding problems can be caused by poor positioning or feeder technique rather than a feeding problem intrinsic to the infant. A note should be made of the feeder, position and any supplements or thickeners added. If the infant is bottle-fed, the type of milk given, type of teat and bottle used should be recorded. If the baby is being breast-fed, the breast and nipple size, shape and health and maternal lactation must be considered.

Mild difficulties with coordination during a feed may not be observed unless there is significant cyanosis or breathing difficulties.[70,88] Therefore, infants need to stay on cardiorespiratory monitors during feeds to enable accurate monitoring of changes in heart rate and respiration.

Monitoring is useful in infants but should not replace careful observation of behavioural cues. State and motor change are sensitive indicators of the infant's ability to integrate sucking, swallowing and breathing and are routinely present prior to more obvious signs of distress.[89] Physiologic distress signals such as changes in tone or colour, hiccups, nasal flaring and facial grimaces need to be noted as well as more obvious signs, as they can indicate underlying physiologic instability with subsequent impact on feeding performance.

In an infant with disruptions in gag reflex, tachypnoea, drooling or frequent suction requirements, it is safer to start a feeding assessment with sterile water as it will be less harmful to the lungs if aspirated. With such a high-risk swallow evaluation the infant should only be assessed if suction equipment and the appropriate staff are available.[54]

When assessing sucking, comments need to be made on the ability to initiate suck, the rate, rhythm and the pattern of the bursts and pauses. These patterns can then be evaluated against patterns in the normal development of sucking co-ordination.

Milk loss around the teat or nipple may indicate poor sucking, particularly weak suction, or poor coordination, leading to milk being pushed back out rather than swallowed.

Nasal regurgitation may indicate problems with palatal closure which may be due to co-ordination or structural problems.

Coughing, choking, increased congestion, desaturation, breathlessness or colour changes during feeds may be indicative of aspiration and warrant further swallow investigation.

The length of feed times can give an idea of feeding efficiency. The entire feed time should take no longer than 30 min. Feeding beyond this time is fatiguing to the infant and calorific expenditure may be in excess of calorific value of feed consumed.[4,89] The average infant takes 0.2 ml per suck at a rate of one suck per second.[90] This means that an infant should be able to consume 60 ml in about 5 min if sucking efficiently without long pauses. Most preterm infants are not able to feed at this level of efficiency while on SCBU due to their immature feeding patterns.

It is important not to intervene during a feeding assessment. This is often difficult for the experienced feeder who is used to employing techniques such as jiggling the teat, pacing or giving jaw support to alter the infant's feeding performance. Such techniques may not be a spontaneous intervention for the next feeder. Therefore, in order to recommend strategies objectively it is important that they are tried in response to assessment, not during it.

Cervical auscultation

The use of cervical auscultation in the evaluation of pharyngeal swallow has become a part of adult bedside dysphagia assessment but agreement over technique has not been reached.[91] A small stethoscope is placed adjacent to the lateral aspect of the larynx.[92] Breath sounds are listened to before, during and after the swallow. This is a subjective evaluation and relies on clinical experience. It demonstrates the bolus transit sounds and abrupt brief actions of the larynx and pharynx preceding and succeeding the bolus transit sounds. The acoustic analysis it gives of swallow sounds may enable detection of swallowing difficulties. It may demonstrate the occasion or absence of a swallow, increased congestion, wheezes or stridor, which may indicate an unswallowed bolus or secretions or aspiration in the airway. This information can then be used to inform further investigations required. It is a screening rather than a diagnostic tool. It cannot currently detect precise physiologic events during the swallow and there is still debate as to what aspects of the swallow are represented by particular sounds. In a recent study by Reynolds et al.,[93] acoustic data were recorded and displayed graphically with the aim of making the interpretation of cervical auscultation data less subjective by replacing the verbal description of the sounds of feeding with quantitative numeric values. This has subsequently been used as a research tool but may provide a more objective assessment tool for clinicians in the future.

Neonatal oral motor assessment scale

Palmer and colleagues[94,95] have developed a clinical assessment tool to categorize the oral motor patterns in the neonatal period.[96] The test has interrater reliability[95] and the user needs training in its administration.

The neonatal oral motor assessment scale (NOMAS) separates characteristics of jaw and tongue movement into categories of normal, disorganized/transitional and dysfunctional. A disorganized suck refers to a lack of rhythm of total sucking activity whereas dysfunction refers to the interruption of the feeding process by abnormal movements. First, sucking is assessed non-nutritively on a pacifier then with a bottle for 2 minutes.

From their assessment and research literature the researchers conclude that the preterm infant initially presents with an immature suck pattern of 3–5 sucks per burst. Due to immature co-ordination, the infant breathes during the pauses. Mature sucking has between 10 and 30 sucks per burst with only brief pauses between bursts. Swallows and respirations occur during the bursts in a coordinated 1:1:1 ratio. A transitional suck can be identified by characteristics of both immature and mature suck patterns (Fig 11.1).

Braun & Palmer[96] found that disorganized preterm infants lacked the ability to make a rate change between rapid non-nutritive (2 per second) and the slower nutritive sucking (1 per second). If infants are not able to make the rate change and continue to suck too quickly, it results in gulping the milk too fast, gagging and choking.[18] Braun & Palmer also observed that a transitional sucking pattern was persistent, post term, in infants who were suffering other complications in addition to their prematurity.

Dysfunctional or abnormal oral motor features are identified, such as excessive jaw excursions, clenching, asymmetrical movements or hypo- or hypertonia. These may indicate specific neurological impairment rather than

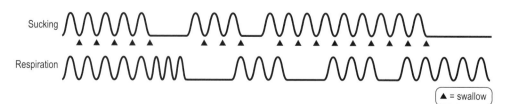

Sucking

Respiration

▲ = swallow

Figure 11.1   Transitional suck pattern.

immaturity and correlate with a poor neurological outcome in the longer term.[96]

The use of the NOMAS to assess breastfeeding behaviour has been questioned. Meier[97] drew attention to the fact that the NOMAS had only been used with bottle-fed infants and therefore the finding that bottle-fed infants have a transitional suck pattern could not be generalized to an infant's breastfeeding behaviour. She highlighted that the patterns of sucking are not interchangeable. Specifically, the rating as dysfunctional or wide jaw excursions that interrupt the seal on the bottle should not apply to breast-fed infants where a wide jaw excursion is essential for effective nipple attachment.

Whether applied in full or used as an adjunct, counting sucks per burst and hypothesizing about what is occurring with swallowing and respiration coordination is a helpful screen to distinguish between the immature, transitional/disorganized and dysfunctional feeder.

Videofluoroscopic swallow study (VFSS)

Videofluoroscopy remains the gold standard for objective swallow assessment. It is a modified barium-swallow study. The infant is positioned upright in supportive seating and is screened swallowing thin barium from a bottle in the lateral plane. Screening focuses on the oral and pharyngeal phase of swallowing and can also assess for penetration or aspiration of contrast into the airway. The study also provides an opportunity to evaluate the effect of intervention techniques on swallow function. The therapist is able to adapt the feeding utensils, position of the infant, consistency of liquid or food given and use feeding techniques such as pacing. Videofluoroscopy is possible with even the smallest infant but certain factors need to be considered and adaptations made.[98] The anatomy and physiology of infant swallowing are different from adult swallowing[99] and interpretation by someone educated in these differences is essential for accurate interpretation.

A VFSS gives a snapshot of the infant's swallowing ability and does not reflect swallow performance throughout an entire feed. Results must therefore be interpreted along with other available clinical data about the child when making management decisions.

The decision to refer for VFSS is taken after clinical evaluation has demonstrated indicators of swallow dysfunction or the infant's clinical picture is indicative of aspiration. It is a team decision and based on a risk-benefit discussion.

MANAGEMENT OPTIONS

The management of feeding difficulties must be done as a multidisciplinary team. The most important factor for an infant's development is sufficient nutrition to facilitate growth and recovery. Oral feeding encouragement must never compromise provision of adequate nutrition.

Oral stimulation

Alerting techniques in the form of oral stimulation can be useful in hyporeactive infants to help them initiate sucking. Perioral stroking or encouragement of NNS prior to a feed may alert the infant to sucking and encourage tongue movements for feeding.[54] Similarly, sweet tastes stimulate sucking, therefore dripping some breast milk on to the lips before a feed may encourage the initiation of sucking.

There is some evidence that oral stimulation through NNS or sensorimotor input to the oral structures has beneficial effects on oral feeding performance when applied before or during oral feeding in medically stable infants over 30 weeks' gestation. Leonard et al.[100] reported an enhanced sucking rate when the cheeks were stroked during an oral feeding session.

Gaebler & Hanzlik[101] demonstrated that infants receiving perioral and intraoral stimulation just before oral feedings scored better on the NOMAS scale[95] and had greater weight gain and fewer days of hospitalization.

Fucile et al.[102] recently published a study detailing an oral stimulation programme used with infants between 26 and 29 weeks' gestation. Infants who were randomized to the programme attained independent oral bottle-feeding earlier and had greater intake and rate of milk transfer than controls. The authors hypothesized that the oral stimulation may have strengthened oral musculature for sucking and may have enhanced the maturation of the central and/or peripheral neural structures, leading to improved sucking skills and co-ordination. Further studies are needed to con-firm the possibility that infants can be trained to improve their sucking skills. As discussed in Chapter 9, sucking skills and suck–swallow–breathe coordination develop with neurological maturity and it remains a topic for debate as to whether this maturity can be speeded up by mechanical intervention programmes.

In units adopting a developmental care approach, interventions take into account cues from the infant about tolerance of a procedure and care is planned accordingly. Stimulation programmes reported in the literature appear to be more prescriptive than reactive and as such may be difficult to adopt in some units. Their use should be after assessing and considering each infant's individual needs.

Positioning

Good positioning for feeding can be critical to feeding success.

When breastfeeding, an infant is usually on the side, with body and head supported by the mother's hand and arm or a pillow. When bottle-fed the infant is often held upright with the head and back supported in the midline, and shoulders forward in flexion. This position can be difficult for small preterm infants (Fig. 11.2).

Preterm infants need support to maintain flexion as they tend to adopt an extended pos-ture. Extension of the neck during feeding can lead to poor airway protection.[4]

Some preterm infants bottle-feed well when upright and flexed. However, some appear to be able to feed better when in side-lying, much like the position an infant is in during a breastfeed (Fig. 11.3). This technique is cur-rently being studied but the hypothesis is that, just as infants experience less desaturation when breastfeeding in the side-lying position, they may be more stable in terms of saturation when bottle-fed in a similar position. This may

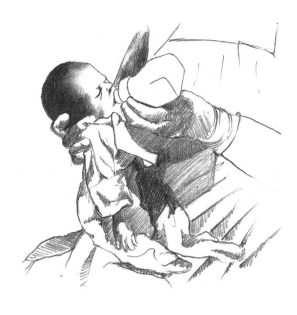

Figure 11.2 Poor upright positioning of a preterm infant.

be due to less hyperflexion and consequently better diaphragmatic movement during feeding, enabling better respiratory function during feeding. It may also avoid milk being poured straight into the throat before a swallow is triggered. Instead milk collects in the cheek until the oral phase of sucking is initiated to move it in a controlled way into the throat. By being on their side, gravity may also encourage the tongue to come away from the hard palate and make introduction of the teat easier.

Side-lying is a useful technique to try with the disorganized feeder who finds coordination of suck, swallow and breathe difficult.

En-face feeding (Fig. 11.4) enables closer observation of infants during bottle-feeding and can mean it is easier to watch for cues on when to pace them to aid coordination with feeds. It can also enable the feeder to have both hands free to give oral support, rewarm a bottle and turn up the oxygen if required during a feed. The 'football hold' enables the mother to visualize the baby's mouth and tongue when rooting to ensure a good attachment.[89]

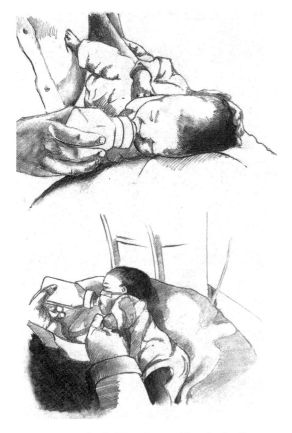

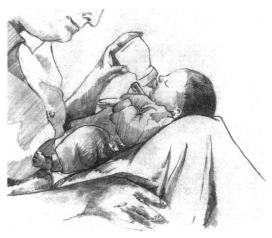

Figure 11.4   En face positioning for feeding.

Figure 11.3   (a, b) Side-lying position for feeding.

Swaddling an infant during a feed may aid organization as it assists in flexion and midline alignment and may allow the infant's gross motor activity to be suppressed, thereby allowing the baby to focus on fine-motor feeding tasks[103] (Fig. 11.5).

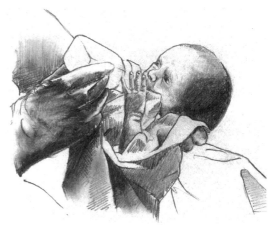

Figure 11.5   Swaddling an infant for feeding.

Support techniques

In general, infants should be allowed to establish their own pace for feeding and should not be coaxed by jiggling the nipple or frequent change in body position.[89] Minimizing stimulation and handling such as bathing, play or tube changes before feed attempts will reserve energy for the work of feeding.[18] However some infants do benefit from specific interventions and support techniques during a feed.

Cheek and jaw support

In an infant with an unstable jaw or weak suction, jaw support can aid feeding performance. Placing a finger halfway between the infant's chin and neck offers support to the base of the tongue (Fig. 11.6). This gentle, even pressure helps the infant to maintain intraoral pressure by lifting the jaw and tongue up to seal against the nipple.[89]

Cheek support with light touch of both cheeks using the thumb and finger (Fig. 11.7)

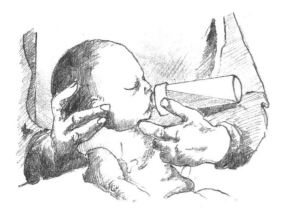

Figure 11.6 Jaw support.

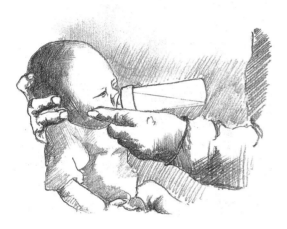

Figure 11.7 Cheek support.

can compensate for the lack of fat/sucking pads and aid in intraoral pressure generation.

An increase in feeding efficiency with jaw and cheek support has been reported.[104] It has not been found to interfere with cardiorespiratory function during bottle-feeding in preterm infants.[105]

In breastfeeding the 'dancer's hand position' (see Chapter 10, Fig. 10.6) can be used to give lower jaw support and provide inward pressure to the cheeks. The breast is supported by the last three fingers of the hand while the thumb and index finger surround the infant's

jaw and rest against the cheeks, providing gentle pressure. This can be particularly helpful with a hypotonic child or a neurologically impaired child with unstable/wide jaw excursions.

It is vital however that the feeder be aware that breaks in suction may be a purposeful act on the part of the infant. The baby may need to catch up on respiratory demands and increase respiration by letting air pass around the nipple. The overzealous feeder may increase the pressure on the cheeks and tongue base as the infant attempts to breathe, exacerbating the infant's distress until the baby is pushed into apnoea and bradycardia.[89]

Pacing

Mature infants adapt the number of sucks per burst to compensate for poor co-ordination. However some immature infants are unable to override the reflex to suck to enable them to stop and take a breath. If infants continue to suck when they need to pause for breath they will eventually desaturate with prolonged swallow apnoea or take a breath during a swallow, resulting in coughing or aspiration. This poorly co-ordinated pattern of feeding is frequently seen in immature preterm infants and, unless supported, the infant will continue to present with co-ordination problems and often fatigue after a short initial feeding attempt.

Pacing the infant by imposing shorter sucking bursts and allowing time for respiratory recovery in the pauses can support immature feeding patterns.[94] The number of sucks the infant can safely do before pausing is assessed and the teat removed to allow for respiratory recovery. If the infant does not allow the bottle to be easily reintroduced then a Haberman feeder or another variable-flow teat could be used, where the bottle can be twisted, allowing alteration in rate of milk flow. The teat can also be tipped so that there is no milk in the nipple.[103]

In two studies, desaturations and irregular respirations during feeding resolved when the bottle was removed in this way.[70,106] There is a need to observe the infant's reaction to differences in flow rates to best support their development of coordination.[103]

Feeding equipment

There is a vast array of feeding equipment available. A sound knowledge of feeding development, difficulties and supportive interventions will enable assessment of a piece of equipment's potential benefits and uses.

Some methods of feeding that are sometimes employed initially to give small amounts of medicine or fluids to a baby, e.g. dropper, spoon or syringe, are not functional as a long-term feeding method and the use of such techniques for large volumes can be time-consuming. They also bypass the need to develop good feeding skills and as such may not be useful techniques.

Different teats/nipples

A single-use nipple that screws directly on to the bottle is usually used on the SCBU as this reduces infection risk and the need for sterilization. A range of teats are produced by various milk companies; however the preterm teats available have a fundamental design error. They are typically fast-flow.[107] The manufacturers have presupposed that a preterm infant has a weak suck and therefore requires a rapid milk flow to compensate and minimize the work of sucking. However, an immature suck is not weak but rather poorly coordinated. Specially manufactured small-sized, high-flow preterm nipples may bypass the oral phase and flood the nasopharynx. If the infant is unprepared for swallowing, the result may be gulping or choking. This may offer a good explanation of the distress that often accompanies early feeding experiences.[89] Some feeding problems may arise specifically due to inappropriate nipple use.[89,108] Reduction of milk flow may reduce the incidence of apnoea or bradycardia during suck-feeding in preterm infants.[107]

The hydrostatic pressure of the milk present in an inverted bottle represents a sustained positive pressure which, independently of the size of the nipple hole, leads to continuous dripping of milk. Even if the infant is resting, the milk continues to flow and the infant will have to keep swallowing to avoid choking.[109–111] Lau et al.[110] advocate the use of a restrictive pattern of milk flow to facilitate earlier oral feeding in infants born at 30 weeks' gestation or earlier. It is likely to mimic the behaviour of blocking of the teat with the tongue that is seen in infants with an immature suck pattern to give time to rest without choking or to catch up with breathing bursts.[112]

Schrank et al.[113] studied a small group of preterm and term infants, looking at the effect of increasing and decreasing milk flow rates on infants' feeding. They found that increasing flow caused rapid increases in suck and swallow frequency in term and preterm infants and increased ingestion rates in term infants. Drooling increased during increased flow and was more prominent in preterm infants but there was no apnoea or other adverse behaviours associated with the increased flow, reflecting the ability of the infant to divert excess formula flow as an efficient airway-protective behaviour. However, the study was limited in not giving fast flow for an entire feed. It may be that a preterm infant would not be able to maintain co-ordination with the fast flow for an entire feed.

Milk flow from a nipple not only depends on the features of the teat but also on the sucking pressures exerted by the infant. These are known to be very variable, particularly in preterm infants who have a limited ability to increase or decrease their sucking pressures in relation to milk flow.[89]

Orthodontic teat advertising claims that the teat resembles the shape of the breast when a baby is attached and therefore mimics the action of breastfeeding more closely and aids orofacial development. However, there is not empirical evidence to support these claims.[114,115] NUK™ teats are widely used on SCBUs in the UK as they are not fast-flow and are a smaller size than the regular-shape teats.

An individualized approach to teat selection is sometimes required. However SCBUs may benefit from a review of the teats routinely used with their preterm babies to avoid the problems discussed above as a result of inappropriate flow rate.

SUMMARY

Feeding problems are multifactorial and require detailed multidisciplinary assessment to provide appropriate support and intervention.

Awareness of the mechanisms that may cause feeding problems can enable preventive measures to be routinely put in place. Supporting the preterm infant in mastery of its most coordinated and complex activity can prevent feeding problems.

It is important that feeding difficulties are assessed individually and appropriately to enable realistic goals to be set and specific interventions to be applied effectively.

References

1. Douglas JE, Bryon M. Interview data on severe behavioural eating difficulties in young children. Arch Dis Child 1996; 75:304–308.
2. Burklow KA, Phelps AN, Schultz JR et al. Classifying complex pediatric feeding disorders. J Pediatr Gastroenterol Nutr 1998; 27:143–147.
3. Bosma JF. Fourth symposium on oral sensation and perception. Prologue to the symposium. Symp Oral Sens Percept 1973; 4:3–8.
4. Jones MW, Morgan E, Shelton JE. Dysphagia and oral feeding problems in the premature infant. Neonatal Netw 2002; 212:51–57.
5. Bier JA, Ferguson A, Cho C et al. The oral motor development of low-birth-weight infants who underwent orotracheal intubation during the neonatal period. Am J Dis Child 1993; 147:858–862.
6. Blaymore Bier JA, Ferguson AE, Morales Y et al. Breastfeeding infants who were extremely low birth weight. Pediatrics 1997; 100:E3.
7. Erenberg A, Nowak AJ. Palatal groove formation in neonates and infants with orotracheal tubes. Am J Dis Child 1984; 138:974–975.
8. Kennedy C, Lipsitt LP. Temporal characteristics of non-oral feedings and chronic feeding problems in premature infants. J Perinat Neonatal Nurs 1993; 7:77–89.
9. Heldt GP. The effect of gavage feeding on the mechanics of the lung, chest wall, and diaphragm of preterm infants. Pediatr Res 1988; 24:55–58.
10. Greenspan JS, Wolfson MR, Holt WJ et al. Neonatal gastric intubation: differential respiratory effects between nasogastric and orogastric tubes. Pediatr Pulmonol 1990; 8:254–258.
11. Chant T. Oro and nasogastric feeding techniques for very low birthweight infants. J Neonatal Nurs 1998; 5:23–25.
12. Huggins PS, Tuomi SK, Young C. Effects of nasogastric tubes on the young, normal swallowing mechanism. Dysphagia 1999; 14:157–161.
13. Shiao SY, Brooker J, DiFiore T. Desaturation events during oral feedings with and without a nasogastric tube in very low birth weight infants. Heart Lung 1996; 25:236–245.
14. Kirby DF, Delegge MH, Fleming CR. American Gastroenterological Association technical review on tube-feeding for enteral nutrition. Gastroenterology 1995; 108:1282–1301.
15. Palmer MM, Heyman MB. Assessment and treatment of sensory-versus motor-based feeding problems in very young children. Inf Young Children 1993; 6:67–73.
16. Di Scipio WJ, Kaslon K, Ruben RJ. Traumatically acquired conditioned dysphagia in children. Ann Otol Rhinol Laryngol 1978; 87:509–514.
17. Blackman J. Children who refuse food. Contemp Pediatr 1998; 15:123–132.
18. VandenBerg KA. Nippling management of the sick neonate in the NICU: the disorganized feeder. Neonatal Netw 1990; 9:9–16.
19. DiPietro JA, Cusson RM, Caughy MO et al. Behavioral and physiologic effects of nonnutritive sucking during gavage feeding in preterm infants. Pediatr Res 1994; 36:207–214.
20. Field T, Ignatoff E, Stringer S et al. Nonnutritive sucking during tube-feedings: effects on preterm neonates in an intensive care unit. Pediatrics 1982; 70:381–384.
21. Field TM. Stimulation of preterm infants. Pediatr Rev 2003; 24:4–11.
22. Gill NE, Behnke M, Conlon M et al. Effect of nonnutritive sucking on behavioral state in preterm infants before feeding. Nurs Res 1988; 37:347–350.
23. Kimble C. Nonnutritive sucking: adaptation and health for the neonate. Neonatal Netw 1992; 11:29–33.
24. Pickler RH, Higgins KE, Crummette BD. The effect of nonnutritive sucking on bottle-feeding stress in preterm infants. J Obstet Gynecol Neonatal Nurs 1993; 22:230–234.
25. Pickler RH, Frankel HB, Walsh KM et al. Effects of nonnutritive sucking on behavioral organization and feeding performance in preterm infants. Nurs Res 1996; 45:132–135.
26. Pinelli J, Symington A, Ciliska D. Nonnutritive sucking in high-risk infants: benign intervention or legitimate therapy? J Obstet Gynecol Neonatal Nurs 2002; 31:582–591.

27. Rochat P, Goubet N, Shah BL. Enhanced sucking engagement by preterm infants during intermittent gavage feedings. J Dev Behav Pediatr 1997; 18:22–26.

28. Winberg J. Pacifier – partner or peril? Acta Paediatr 1999; 88:1177–1179.

29. Webster E. The use of pacifiers for non-nutritive sucking by babies in a neonatal unit. J Neonatal Nurs 1999; 5:23–29.

30. Bernbaum JC, Pereira GR, Watkins JB et al. Nonnutritive sucking during gavage feeding enhances growth and maturation in premature infants. Pediatrics 1983; 71:41–45.

31. Measel CP, Anderson GC. Nonnutritive sucking during tube-feedings: effect on clinical course in premature infants. JOGN Nurs 1979; 8:265–272.

32. Schwartz R, Moody L, Yarandi H et al. A meta-analysis of critical outcome variables in nonnutritive sucking in preterm infants. Nurs Res 1987; 36:292–295.

33. Sehgal SK, Prakash O, Gupta A et al. Evaluation of beneficial effects of nonnutritive sucking in preterm infants. Ind Pediatr 1990; 27:263–266.

34. Widstrom AM, Marchini G, Matthiesen AS et al. Nonnutritive sucking in tube-fed preterm infants: effects on gastric motility and gastric contents of somatostatin. J Pediatr Gastroenterol Nutr 1988; 7:517–523.

35. Dumont RC, Rudolph CD. Development of gastrointestinal motility in the infant and child. Gastroenterol Clin North Am 1994; 23:655–671.

36. De Curtis M, McIntosh N, Ventura V et al. Effect of nonnutritive sucking on nutrient retention in preterm infants. J Pediatr 1986; 109:888–890.

37. Ernst JA, Rickard KA, Neal PR et al. Lack of improved growth outcome related to nonnutritive sucking in very low birth weight premature infants fed a controlled nutrient intake: a randomized prospective study. Pediatrics 1989; 83:706–716.

38. Szabo JS, Hillemeier AC, Oh W. Effect of non-nutritive and nutritive suck on gastric emptying in premature infants. J Pediatr Gastroenterol Nutr 1985; 4:348–351.

39. Pinelli J, Symington A. Non-nutritive sucking for promoting physiological stability and nutrition in preterm infants. Cochrane Database Syst Rev 2001; (3):CD001071 Review.

40. Aarts C, Hornell A, Kylberg E et al. Breast-feeding patterns in relation to thumb sucking and pacifier use. Pediatrics 1999; 104:e50.

41. Howard CR, Howard FM, Lanphear B et al. The effects of early pacifier use on breast-feeding duration. Pediatrics 1999; 103:E33.

42. Kramer MS, Barr RG, Dagenais S et al. Pacifier use, early weaning, and cry/fuss behavior: a randomized controlled trial. JAMA 2001; 286:322–326.

43. Victora CG, Behague DP, Barros FC et al. Pacifier use and short breast-feeding duration: cause, consequence, or coincidence? Pediatrics 1997; 99:445–453.

44. Vogel AM, Hutchison BL, Mitchell EA. The impact of pacifier use on breast-feeding: a prospective cohort study. J Paediatr Child Health 2001; 37:58–63.

45. Schubiger G, Schwarz U, Tonz O. UNICEF/WHO baby-friendly hospital initiative: does the use of bottles and pacifiers in the neonatal nursery prevent successful breast-feeding? Neonatal Study Group. Eur J Pediatr 1997; 156:874–877.

46. Saadeh R, Akre J. Ten steps to successful breast-feeding: a summary of the rationale and scientific evidence. Birth 1996; 23:154–160.

47. Collins CT, Ryan P, Crowther CA et al. Effect of bottles, cups, and dummies on breast feeding in preterm infants: a randomised controlled trial. Br Med J 2004; 329:193–198.

48. Drosten F. Pacifiers in the NICU: a lactation consultant's view. Neonatal Netw 1997; 16:47, 50.

49. Bingham PM, Abassi S, Sivieri E. A pilot study of milk odor effect on nonnutritive sucking by premature newborns. Arch Pediatr Adolesc Med 2003; 157:72–75.

50. Millunchick EW, McArtor RD. Fatal aspiration of a makeshift pacifier. Pediatrics 1986; 77:369–370.

51. Costeloe K, Hennessy E, Gibson AT et al. The EPICure study: outcomes to discharge from hospital for infants born at the threshold of viability. Pediatrics 2000; 106:659–671.

52. Wood NS, Marlow N, Costeloe K et al. Neurologic and developmental disability after extremely preterm birth. EPICure Study Group. N Engl J Med 2000; 343:378–384.

53. Wolff PH. The serial organization of sucking in the young infant. Pediatrics 1968; 42:943-956.

54. McBride MC, Danner SC. Sucking disorders in neurologically impaired infants: assessment and facilitation of breast-feeding. Clin Perinatol 1987; 14:109–130.

55. Wilson DC, McClure G, Halliday HL et al. Nutrition and bronchopulmonary dysplasia. Arch Dis Child 1991; 66:37–38.

56. Kurzner SI, Garg M, Bautista DB et al. Growth failure in infants with bronchopulmonary dysplasia: nutrition and elevated resting metabolic expenditure. Pediatrics 1988; 81:379–384.

57. Yeh TF, McClenan DA, Ajayi OA et al. Metabolic rate and energy balance in infants with bronchopulmonary dysplasia. J Pediatr 1989; 114:448–451.

58. Frank L, Sosenko IR. Undernutrition as a major contributing factor in the pathogenesis of bronchopulmonary dysplasia. Am Rev Respir Dis 1988; 138:725–729.

59. Sindel BD, Maisels MJ, Ballantine TV. Gastroesophageal reflux to the proximal esophagus in infants with bronchopulmonary dysplasia. Am J Dis Child 1989; 143:1103–1106.

60. Bazyk S. Factors associated with the transition to oral feeding in infants fed by nasogastric tubes. Am J Occup Ther 1990; 44:1070–1078.

61. Pridham K, Brown R, Sondel S et al. Transition time to full nipple feeding for premature infants with a history of lung disease. J Obstet Gynecol Neonatal Nurs 1998; 27:533–545.

62. Craig CM, Lee DN, Freer YN et al. Modulations in breathing patterns during intermittent feeding in term infants and preterm infants with bronchopulmonary dysplasia. Dev Med Child Neurol 1999; 41:616–624.

63. Johnson DB, Cheney C, Monsen ER. Nutrition and feeding in infants with bronchopulmonary dysplasia after initial hospital discharge: risk factors for growth failure. J Am Diet Assoc 1998; 98:649–656.

64. Lifschitz MH, Seilheimer DK, Wilson GS et al. Neurodevelopmental status of low birth weight infants with bronchopulmonary dysplasia requiring prolonged oxygen supplementation. J Perinatol 1987; 7:127–132.

65. Yu VY, Orgill AA, Lim SB et al. Growth and development of very low birthweight infants recovering from bronchopulmonary dysplasia. Arch Dis Child 1983; 58:791–794.

66. Timms BJ, DiFiore JM, Martin RJ et al. Increased respiratory drive as an inhibitor of oral feeding of preterm infants. J Pediatr 1993; 123:127–131.

67. Garg M, Kurzner SI, Bautista DB et al. Clinically unsuspected hypoxia during sleep and feeding in infants with bronchopulmonary dysplasia. Pediatrics 1988; 81:635–642.

68. Gewolb IH, Bosma JF, Reynolds EW et al. Integration of suck and swallow rhythms during feeding in preterm infants with and without bronchopulmonary dysplasia. Dev Med Child Neurol 2003; 45:344–348.

69. Singer LT, Davillier M, Preuss L et al. Feeding interactions in infants with very low birth weight and bronchopulmonary dysplasia. J Dev Behav Pediatr 1996; 17:69–76.

70. Rosen CL, Glaze DG, Frost JD Jr. Hypoxemia associated with feeding in the preterm infant and full-term neonate. Am J Dis Child 1984; 138:623–628.

71. Thoyre SM, Carlson JR. Preterm infants' behavioural indicators of oxygen decline during bottle feeding. J Adv Nurs 2003; 43:631–641.

72. Thoyre SM, Carlson J. Occurrence of oxygen desaturation events during preterm infant bottle feeding near discharge. Early Hum Dev 2003; 72:25–36.

73. Hyman PE. Gastroesophageal reflux: one reason why baby won't eat. J Pediatr 1994; 125:S103–S109.

74. Newell SJ, Booth IW, Morgan ME et al. Gastro-oesophageal reflux in preterm infants. Arch Dis Child 1989; 64:780–786.

75. Thach BT. Maturation and transformation of reflexes that protect the laryngeal airway from liquid aspiration from fetal to adult life. Am J Med 2001; 111 (suppl. 8A):69S–77S.

76. Malfroot A, Vandenplas Y, Verlinden M et al. Gastroesophageal reflux and unexplained chronic respiratory disease in infants and children. Pediatr Pulmonol 1987; 3:208–213.

77. Orenstein SR, Orenstein DM. Gastroesophageal reflux and respiratory disease in children. J Pediatr 1988; 112:847–858.

78. Borowitz SM, Borowitz KC. Gastroesophageal reflux in babies: impact on growth and development. Inf Young Children 1997; 10:14–26.

79. Mittal RK, Stewart WR, Schirmer BD. Effect of a catheter in the pharynx on the frequency of transient lower esophageal sphincter relaxations. Gastroenterology 1992; 103:1236–1240.

80. Mathisen B, Worrall L, Masel J et al. Feeding problems in infants with gastro-oesophageal reflux disease: a controlled study. J Paediatr Child Health 1999; 35:163–169.

81. Grant L, Cochran D. Can pH monitoring reliably detect gastro-oesophageal reflux in preterm infants? Arch Dis Child Fetal Neonatal Ed 2001; 85:F155–F157.

82. Orenstein SR, Shalaby TM, Putnam PE. Thickened feedings as a cause of increased coughing when used as therapy for gastroesophageal reflux in infants. J Pediatr 1992; 121:913–915.

83. Dhillon AS, Ewer AK. Diagnosis and management of gastro-oesophageal reflux in preterm infants in neonatal intensive care units. Acta Paediatr 2004; 93:88–93.

84. Lemons PK. From gavage to oral feedings: just a matter of time. Neonatal Netw 2001; 20:7–14.

85. Otamiri G, Berg G, Finnstrom O et al. Neurological adaptation of infants delivered by emergency or elective cesarean section. Acta Paediatr 1992; 81:797–801.

86. Lau C, Hurst N. Oral feeding in infants. Curr Probl Pediatr 1999; 29:105–124.

87. Lau C, Kusnierczyk I. Quantitative evaluation of infant's nonnutritive and nutritive sucking. Dysphagia 2001; 16:58–67.

88. Mathew OP. Respiratory control during nipple feeding in preterm infants. Pediatr Pulmonol 1988; 5:220–224.

89. Lemons PK, Lemons JA. Transition to breast/bottle feedings: the premature infant. J Am Coll Nutr 1996; 15:126–135.

90. Selley WG, Ellis RE, Flack FC et al. Coordination of sucking, swallowing and breathing in the newborn: its relationship to infant feeding and normal development. Br J Disord Commun 1990; 25:311–327.

91. Takahashi K, Groher ME, Michi K. Methodology for detecting swallowing sounds. Dysphagia 1994; 9:54–62.

92. Vice FL, Heinz JM, Giuriati G et al. Cervical auscultation of suckle feeding in newborn infants. Dev Med Child Neurol 1990; 32:760–768.

93. Reynolds EW, Vice FL, Bosma JF et al. Cervical accelerometry in preterm infants. Dev Med Child Neurol 2002; 44:587–592.

94. Palmer MM, Palmer MM, Crawley K et al. Identification and management of the transitional

suck pattern in premature infants. Neonatal oral-motor assessment scale: a reliability study. J Perinat Neonatal Nurs 1993; 7:66–75.

95. Palmer MM, Crawley K, Blanco IA. Neonatal oral-motor assessment scale: a reliability study. J Perinatol 1993; 13:28–35.

96. Braun MA, Palmer MM. A pilot study of oral-motor dysfunction in "at-risk" infants. Phys Occ Ther Pediatr 1985; 5:13–25.

97. Meier PP. Transitional suck patterns in premature infants. J Perinat Neonatal Nurs 1994; 8:vii–viii.

98. O'Donoghue S, Bagnall A. Videofluoroscopic evaluation in the assessment of swallowing disorders in paediatric and adult populations. Folia Phoniatr Logop 1999; 51:158–171.

99. Newman LA, Cleveland RH, Blickman JG et al. Videofluoroscopic analysis of the infant swallow. Invest Radiol 1991; 26:870–873.

100. Leonard EL, Trykowski LE, Kirkpatrick BV. Nutritive sucking in high risk neonates after perioral stimulation. Phys Ther 1980; 60:229–302.

101. Gaebler CP, Hanzlik JR. The effects of a prefeeding stimulation programme on preterm infants. Am J Occ Ther 1996; 50:184–192.

102. Fucile S, Gisel E, Lau C. Oral stimulation accelerates the transition from tube to oral feeding in preterm infants. J Pediatr 2002; 141:230–236.

103. Shaker CS. Nipple feeding preterm infants: an individualized, developmentally supportive approach. Neonatal Netw 1999; 18:15–22.

104. Einarsson-Backes LM, Deitz J, Price R et al. The effect of oral support on sucking efficiency in preterm infants. Am J Occup Ther 1994; 48:490–498.

105. Hill AS, Kurkowski TB, Garcia J. Oral support measures used in feeding the preterm infant. Nurs Res 2000; 49:2–10.

106. Guilleminault C, Coons S. Apnea and bradycardia during feeding in infants weighing greater than 2000 gm. J Pediatr 1984; 104:932–935.

107. Mathew OP. Determinants of milk flow through nipple units. Role of hole size and nipple thickness. Am J Dis Child 1990; 144:222–224.

108. Jain L, Sivieri E, Abbasi S et al. Energetics and mechanics of nutritive sucking in the preterm and term neonate. J Pediatr 1987; 111:894–898.

109. Lau C, Schanler RJ. Oral motor function in the neonate. Clin Perinatol 1996; 23:161–178.

110. Lau C, Sheena HR, Shulman RJ et al. Oral feeding in low birth weight infants. J Pediatr 1997; 130:561–569.

111. Lau C, Alagugurusamy R, Schanler RJ et al. Characterization of the developmental stages of sucking in preterm infants during bottle feeding. Acta Paediatr 2000; 89:846–852.

112. Bu'Lock F, Woolridge MW, Baum JD. Development of co-ordination of sucking, swallowing and breathing: ultrasound study of term and preterm infants. Dev Med Child Neurol 1990; 32:669–678.

113. Schrank W, Al Sayed LE, Beahm PH et al. Feeding responses to free-flow formula in term and preterm infants. J Pediatr 1998; 132:426–430.

114. Drane D. The effect of use of dummies and teats on orofacial development. Breastfeed Rev 1996; 4:59–64.

115. Nowak AJ, Smith WL, Erenberg A. Imaging evaluation of artificial nipples during bottle feeding. Arch Pediatr Adolesc Med 1994; 148:40–42.

116. Protecting, promoting and supporting breastfeeding: the special role of maternity services. A joint WHO/UNICEF statement, Geneva: WHO, 1989.

Chapter 12

Benchmarking and education

Sue C Bell

SUMMARY OF RECOMMENDATIONS

- Nutritional outcome measures should be an integral aspect of medical and nursing management of the premature infant
- Written standards should be set
- Practice should be regularly audited and the results fed back to neonatal staff
- Benchmarking of nutritional outcomes needs to be developed within neonatal units and shared locally and internationally
- Standards should be reappraised following audit and the appropriate action taken
- There should be regular education of neonatal and community staff on optimizing lactation, breast-feeding and nutritional care

BENCHMARKING

In the UK, the National Health Service (NHS) defines benchmarking as: 'the continuous, systematic search for and the implementation of best practices, which will lead to superior performance'.

Essence of care

This is a UK initiative aimed at improving standards of care nationally. This initiative is a patient-focused system and is called 'clinical practice benchmarking' or CPBM.

Clinical practice benchmarking

CPBM is defined as a process through which best practice is identified and continuous improvement is pursued through comparison and sharing.

Standards

Standards are achieved as a result of best practice, elicited by benchmarking.

Audit

The term 'audit' means to monitor whether standards are met by a systematic process that ensures best practice is evaluated regularly.

Benchmarking was originally a surveyor's term, used to describe distinctive landmarks on a map; the term 'benchmarking' is now more frequently used to describe a standard against which others are measured. Benchmarking is the continuous process of measuring one's products, services and practices against leaders, allowing one to identify best practice, and that will lead to superior performance. Benchmarking is used to attain continuous improvement and superior performance in the NHS in the UK. Neonatal units have become involved with this practice, which has led to national and international collaborative work.

Benchmarking can be useful in neonatal units by encouraging practitioners:

- to establish effective goals and objectives for neonatal nutrition in order to become comparable to other units of excellence
- to develop research-based practice
- to provide a forum for the exchange of ideas

An excellent example of benchmarking is the Vermont-Oxford Network that was established in the USA. Neonatologists were inspired by the Cochrane Collaboration in the UK to set up a network through which the collection of systematic data would support research and quality improvement in neonatal care. Girish & Leaf[1] explain how benchmarking has led to clinical improvements in neonatal care. Crabtree[2] dis-cusses the impact of benchmarking in the UK in the Trent region. This paper describes how 13 neonatal units initiated benchmarking in five areas of practice: (1) naso- and orogastric feeding; (2) endotracheal suctioning; (3) the assessment and management of pain; (4) expressing and storing breast milk; and (5) breastfeeding. It is hoped that this will result in improved quality of care in neonatal units in the UK.

In the USA, Kuzma-Reilly[3] discusses how benchmarking was used to implement evidence-based nutritional outcomes in neonatal units. This practice has led to an improvement in nutrient intake and growth, with a reduction in the length of hospital stay and related costs in the hospitals studied.

In order to implement benchmarking in neonatal units, Field[4] discusses how it should become a core-funded clinical service. Field[4] suggests that the work should be collated and evaluated by trained public health doctors. These doctors would need training in perinatal and paediatric issues with a mandatory set of data to review. The data should also include a follow-on assessment of children at 2 years.

BENCHMARKING OF NUTRITION AND BREASTFEEDING IN PRETERM INFANTS

Research has suggested that close nutritional monitoring according to agreed protocols is needed to improve nutritional outcomes for preterm infants. A dietician or a nutritionist should provide the monitoring.[3,5–12]

Nutritional management should be an integral aspect of medical and nursing care of the premature infant:

- to ensure that the standards for the best nutritional care for preterm infants can be developed and audited
- to provide information on current practice with respect to feeding and growth
- to help ensure that nutritional care becomes part of medical and nursing practice
- to improve nutritional status by reducing morbidity and promoting earlier discharge

- to find optimal ways of delivering an improved service (e.g. a multidisciplinary team, including a dietician/nutritionist focusing on nutritional outcomes)

OUTCOME MEASURES IN PROVISION OF OPTIMUM NUTRITION

- improved growth
- earlier discharge
- reduced sepsis rates
- reduced readmission rates
- improved cognitive development (see Chapter 8)

Nutrition in preterm infants

Best practice for nutritional standards, based on evidence from the published papers discussed above, has been divided into eight factors. Each factor needs to be considered individually to attain best practice for the nutrition of preterm infants.

Table 12.1 lists each of the eight factors together with their relevant benchmarks of best practice, thus providing an initial review of best practice for enteral nutrition in neonates.

Each factor is discussed in more detail in Table 12.2 to enable an outline of best practice for enteral neonatal nutrition to be achieved.

The best-practice benchmarking indicated in Tables 12.1 and 12.2 can be developed by units to monitor practice and compare with other neonatal intensive care units to improve outcome measures for the nutritional needs of these vulnerable infants.

IN–SERVICE TRAINING

In-service training is essential for maintaining and communicating best practice. A training programme should be mandatory for all neonatal and community health professionals.

Written information needs to be reviewed regularly to ensure that current practice information is up to date.

Table 12.1 The eight factors comprising best practice for nutritional standards

Factor	Benchmark of best practice
1. Type of feed	Feed provided meets nutritional requirements, including review for the need for supplementation in cases where a chosen feed does not provide adequate nutrients
2. Support for lactation and breast-feeding	Mothers are given correct information on methods to express and store their milk and later to breastfeed their infant
3. Route of feeding	Feeds are given according to an infant's clinical and developmental stage of feeding, e.g. orogastric, nasogastric, cup-feeding, breastfeeding and bottlefeeding
4. Method of feeding	Feeds are given according to the clinical condition and developmental stage of infant, e.g. nasogastric, cup, breast, bottle
5. Monitoring growth	Weight, length, head circumference, feed type, volume and serum biochemistry. Action is taken when growth is suboptimal
6. Screening and assessment to identify infant's nutritional needs	All patients identified as at risk are reviewed on a regular basis
7. Planning, implementation and evaluation of care for those infants at nutritional risk	Plans of care based on nutritional assessments are devised, implemented and evaluated
8. Discharge nutrition and promotion for long-term health	An ongoing assessment of growth and nutritional status is provided

Table 12.2

Factor 1	Benchmark of best practice
Type of feed	Feed gives optimal outcome with respect to morbidity as well as meeting nutritional requirements, with review for the need for extra nutrients in cases where growth and nutritional status are suboptimal

Indicators of best practice	Source of information	Y/N
• Wherever possible, breast milk is given		
• Current nutrient guidelines are used to ensure nutrient requirements are met from milk available	Dietician /nutritionist	
• Guidelines on the nutritional needs of the preterm infant are available at ward level and updated annually	Doctor, dietician/nutritionist	
• Mother's own breast milk may need to be fortified to meet nutritional requirements as indicated		
• Regular review of commercial vitamins, minerals and breast-milk fortifiers to ensure appropriate dose and type are given	Dietician/nutritionist, pharmacist, doctor	
• Training is provided on the use of breast milk and formula milk to the multidisciplinary team to ensure parents/carers receive correct and appropriate information	Neonatal midwife, dietician/nutritionist	
• Leaflets are available to parents on milk-handling and storage and the preparation of feeds (see factor 2 for breast-feeding)	Neonatal midwife/neonatal nurse	

Factor 2	Benchmark of best practice
Support for lactation and breast-feeding	There is active promotion of breast-feeding and support for mothers to maintain lactation

Indicators of best practice	Source of information	Y/N
• All infants exclusively receive mother's own milk	Neonatal midwife/neonatal nurse	
• Dedicated expressing facilities are available on unit		
• There is a selection of suitable pumps and milk shields available for individual choice		
• Staff adhere to the breastfeeding policy, which is updated and evidence-based		
• Storage facilities meet standards (see Chapter 6)		
• All mothers receive and understand individualized verbal and written evidence-based information, which is consistent and documented in the appropriate place		
• All staff receive breastfeeding training within 6 months of taking up post, with annual updates		
• Breastfeeding mothers will receive continuity of support from breastfeeding advisors/neonatal community team who will have been involved in their care prior to discharge		

(Continued)

Table 12.2 Continued

Factor 3	Benchmark of best practice
Route of feeding	Feeds are given according to an infant's clinical and developmental stage of feeding, e.g. orogastric, nasogastric, cup-feeding, bottle-feeding (see Factor 2 for breastfeeding)

Indicators of best practice	Source of information	Y/N
• Route of feeding assessed regularly	Doctor/nurse	
• Educational training on different methods of feeding given regularly on unit	Gastroenterology nurse specialist	
• Types of feeding tube reviewed in respect to quality assurance	Gastroenterology nurse specialist	
• The development of infant feeding included in mandatory in-service training	Speech therapist	
• Standards for all feeding methods available at ward level	Neonatal breast-feeding nurse	

Factor 4	Benchmark of best practice
Method of feeding	Feeds are given according to the clinical condition and developmental stage of infant Nasogastric feeding (bolus continuous) oral feeding

Indicators of best practice	Source of information	Y/N
• Volume and type of feed are increased at appropriate rate, depending on clinical needs of neonate	Doctor	
• Training of staff on all aspects of infant feeding	Gastroenterology nurse specialist	
• Different feeding methods are assessed regularly to ensure they are in line with the maturation and the development of feeding skills	Speech therapist Neonatal nurse	

Factor 5	Benchmark of best practice
Monitoring growth	Weight, length, head circumference, feed type and volume are recorded and action taken when there is cause for concern

Indicators of best practice	Source of information	Y/N
A nutrition chart records the following:		
• Centile of current weight/length and weight/length to be aimed for	Doctor, nursing staff	
• Feed volume (ml/kg) prescribed plus actual daily intake of kcal/kg and protein/kg	Dietician/nutritionist	
• Weight gain recorded as g/kg per day over 7 days		
• Length in cm weekly		
• Head circumference in cm weekly		
• Weight, length and head circumference are plotted on a growth chart weekly	Nurse/doctor, dietician/nutritionist	
• Growth charts monitored and referral/action put in place as indicated by nutrition screening tool	Dietician /nutritionist	
• Multidisciplinary training on monitoring to ensure growth is documented appropriately	Dietician /nutritionist	

(Continued)

Table 12.2 Continued

Factor 6	Benchmark of best practice
Screening and assessment to identify infant's nutritional needs	Nutritional screening is conducted regularly for all patients identified as at risk

Indicators of best practice	Source of information	Y/N

A nutrition screen is carried out on all preterm infants weekly and the following are plotted on the most appropriate growth chart:

- Weight
- Length
- Head circumference

Blood tests are done weekly on :

- Sodium, potassium, albumin, urea, full blood count, calcium, phosphate, alkaline phosphatase, albumin, C-reactive protein
- Record of steroid use
- Record of sepsis
- Record patent ductus arteriosus

Action/assessment taken if growth failing as follows:

- Weight gain falling away from centile (N.B.: when diuresis is not expected)
- Length velocity decreases over 1–2 weeks
- Abnormal blood tests

Action taken if specialized feeding is needed, e.g.:

- Addition of breast-milk fortifier
- Change in breast milk or preterm formula
- Syndromes/inborn errors of metabolism
- Uncertainty about addition of vitamins or mineral supplements

Referrals and action taken if infant is at nutritional risk

At-risk infants are reviewed regularly

Audit of screening tool

Training given on nutrition screening to multidisciplinary team

Source of information (right column): Doctor / Dietician /nutritionist / Nursing staff

Factor 7	Benchmark of best practice
Planning, implementation and evaluation of care for those infants at nutritional risk	Care plans based on ongoing nutritional assessments are devised, implemented and evaluated

Indicators of best practice	Source of information	Y/N

- Screened infants are reassessed weekly
- Individualized care plans written for infants are reviewed daily
- Nutrition flow charts are reviewed by staff and dieticians
- Nutrition care plans are followed as specified
- Growth charts are reviewed weekly by staff and dieticians
- Audit review of monitoring

Source of information: Doctor / Nursing staff / Dietician/nutritionist

(Continued)

Table 12.2 Continued

Factor 8	Benchmark of best practice
Discharge nutrition for optimal nutritional status	Provision of information to enable infant to have appropriate nutrition for growth and optimal nutritional status

Indicators of best practice	Source of information	Y/N
• Provision of information leaflets on preterm feeding given to parents/carers	Neonatal midwife	
• Provision of information leaflets on preterm weaning given to parents/carers	Dietician /nutritionist	

Indicators of best practice	Source of information	Y/N
• Parents/carers given information on formula composition to ensure informed choice regarding feeding	Neonatal midwife	
• Advise on use of vitamins or other supplements that may be needed during the first year postdischarge	Dietician/nutritionist	

METHODS FOR DISSEMINATING STANDARDS OF NUTRITIONAL CARE

- daily ward rounds
- weekly nutrition round
- monthly journal club for neonatal nutrition
- regular updates regarding preterm nutrition should be in place for the multidisciplinary team, including the community team
- annual review of parent information leaflets relating to infant feeding

In the UK a nutritional neonatal interest group has been set up by state-registered paediatric dieticians. The aims of this group are:

- to undertake joint audit and research to develop formalized standards for dissemination
- to create a forum for review and discussion of current issues and journals
- to formulate a network of neonatal dieticians within neonatology to share practice
- to provide evidence-based education and advice to non-specialists and specialists in the field of neonatal nutrition

This group will help to enable the development of a coordinated approach to the management of nutrition within neonatal intensive care units in the UK. In the USA neonatal issues of benchmarking are linked to the Vermont-Oxford Network.[13] The American Association of Dietetics has a website for information exchange on neonatal nutrition.[14] An Australian website is also available for general advice.[15]

References

1. Girish S, Leaf AA. International benchmarking in neonatal intensive care :the Vermont-Oxford network. Clin Govern Bull 2003; 5:8–10.
2. Crabtree L. Clinical practice benchmarking: putting it to the test. J Neonatal Nurs 2002 ; 8:156–159.
3. Kuzma-O'Reilly B, Duenas M, Greecher C, et al. Evaluation, development, and implementation of potentially better practices in neonatal intensive care nutrition. Pediatrics 2003; 111 (suppl. E):e461–e470.
4. Field D, Manktelow E, Draper S. Bench marking and performance management in neonatal care: easier said than done! Arch Dis Child Fetal Neonatal Ed 2002; 87:F163–F164.

5. Premji S, Chessell L, Paes B et al. Variation in feeding practices for premature infants <1500g : impetus for clinical practice guidelines. Pediatr Res 1999; 45:1702 (abstract).

6. Olsen I, Richardson D, Schmid C. Intersite differences in weight growth velocity of extremely premature infants. Pediatrics 2002; 110:1125–1132.

7. Michel SH, Silver J, Pleasure J. Nutrition risk in children participating in a NICU follow up clinic. Pediatr Res 1997; 41:1213 (abstract).

8. Marriott J, Bishop K. Feeding practices in special care baby units in the UK. Bournemouth: Clinical Nutrition and Metabolism Group of the Nutrition Society; 1998 (abstract).

9. Elsaesser K. Dietitian intervention in neonatal intensive care reduces error and improves clinical outcomes. J Am Dietet Assoc 1998;98:A21 (abstract).

10. Georgieff M, Mills MM. Changes in nutritional management and outcome of VLBW infants. Am J Dis Child 1989;143:82–85.

11. Stave V, Robbins S, Fletcher A. A comparison of growth rates of premature infants prior to and after close nutritional monitoring. Clin Proc CHNMC1979; 35:171–180.

12. Fenton T, Geggie J, Warner J et al. Nutrition services in Canadian neonatal intensive care. Can J Diet Pract Res 2000; 61:172–175.

13. http://www.webmaster@vtoxford.org. Information on the Vermont Oxford network for best practice in neonatalogy.

14. http://www.pedi-rd. American dietetic website for information exchange on nutrition.

15. http://www.nhmrc.gov.au/publications/synopses/dietsyn.htm. Dietary guidelines for Australia.

Glossary

ACIDOSIS   A metabolic condition, characterized by an increase in hydrogen ion concentration, that occurs when the body is no longer able to buffer free hydrogen ions in the blood, resulting from either the accumulation of acid or depletion of the alkaline reserve (bicarbonate) in the blood and body tissues. This usually causes the pH of the blood to drop (and become more acidic).

ANTENATAL (ANTEPARTUM)   Before the onset of labour.

ANTIBODY   An immunoglobulin formed in response to an antigen, including bacteria and viruses. (Breast milk contains antibodies to antigens to which either the infant or the mother have been exposed.)

APGAR SCORE   An index of physiological status or depression at birth.

APNOEA   Cessation of breathing.

ARTIFICIAL INFANT MILK (FORMULA)   Any milk preparation, other than human milk, that is intended to be a source of nourishment for infants.

ASPIRATION   Inhalation of a substance into the lungs by accident.

AUDIT   To monitor if standards are met by a systematic process that ensures best practice is evaluated regularly.

AUTOCRINE   A bioactive substance produced by a cell that regulates metabolic pathways within the same cell.

BENCHMARKING   The continuous, systematic search for and implementation of best practices that will lead to superior performance.

BIRTH WEIGHT (WORLD HEALTH ORGANIZATION–RECOMMENDED DEFINITION)   The first weight of the fetus or newborn obtained after birth. This weight should preferably be measured within the first hour of life, before significant weight loss has occurred. Definitions are as follows:
- low birth weight (LBW): < 2500 g
- very low birth weight (VLBW): < 1500 g
- extremely low birth weight (ELBW): < 1000 g

BANKED HUMAN MILK   *See:* Donor milk.

BLINDING   Ensuring the conditions of an experiment are 'blinded' so that the subject (or person administering a treatment) does not know which treatment is being administered.

BODY MASS INDEX   Weight (in kg) divided by height (in metres) squared. A measure of appropriateness of body size.

BOLUS   A mass of food or liquid that is ready to swallow or travel through a tube.

BRADYCARDIA   A slowness of the heart beat, as evidenced by slowing of the pulse rate.

BREAST-MILK FORTIFICATION   The addition of specific supplements to breast milk to increase its nutrient level for preterm infants.

BUCCAL PADS   Also known as fat or sucking pads. Fat pads sheathed by the masseter muscles in an infant's cheeks. The buccal pads touch and provide stability for the tongue, which enhances the tongue's ability to compress breast tissue during suckling.

CASE-CONTROL STUDIES   Case-control studies compare risk factors in people who have a particular disease or outcome with a sample from the same population who do not. Controls may be matched to the cases by age, sex or other factors. The means of selecting controls aims to ensure that differences between controls and cases reflect exposure to suspected causes, rather than to confounding factors. Confounding factors such as age prevent the logical separation of causal events/exposures from other influences on the outcome.

CHOANAL ATRESIA   Congenital bony or membranous occlusion of one or both nasal choanae, due to failure of the embryonic bucconasal membrane to rupture.

CHOLECYSTOKININ   A hormone secreted mainly by the duodenal mucosa. The main function of cholecystokinin is to regulate the emptying of the gallbladder and secretion of enzymes from the pancreas.

CHRONIC LUNG DISEASE (PREVIOUSLY KNOWN AS BRONCHOPULMONARY DYSPLASIA OR BPD)   A respiratory disease seen in infants who have received mechanical respiratory support (with high oxygenation) in the neonatal period. Often associated with those infants who have been treated for hyaline membrane disease, due to prematurity.

CHRONOLOGICAL AGE   A term that is used to indicate the age from the actual day the baby was born.

CLEFT PALATE   A congenital fissure in the roof of the mouth forming a communication between the nasal passages and the oral cavity.

COLOSTRUM   Colostrum is stored in the breast during pregnancy and in the early postpartum period. It is thicker than mature milk, reflecting a higher content of proteins, many of which are immunoglobulins.

CONFIDENCE INTERVALS (CI)   A range of values of a variable, constructed so that the interval has a specified probability of including the population mean or rate for that variable. For example, perinatal mortality rate in 1994 in district X is 8.9 per 1000 total births (95% CI 6.5–11.4).

CONTROL   As used in a case-control study or randomized controlled trial, control means persons in a comparison group that differ in the disease or other outcome in question. If matched controls are used they are selected so that they are similar to the study group, or cases, in specific characteristics, e.g. age, sex, weight.

CORTISOL   A hormone secreted by the adrenal glands in response to stress. It actions result in raising blood sugar levels and assists in glycogen storage in the liver.

CORRECTED AGE   The corrected age is based on the age the child would be if the pregnancy had actually gone to term (age of the baby minus the weeks born premature). Example:
- Baby B was born at 28 weeks' gestations
- He was 12 weeks premature (40 weeks – 28 weeks = 12 weeks = 3 months)
- Today it is 6 months past the day he was actually born
- Corrected age = 6 months – 3 months
- Baby B is 3 months corrected age.

CREAMATOCRIT   The proportion of fat in a milk sample determined by using a centrifuged sample. The creamatocrit, or the percentage of total volume in the capillary tube which is equivalent to lipid, can be converted to a rough estimate of lipid and caloric content by using a published regression graph.

CYANOSIS   A bluish discoloration of the skin and mucous membranes due to excessive concentration of reduced haemoglobin in the capillaries.

DESATURATION   A drop in the concentration of oxygen in the blood.

DONOR MILK   Human milk voluntarily contributed to a human milk bank by women unrelated to the recipient.

DONOR EXPRESSED BREAST MILK (DEBM)   Donor milk which has been expressed from the breast, as opposed to the collection of milk which has dripped from one breast while the other is being expressed (known as drip milk).

DYSPHAGIA   Difficulty in swallowing.

ENERGY EXPENDITURE   Amount of calories used in daily activities.

ENTERAL FEED   A feed that goes into the gastrointestinal tract.

EPIDEMIOLOGY   The study of the distribution and determinants of health-related states and events in populations, and the application of this to the control of health problems.

EXPECTED DUE DATE/EXPECTED DATE OF DELIVERY (EDD)   The calculated date 40 weeks and 0 days after the actual or presumed first day of the last menstrual period (*see* Gestational age). This is close to the date by which 50% of normal human pregnancies will have delivered, but the scatter of spontaneous onset of labour with normal outcome around this date is at least 2 weeks either side.

EXTREMELY LOW BIRTH WEIGHT (ELBW)   *See* Birth weight.

FETUS   The unborn infant in the postembryonic period, after major structures have been outlined, from 9 weeks after fertilization until birth.

FOREMILK   Foremilk is the first milk or the milk at the beginning of either a breastfeed or breast expression. It is lower in fat than the milk at the end of the breastfeed or expression period (hindmilk). The fat content in foremilk is dependent on how much milk is in the breast. The more milk in the breast, the less fat in the foremilk.

GALACTOGOGUE   Any food or groups of foods thought to possess qualities that increase the volume or quality of milk produced by the lactating woman who eats such foods.

GASTRO-OESOPHAGEAL REFLUX (GOR)   The return of stomach contents back up into the oesophagus. This can cause heartburn if the refluxed liquid is acidic.

GESTATIONAL AGE   The duration of pregnancy (gestational age) is measured from the first day of the actual or presumed last (most recent) normal menstrual period (LMP). Gestational age is commonly expressed in completed weeks or completed days or weeks and days. Thus, events occurring 280–286 days (40 weeks + 0 days to 40 weeks + 6 days) after the onset of the LMP are considered to have occurred at 40 weeks' gestation (during the 41st week). The current definition of duration of pregnancy does not formally recognize modern accurate methods for estimating the duration of pregnancy, which are independent of knowledge of the date of the start of the last period. The use of such measures in current practice is therefore inconsistent. Ultrasound scan in the first half of pregnancy is by far the most important and widely available method of dating a pregnancy in the absence of menstrual history. As an interim position, calculations should be based on menstrual history when there is less than 7 days' difference between estimates of gestational age, but ultrasound scan measures dates should be used for differences of 7 days or more. Such a revision of dates should be indicated by the addition of the term, 'by scan' or 'scan dates'. As ovulation does not usually occur until 2 weeks after the first day of the last period, and fertilization within 2 days of that, the traditional calculation of gestational age always includes approximately 2 weeks during which a mother could not have been pregnant. This method of measuring should more correctly be called postmenstrual age. Accurate durations from fertilization or conception should be referred to as postfertilization age or postconception age.

GOLGI A cytoplasmic organelle within the cell that forms vesicles, particularly for the transport of proteins and other constituents (e.g. lactose) to the extracellular environment.

HINDMILK The milk at the end of either a breast feed or breast-milk expression period. Hindmilk is higher in fat than foremilk. As with foremilk, the amount of fat in the hindmilk indicates how much milk is left in the breast. Therefore the higher the fat, the less milk remains in the breast.

HUMAN MILK BANK A service that collects, screens, processes, stores and distributes donated human milk.

HYPERCARBIA An excess of carbon dioxide in the blood.

HYPOVENTILATION A state in which there is a reduced amount of air entering the pulmonary alveoli.

HYPOXAEMIA Below-normal oxygen content in arterial blood due to deficient oxygenation of the blood and resulting in hypoxia.

HYPOXIA Reduction of oxygen supply to tissue below physiological levels despite adequate perfusion of the tissue by blood.

INSULIN A hormone synthesized in the pancreas and then secreted by the beta cells of the islets of Langerhans into the blood. Insulin is necessary for the metabolism of carbohydrates, lipids and proteins. It regulates blood sugar levels by facilitating the uptake of glucose into tissues and by reducing the release of glucose from the liver. When insulin is deficient or when insulin resistance occurs, diabetes mellitus can result.

INTRAORAL Inside the oral cavity/mouth.

INTUBATION The insertion of a tube into a body canal or hollow organ, such as into the trachea or stomach. Usually referring to the insertion of a tube to aid ventilation in sick neonates. This can be nasal or endotracheal.

LACTOCYTE The mammary secretory epithelial cell.

LACTOGENESIS I The stage of breast development during pregnancy in which the mammary epithelial cells differentiate into lactocytes. The lactocytes are able to secrete milk-specific components such as lactose, casein and α-lactalbumin that can be detected in milk secretion, blood or urine.

LACTOGENESIS II The onset of copious milk secretion. Lactogenesis II can be identified by either an increase in milk production or acute changes in milk (colostrum) composition and these often precede the mother sensing milk 'coming in'. The initiation of lactation is caused by a sharp decrease in progesterone in the maternal blood and occurs between 30 and 40 h postpartum, whereas the sensation of the milk 'coming in' occurs between 24 and 102 h after birth, with a mean of 59–64 h.

LETDOWN *See* Milk ejection.

LENGTH Length is measured supine (= lying on back) in infants, usually up to 2 years of age. It is close to, but not exactly the same as, height, which is measured standing. Length cannot be accurately measured by a single observer or without appropriate equipment.

LOGISTIC REGRESSION This analysis involves the creation of a model relating a dichotomous outcome variable of interest to other explanatory variables. The explanatory variables may be continuous or dichotomous.

LOW BIRTH WEIGHT (LBW)   *See* Birth weight.

MACROGLOSSIA   Excessively large tongue.

MAMMOGENESIS   The growth of the mammary gland that occurs by extension and branching of the ductal system. It is followed by extensive lobular-alveolar growth in the first half of pregnancy, by which time some secretions may be present. In the last trimester there is a further increase in lobular size and secretion in the alveoli. Mammogenesis generally results in a marked increase in breast size during pregnancy, although it is possible for the secretory tissue to replace fatty tissues without a marked increase in breast size.

MECHANICAL VENTILATION   Mechanically assisted breathing using an electrically powered device that forces oxygenated air into the lungs and then allows time for passive exhalation of air.

MICROGNATHIA   Abnormal smallness of the jaws, especially of the mandible.

MILK EJECTION   The period of time in which there is an increased availability of the milk from the nipple as a result of stimulation of the milk ejection reflex.

MILK EJECTION REFLEX   The neurohormonal reflex resulting from the tactile stimulation of the nipple sending neural impulses to the hypothalamus and posterior pituitary, resulting in the release of oxytocin into the systemic circulation. Oxytocin causes the contraction of myoepithelial cells surrounding the alveoli in the breast, moving milk into the collecting ducts and expanding these ducts as the milk flows forward to the nipple.

MINUTE VENTILATION   The total amount of gas expelled from the lungs per minute.

MORBIDITY   This term refers to illness and disability, and is often used to refer to non-fatal outcomes of disease, such as handicap, chronic illness or disability.

NASOGASTRIC (NG) TUBE   A flexible plastic tube that is introduced through the nostril to the nasopharynx and advanced to the stomach.

NECROTIZING ENTEROCOLITIS (NEC)   Inflammation of the intestinal tract which may cause tissue to die (necrose). Most commonly occurring around the junction of the small and large bowel. It is predominantly a disease of the preterm neonate and appears to involve prematurity, gut flora disturbance and poor gut blood flow.

NEONATAL   Referring to the newborn (up to 28 days old).

NEONATAL PERIOD   The first 28 days after live birth (0–27 days inclusive); the early neonatal period covers 0-6 days inclusive after live birth.

NIPPLE   (Also used in Chapters 9 and 11 to refer to a teat on a bottle.)

Cylindrical pigmented protuberance on the breast. The human nipple contains 15–20 nipple pores through which milk flows.

OEDEMA   Swelling.

OESOPHAGITIS   Inflammation of the oesophagus.

OLIGOHYDRAMNIOS   The presence of less than the normal amount of amniotic fluid.

OROFACIAL   Referring to the face and mouth region.

OROGASTRIC (OG) TUBE   A flexible plastic tube that is introduced through the mouth to the oropharynx and advanced to the stomach.

OXYTOCIN   A small peptide hormone comprising nine amino acids. It is synthesized in the supraoptic and paraventricular neurons in the hypothalamus. It then passes to the posterior pituitary gland and is stored in terminal neurones before being secreted into the blood. During suckling, oxytocin is released and causes contraction of the myoepithelial cells that surround the milk-filled alveoli, thereby forcing the milk into the milk ducts so that it is available to be removed. In addition to milk ejection, oxytocin has many diverse physiological effects, such as the contraction of the uterus.

PACIFIER Artificial teat or dummy used to calm an infant or practice non-nutritive sucking.

PARITY Number of previous pregnancies a woman has had which resulted in either live birth or stillbirth.

PASTEURIZATION The heating of milk to destroy pathogens.

PATHOGEN Substance or organism capable of producing illness.

PERINATAL Around the time of birth.

PERIORAL Around the mouth

POLYHYDRAMNIOS The presence of more than the normal amount of amniotic fluid.

PHARYNX The musculomembranous passage between the mouth and posterior nares and the larynx and oesophagus. Above the soft palate is the nasopharynx; the oropharynx lies between the soft palate and epiglottis and the hypopharynx between the epiglottis and oesophagus and larynx.

POSTMENSTRUAL AGE Gestational age plus the weeks since birth (corrected age).

POSTPARTUM After birth.

PRETERM A preterm birth is one less than 37 completed weeks (259 days) from the first day of the last menstrual period. A term birth is one from 37 to less than 42 completed weeks (259–293 days). A later birth is referred to as postterm.

PROLACTIN A hormone produced by the anterior pituitary gland. It is involved in the regulation of breast growth during pregnancy and the maintenance of lactation.

PULMONARY RESISTANCE The opposition of the tracheobronchial tree to air flow: the mouth to alveoli pressure difference divided by the air flow.

PYLORIC SPHINCTER The circular fold of mucous membrane containing a ring of circular muscle fibres that closes the pylorus of the stomach. It is also referred to as the pyloric valve.

RANDOMIZED CONTROLLED TRIAL (RCT) A clinical trial that involves at least one test treatment and one control treatment: concurrent enrolment and follow-up of the test- and control-treated groups, and in which the treatments to be administered are selected by a random process.

RESPIRATORY DISTRESS SYNDROME A condition of the newborn marked by dyspnoea with cyanosis, expiratory grunt and retraction of the suprasternal notch or costal margins, frequently occurring in premature infants, children of diabetic mothers and infants delivered by caesarean section, and sometimes with no apparent predisposing cause.

SAMPLE A subset of the population selected for study.

SCBU Special care baby unit.

SEDATIVE An agent causing relaxation.

SGA Small-for-gestational age.

STANDARDS Standards are a result of best practice elicited by benchmarking (*see* Benchmarking).

STORAGE CAPACITY The storage capacity of a breast is defined as the maximum amount of milk that can be stored in the breast and is available to the infant under normal patterns of breast-feeding. The breast storage capacity can be determined by subtracting the minimum breast volume from the maximum breast volume observed over the 24-h period. There is a wide variation in the storage capacity of a woman's breast, ranging from 60 to 600 ml, and breasts with larger storage capacities have the potential to deliver more milk at either a breast feed or a pumping session.

SUBGLOTTIC STENOSIS   Narrowing or stricture below the glottis/vocal folds.

SUCKING, NON–NUTRITIVE (NNS)   Sucking on a dummy (pacifier) or emptied breast, or fingers for comfort, but not to receive nutrition. NNS usually occurs at a faster rate than nutritive sucking

SUCKING, NUTRITIVE   Steady rhythmic sucking during continuous milk flow which enables an infant to obtain liquid nutrition.

SUPPLEMENTAL OXYGEN   Oxygen-enriched air delivered into the respiratory tract.

TACHYPNOEA   An abnormally rapid (usually shallow) respiratory rate.

TERM   The culmination of pregnancy at the end of 40 weeks from the last menstrual period or 38 weeks from conception.

TONGUE TIE   Impeded motion of the tongue because of the shortness of the frenulum, or of the adhesion of its margins to the gums.

TRACHEOBRONCHOMALACIA   Degeneration of elastic and connective tissue of the bronchi and trachea.

TRIMESTER   The three trimesters of pregnancy are the first 3 months; months 4–6; and the last 3 months.

VERY LOW BIRTH WEIGHT (VLBW)   *See* Birth weight.

Resources

Support organizations

UK

Association of Breastfeeding Mothers (ABM)
PO Box 207, Bridgewater, Somerset TA6 7YT
http: home.clara.net/abm

BLISS – the premature charity
www.bliss.org.uk

BLISS parent information leaflets
- BPD/chronic lung disease
- Breastfeeding your premature baby
- Containment holding
- Parent information guide
- RSV (respiratory syncytial virus)
- Ventilation
- Weaning your premature baby

Breastfeeding Network
PO Box 11126, Paisley, Scotland PA2 8YB
e-mail: email@breastfeedingnetwork.org.uk
www.breastfeeding.co.uk/bfn
www.clapa.com

Cleft Lip and Palate Association (CLAPA)
Hospital for Sick Children, Great Ormond
Street, London WC1N 3JH
Tel: 0207 4059200

Lactation Consultants of Great Britain
PO Box 56, Virginia Water GU25 4WB
www.lcgb.org

La Lèche League – breastfeeding help and information
BM 3424, London WC1N 3XX
www.laleche.org.uk

Multiple Birth Foundation
Hammersmith House Level 4, Queen
Charlotte's and Chelsea Hospital, Du Cane
Road, London W12 0HS
e-mail: info@multiplebirths.org.uk
www.multiplebirths.org.uk

National Childbirth Trust
Alexandra House, Oldham Terrace, Acton,
London W3 6NH
www.nctpregnancyandbabycare.com

Twins and Multiple Births Association (TAMBA)
PO Box 30, Little Sutton, South Wirral LI66
1TH
Tel: 0870 121 4000
www.tamba.org.uk

UNICEF Baby Friendly Initiative
Africa House, 64–78 Kingsway, London WC2B
6NB
www.babyfriendly.org.uk

International

Academy of Breastfeeding Medicine
www.bfmed.org/board.html

International Confederation of Midwives
Eisenhowerlaan 138, 2517 KN The Hague, The
Netherlands
Tel: + 31 70 3060520
Fax: + 31 70 3555651
e-mail: info@internationalmidwives.org
www.internationalmidwives.org

**International Lactation Consultants
Association**
www.ilca.org

La Lèche League International
www.lalecheleague.org

UNICEF
www.unicef.org

World Health Organization (WHO)
www.who.int

Expressing and feeding equipment

UK

Ameda-Egnell
www.ameda.com/international/asp

AVENT
www.aventbaby.com

**CLAPA – stocks Haberman feeder, soft
bottles** and orthodontic teats
www.clapa.com

Easy Expression Halterneck Bra
www.expressyourselfbras.co.uk

Expressions Breastfeeding
www.breastpumps.co.uk

NUK teats and pacifiers
Helpline (UK): 0845 300 2467
Mail order: 0879 787 6220 or 0870 199 3593
www.nukbaby.co.uk

Wee Thumbie Premie baby pacifier
www.homeforebabies.com

International

Hollister
www.hollister.com

Lact-Aid International
www.lact-aid.com

Medela
www.medela.com

Growth charts and growth-measuring equipment

UK

Castlemead Publications
Raynham House, Broadmeads, Ware, Herts
SG12 9HY
Tel: 01920 465525

Child Growth Foundation
2 Mayfield Avenue, Chiswick, London W4 1PW
Tel: +44(0)20 8995 0257/8994 7625
email: cgflondon@aol.com

Harlow Printing
Maxwell Street, South Shields, Tyne and Wear
NE33 4PX
Tel: 0191 4554286
email: sales@harlowprinting.co.uk

USA

Fenton TR. A new growth chart for preterm
babies: Babson and Benda's chart updated
with recent data and a new format. BMC
Pediatr 2003; 3:13. (This can be printed from
the web free of charge.)

Videos

Calgary Health Region. Side by side:
breastfeeding multiples. Alberta, Canada:
Calgary Health Region: 1992.

Jones E, Spencer SA. Breastfeeding the preterm
infant – a positive approach. Unit 2, Belvedere
Trading Estate, Taunton TA1 1BH, UK: 1997.

Morton J. A premie needs his mother: first steps to breastfeeding your premature infant. Palo Alto, CA: 2002.

CD-ROM

Spencer SA, Jones E. Breastfeeding: multimedia learning resource for healthcare professionals. 1998. Available online at: www.matrixmultimedia.co.uk.

Websites

Breastfeeding Pharmacology
www.neonatal.ttuhsc.edu/lact

Kangaroo Mother Care
www.kangaroomothercare.com

Preemie-L Organisation
www.preemie-l.org/bfaq.html

Professional development and support

UK and international

African Medical and Research Foundation
www.amref.org

American Academy of Pediatrics
www.aap.org

American Dietetic Association
www.eatright.org

Amy Spangler's Feeding Times
www.amysbabycompany.com/newsletter/marchapril2004.html

Association of Women's Health, Obstetric and Neonatal Nurses
www.awhonn.org

Bright Future Lactation Resource Centre
www.bflrc.com

British Association of Perinatal Medicine
www.bapm.org

British Dietetic Association
www.bda.uk.com

Department of Health (UK)
www.doh.gov.uk

Dietary Guidelines for Australia
www.nhmrc.gov.au/publications/synopses/dietsyn.html

Dietitians of Canada
www.dietitians.ca

Human Milk Banking Association of North America
www.hmbana.com

International Pediatric Association
www.ipa-france.net

National Association of Neonatal Nurses
www.nann.org

National Electronic Library for Health (UK)
www.nelh.nhs.uk

Neonatal Nurses Association
www.neonatal-nursing.co.uk

Paediatric and Neonatal Dietetic Information Exchange
Pedi-rd@list.uiowa.edu
To subscribe: Listserv@list.uiowa.edu

Royal College of Midwives
www.rcm.org.uk

Royal College of Paediatricians
www.rcpch.ac.uk

Royal College of Speech and Language Therapists
www.rcslt.org

UK Association for Milk Banking
www.ukamb.org

Index